Common Ear Diseases in Dogs: Diagnosis and Management

Edited by

Tanmoy Rana

Department of Veterinary Clinical Complex
West Bengal University of Animal & Fishery Sciences
Kolkata-700094, India

Common Ear Diseases in Dogs: Diagnosis and Management

Editor: Tanmoy Rana

ISBN (Online): 978-981-5313-59-8

ISBN (Print): 978-981-5313-60-4

ISBN (Paperback): 978-981-5313-61-1

© 2025, Bentham Books imprint.

Published by Bentham Science Publishers Pte. Ltd. Singapore. All Rights Reserved.

First published in 2025.

need for a court order if at any point you breach any terms of this License Agreement. In no event will any delay or failure by Bentham Science Publishers in enforcing your compliance with this License Agreement constitute a waiver of any of its rights.

3. You acknowledge that you have read this License Agreement, and agree to be bound by its terms and conditions. To the extent that any other terms and conditions presented on any website of Bentham Science Publishers conflict with, or are inconsistent with, the terms and conditions set out in this License Agreement, you acknowledge that the terms and conditions set out in this License Agreement shall prevail.

Bentham Science Publishers Pte. Ltd.
80 Robinson Road #02-00
Singapore 068898
Singapore
Email: subscriptions@benthamscience.net

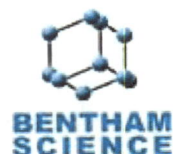

BENTHAM SCIENCE

CONTENTS

PREFACE

Common Ear Diseases in dogs: Diagnosis, and Management 1e book cover otic disease as a serious ailment at the forefront of veterinary medicine. The book covers updated information for practicing veterinarians in identifying small animal ear diseases. It also illustrates the anatomy of the ear, examination techniques, pathophysiology, and treatment strategy to prevent the disease. Various predisposing factors, primary causes, and perpetuating factors associated with ear diseases in dogs are elaborately described in the book. Various therapeutic options with new drugs, and nutritional products may prove to be valuable in the prevention and treatment of ear diseases in dogs. The book covers an extensive study of the diseases of the pinna, external ear canal, middle ear, and inner ear. Various photos are included in the book for easy identification of diseases. The book is an invaluable resource for both veterinarians in training and in practice for gathering knowledge about the ear diseases of dogs. The contributors are specialized in their knowledge for the writing of the individual chapter. This book is especially intended for pet practitioners, academics, researchers, veterinarians, and DVM graduate students engaged with a special interest in pet animal health, and management. I hope that this book serves new paradigms for the stimulus to further research in clarifying the pathomechanisms, diagnosis, and treatment of ear diseases in dogs. I expect that the reader will find this book interesting as well as up-to-date information about ear diseases and will utilize the knowledge in the research and teaching to the new generation. I always welcome constructive feedback and encouragement from my veterinarian colleagues all over the world.

Tanmoy Rana
Department of Veterinary Clinical Complex
West Bengal university of Animal & Fishery Sciences
Kolkata-700094, India

List of Contributors

Apoorva Mishra
Department of Veterinary Surgery and Radiology, College of Veterinary Science and A.H., N.D.V.S.U, Jabalpur (M.P.), 482001, India

Archana Mahapatra
Department of Veterinary Anatomy, Faculty of Veterinary and Animal Sciences, Institute of Agricultural Sciences, Banaras Hindu University, Uttar Pradesh, India

Anju Nayak
Department of Veterinary Microbiology, College of Veterinary Science & A.H., Jabalpur, Nanaji Deshmukh Veterinary Science University, Jabalpur, Madhya Pradesh, India

Ajay Rai
Department of Veterinary Microbiology, College of Veterinary Science & A.H., Jabalpur, Nanaji Deshmukh Veterinary Science University, Jabalpur, Madhya Pradesh, India

Alok Kumar Chaudhary
Department of Veterinary Medicine, DUVASU, Mathura, India

Apra Shahi
Department of Veterinary Surgery and Radiology, College of Veterinary Science and A.H., N.D.V.S.U, Jabalpur (M.P.), 482001, India

Abhishek Kalundia
Cornerstone Pet Clinic, Hyderabad-500089, India

Amitava Roy
Department of Livestock Farm Complex, West Bengal University of Animal & Fishery Sciences, Kolkata, India

Arkaprabha Shee
Subject Matter Specialist (Vet. & Ani. Sc.), Dhaanyaganga Krishi Vigyan Kendra, RKMVERI, Sargachi, Murshidabad, West Bengal, India

Babita Das
Department of Veterinary Surgery and Radiology, College of Veterinary Science and A.H., N.D.V.S.U, Jabalpur (M.P.), 482001, India

B. Prakash Kumar
Department of Veterinary Surgery and Radiology, CVSc, Garividi, Vizianagaram District, Andhra Pradesh-535101, India

Bhavanam Sudhakara Reddy
College of Veterinary Science-Proddatur, Sri Venkateswara Veterinary University, Andhra Pradesh, India

Chinmoy Maji
Subject Matter Specialist (Animal Health), North 24 Parganas Krishi Vigyan Kendra, Ashokenagar, West Bengal University of Animal and Fishery Sciences, West Bengal, India

Dadireddy Narmada Raghavi
College of Veterinary Science-Proddatur, Sri Venkateswara Veterinary University, Andhra Pradesh, India

Dinesh
Department of Veterinary Surgery and Radiology, Lala Lajpat Rai University of Veterinary and Animal Sciences- Hisar, Haryana, India

Diva Dhingra
Department of Veterinary Surgery and Radiology, College of Veterinary Science and A.H., N.D.V.S.U, Jabalpur (M.P.), 482001, India

D. Sai Bhavani
State Institute of Animal Health, Tanuku, West Godavari District, Andhra Pradesh-534211, India

Deepak Kumar
Department of Veterinary Pathology, Bihar Veterinary College, Patna, B, Patna-800014, India, ihar Animal Sciences University, Patna-800014, India

Falguni Mridha	Department of Veterinary Clinical Complex, Faculty of Veterinary & Animal Science, West Bengal University of Veterinary & Animal Sciences, Kolkata-700094, India
G. Saritha	Department of Veterinary Medicine, CVSc, Proddatur, SVVU, India
H. K. Mehta	Department of Veterinary Medicine, College of Veterinary Science and A.H. Mhow, NDVSU Jabalpur (MP), India
Habbu Aishwarya Sunder	Central Institute for Research on Buffaloes (CIRB), Nabha, Punjab, India
Jasvinder Singh Sasan	Division of Veterinary Anatomy, Faculty of Veterinary Sciences and Animal Husbandry, , , Sher-EKashmir University of Agricultural Sciences and Technology of Jammu, Jammu and Kashmir, India
Jigar Raval	National Dairy Development Board, Anand-388001, Gujarat, India
J. Jyothi	Department of Veterinary Medicine, P.V. Narasimharao Telangana Veterinary University, Hyderabad, India
Kamal Sarma	Division of Veterinary Anatomy, Faculty of Veterinary Sciences and Animal Husbandry, , , Sher-EKashmir University of Agricultural Sciences and Technology of Jammu, Jammu and Kashmir, India
K. Manoj Kumar	Department of Veterinary Clinical Complex, CVSc, Garividi, Vizianagaram District, Andhra Pradesh-535101, India
Kambala Swetha	College of Veterinary Science-Proddatur, Sri Venkateswara Veterinary University, Andhra Pradesh, India
Kruti Debnath Mondal	Teaching Veterinary Clinical Complex, Faculty of Veterinary and Animal Sciences, I. Ag. SC., BHU, Mirzapur, UP, India
M. Bhavya Sree	P.V. Narasimharao Telangana Veterinary University, Hyderabad, India
Nidhi S. Choudhary	Department of Veterinary Medicine, College of Veterinary Science and A.H. Mhow, NDVSU Jabalpur (MP), India
Prasanta Kumar Koustasa Mishra	College of Veterinary Science and Animal Husbandry, OUAT, Odisha, India
Poonam Shakya	Department of Veterinary Microbiology, College of Veterinary Science & A.H., Jabalpur, Nanaji Deshmukh Veterinary Science University, Jabalpur, Madhya Pradesh, India
Pranav Anjaria	College of Veterinary Science & Animal Husbandry, Kamdhenu University, Anand-388001, Gujarat, India
Priyanka Pandey	Department of Veterinary Surgery and Radiology, Khalsa College of Veterinary and Animal Sciences, Amritsar Punjab, India
Randhir Singh	Department of Veterinary Surgery and Radiology, College of Veterinary Science and A.H., N.D.V.S.U, Jabalpur (M.P.), 482001, India
Ram Niwas	Department of Veterinary Surgery and Radiology, Lala Lajpat Rai University of Veterinary and Animal Sciences- Hisar, Haryana, India
Randhir Singh	Department of Veterinary Surgery and Radiology, College of Veterinary Science and A.H., N.D.V.S.U, Jabalpur (M.P.), 482001, India

Rakesh Dangi	Department of Veterinary Medicine, College of Veterinary Science and A.H. Mhow, NDVSU Jabalpur (MP), India
Rajesh Kumar	Department of Veterinary Surgery and Radiology, Bihar Veterinary College, Patna-14, Bihar, India
Shobha Jawre	Department of Veterinary Surgery and Radiology, College of Veterinary Science and A.H., N.D.V.S.U, Jabalpur (M.P.), 482001, India
Shalini Suri	Division of Veterinary Anatomy, Faculty of Veterinary Sciences and Animal Husbandry, , , Sher-EKashmir University of Agricultural Sciences and Technology of Jammu, Jammu and Kashmir, India
Satish Kumar Pathak	Department of Veterinary Anatomy, Faculty of Veterinary and Animal Sciences, Institute of Agricultural Sciences, Banaras Hindu University, Uttar Pradesh, India
Sanjiv Kumar	Department of Veterinary Pathology, Bihar Veterinary College, Patna-14, Bihar, India
Savita Kumari	Department of Veterinary Microbiology, Bihar Veterinary College, Patna, Bihar Animal Sciences University, Patna-800014, India
Sirigireddy Sivajothi	College of Veterinary Science-Proddatur, Sri Venkateswara Veterinary University, Andhra Pradesh, India
Sandeep Kumar	Department of Veterinary Surgery and Radiology, Lala Lajpat Rai University of Veterinary and Animal Sciences- Hisar, Haryana, India
Santanu Pal	Indian Veterinary Research Institute, Izatnagar-243122, India
S.K. Maiti	Department of Teaching Veterinary Clinical Complex, Anjora, Durg, Chhattisgarh, India
Shraddha Sinha	Department of Teaching Veterinary Clinical Complex, Anjora, Durg, Chhattisgarh, India
Sumit Gautam	Department of Veterinary Medicine, College of Veterinary Science and A.H. Mhow, NDVSU Jabalpur (MP), India
Sanjay Shukla	Department of Veterinary Microbiology, College of Veterinary Science & A.H., Jabalpur, Nanaji Deshmukh Veterinary Science University, Jabalpur, Madhya Pradesh, India
Sirigireddy Sivajothi	College of Veterinary Science-Proddatur, Sri Venkateswara Veterinary University, Andhra Pradesh, India
Thulasiraman Parkunan	Department of Veterinary Physiology and Biochemistry, Faculty of Veterinary and Animal Sciences, Institute of Agricultural Sciences, Banaras Hindu University, Uttar Pradesh, India
Tanmoy Rana	Department of Veterinary Clinical Complex, West Bengal University of Veterinary & Animal Sciences, Kolkata-700094, India
T. Jayanth Sai Kumar Reddy	P.V. Narasimharao Telangana Veterinary University, Hyderabad, India
Urfeya Mirza	Department of Veterinary Surgery and Radiology, Khalsa College of Veterinary and Animal Sciences, Amritsar Punjab, India
Uiase Bin Farooq	MR College of Veterinary and Animal Sciences, Jhajjar, Haryana, India

Varun Kumar Sarkar Division of Medicine, ICAR-IVRI Izatnagar, Bareilly (UP), India

Vandana Gupta Department of Veterinary Microbiology, College of Veterinary Science & A.H., Jabalpur, Nanaji Deshmukh Veterinary Science University, Jabalpur, Madhya Pradesh, India

V. Agrawal Department of Veterinary Parasitology, College of Veterinary Science and A.H. Mhow, NDVSU Jabalpur (MP), India

CHAPTER 1

Introduction

Apoorva Mishra[1,*], Randhir Singh[1], Babita Das[1] and Shobha Jawre[1]

[1] Department of Veterinary Surgery and Radiology, College of Veterinary Science and A.H., N.D.V.S.U, Jabalpur (M.P.), 482001, India

Abstract: This chapter discussed some common ear illnesses such as otitis, haematoma, tumors *etc.* and establishes the groundwork for understanding the significance of ear health in dogs. We will go more into each ear ailment and examine diagnosis and treatment options in the upcoming chapters. It is crucial for any veterinarian to comprehend the anatomy of a dog's ear, identify common ear illnesses, and know how to diagnose and treat them.

Keywords: Anatomy of ear, Common ear diseases, Diagnosis and prevention.

INTRODUCTION

The ears are a crucial part of a dog's anatomy, serving not only as sensory organs but also playing a significant role in maintaining balance. Otitis externa, or inflammation of the skin lining the ear canal, is the most common cause of canine ear illness and can result in otitis media, a secondary infection of the middle ear chamber. The majority of the time, ear inflammation is a symptom of a more widespread skin condition. As a result, dogs with ear issues frequently lick or chew at their feet or experience irritation elsewhere. In addition to the ear illness, more severely infected dogs may also exhibit obvious signs of skin allergies throughout other body regions. Because of the environment inside the ear, the ears are frequently more seriously impacted by this generalized skin irritation than other parts of the body. The hypersensitivity or skin allergy first results in a mild degree of inflammatory processes, which promotes the growth of bacteria and yeast organisms that are ordinarily found on the skin. Most skin locations in dogs with moderate cases can escape considerable overgrowth of these organisms, but the warm, moist environment inside the ear canal creates the perfect conditions for these organisms to proliferate and subsequently exacerbate inflammation. As the organisms proliferate, more inflammation and skin damage are brought on by

* **Corresponding author Apoorva Mishra:** Department of Veterinary Surgery and Radiology, College of Veterinary Science and A.H., N.D.V.S.U, Jabalpur (M.P.), 482001, India; E-mail: mishra.ap07@gmail.com

their presence, creating a vicious cycle. Unfortunately, due to their unique structure and susceptibility to various environmental factors, dogs are prone to a range of ear diseases. In this chapter, we will delve into the world of canine ear health, exploring the anatomy of a dog's ear, common ear diseases, their causes, symptoms, and preventive measures [1].

ANATOMY OF A DOG'S EAR

Before we delve into the specifics of ear diseases, it's essential to understand the basic anatomy of a dog's ear. A dog's ear consists of three main parts:

Outer Ear (Pinna)

The visible part of the ear is called the pinna, which varies in shape and size among different breeds. It's designed to capture sound waves and funnel them into the ear canal.

Middle Ear

The middle ear begins with the ear canal and includes the eardrum (tympanic membrane) and a system of small bones (ossicles). Sound waves are transmitted through the ear canal to the eardrum, where they are converted into vibrations.

Inner Ear

Beyond the eardrum lies the inner ear, which contains the cochlea, responsible for converting vibrations into electrical signals sent to the brain. The inner ear also plays a crucial role in balance and orientation.

The canine ear canal is more vertical than that of a human, forming an L-shape that tends to hold in fluid. This makes dogs more prone to ear infections. Ear infections are typically caused by bacteria, yeast, or a combination of both. In puppies, ear mites can also be a source of infection.

The pinna, middle ear, inner ear, and external ear canal form the canine ear. The cartilage of the auricle and annulus constitute the external ear. At the external ear canal opening, the pinna's auricular cartilage takes on the appearance of a funnel. After approximately one inch, the auricular and annular cartilage that makes up the horizontal ear canal emerges from the vertical ear canal. The three auditory ossicles, the tympanic membrane, and the air-filled tympanic cavity are part of the middle ear [2]. The pars flaccida and pars tensa make up the semitransparent tympanic membrane. The little epitympanic recess, the huge ventral bulla, and the tympanic bulla proper make up the tympanic cavity. The cochlea is located on the promontory, which is the medial wall of the tympanic cavity. A thin membrane covers the cochlear (round) window, which is situated in the caudolateral section of the promontory. The stapes footplate is linked to a thin diaphragm that covers the vestibular (oval) window, which is situated on the dorsolateral surface of the promontory. The auditory tube is a brief canal that connects the rostral region of the tympanic cavity proper to the nasopharynx. The bones that carry and intensify air vibrations from the tympanic membrane to the inner ear are called auditory ossicles (Fig. **1**). The petrous part of the temporal bone contains a bony labyrinth that houses the inner ear. The membrane labyrinth, with its auditory and vestibular organs, is housed within the bone labyrinth [3].

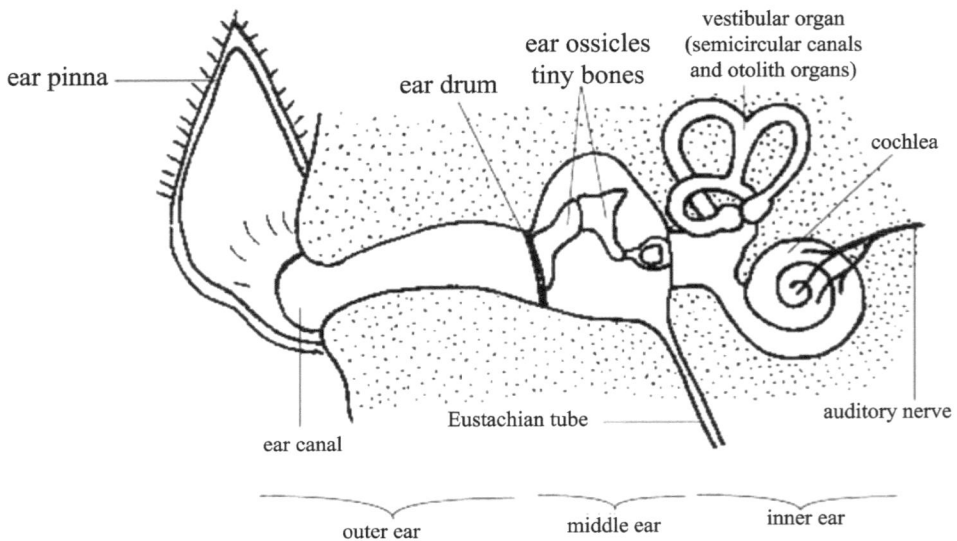

Fig. (1). Internal structure of ear of dog.

COMMON EAR DISEASES IN DOGS

Now, let's explore some of the most common ear diseases that affect dogs. There are three types of ear infections, known formally as otitis externa, media, and interna. The most common is otitis externa, in which inflammation affects the layer of cells lining the external portion of the ear canal. Otitis media and interna refer to infections of the middle and inner ear canal, respectively. These infections often result from the spread of infection from the external ear. Otitis media and interna can be very serious and may result in deafness, facial paralysis, and vestibular signs. That's why it's important to prevent infections and seek early treatment when problems arise [4].

Otitis Externa

This is the inflammation of the external ear canal, often caused by factors such as allergies, moisture, foreign bodies, or ear mites. Symptoms may include redness, itching, discharge, and a foul odor.

Otitis Media

Otitis media refers to inflammation of the middle ear. It's typically a result of untreated otitis externa or the spread of infection. Dogs with otitis media may show signs of pain, head tilting, and a reluctance to chew or open their mouths.

Otitis Interna

This is a severe infection of the inner ear, causing vestibular issues, such as loss of balance, head tilting, and abnormal eye movements. It can be caused by untreated otitis media or systemic infections.

Aural/ Ear Hematomas

Hematomas occur when blood vessels rupture within the ear flap due to vigorous shaking or head scratching. This leads to the accumulation of blood and a swollen, painful ear flap. Surgery is the most common treatment of choice for recurrent or persistent hematoma in dogs and cats (Figs. **2a**, **2b**). The most commonly reported approach is a linear incision with sutures. Dogs with aural hematomas have a decent to excellent prognosis provided the perpetuating causes are removed [5].

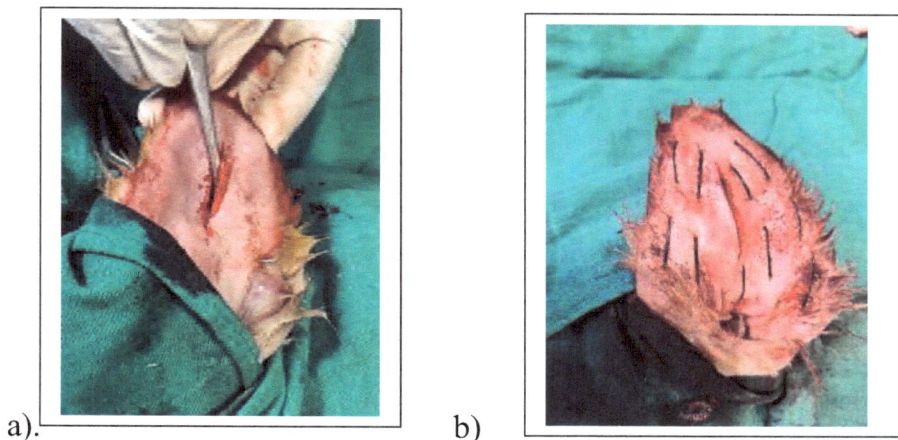

a).   b)

Fig. (2). Aural haematoma in a dog (**a**) linear incision on ear pinna (**b**) horizontal mattress suture placement.

It's crucial to keep in mind that the formation of an aural hematoma is not a primary condition until there has been ear trauma. To successfully resolve the hematoma, the primary, predisposing, and perpetuating factors that lead to the formation of otitis media and/or aural hematomas must be addressed.

As long as the underlying cause is addressed, an aural hematoma may resolve on its own, however, as a result of this, the pinna and ear canal may undergo potentially serious morphological alterations. Recurrent otitis media may be exacerbated by long-term alterations to the pinna's architecture in cases of severe ear deformity.

Ear Tumors

Ear canal tumors are comparatively rare, making up 2–6% of all tumors in dogs. While less common, dogs can develop benign or malignant tumors in their ears, which may require surgical intervention. Tumors may develop from any of the structures lining or supporting the ear canal including the outer layer of skin, the glands that produce earwax and oil, or any of the bones, connective tissues, muscles, or middle layers of the skin. Tumors of the external ear canal and pinna are more common than tumors of the middle or inner ear. Even though the etiology of these tumors remains more as a research topic, it is believed that chronic ear canal inflammation may produce aberrant tissue growth and development, which in turn may result in the creation of an ear canal tumor. The prognosis for dogs with ear canal tumors is not well understood. Furthermore, it is mostly unknown how different treatments (such as surgery, radiotherapy, or chemotherapy) may help with the regression and remission of ear canal tumors [6].

Apart from these common diseases, dogs may also suffer from some less common infections such as traumatic lacerations of ear, ear polyps, vestibular diseases, ruptured eardrum, para-aural abscess *etc.* which are discussed in detail in further chapters of this book.

CAUSES OF EAR DISEASES

Ear diseases in dogs can result from various factors, including allergies, parasites, foreign objects, bacterial or yeast infections, and genetic predispositions. It is crucial that the doctor assess involvement of numerous primary, predisposing, and perpetuating variables that may be contributing to ear ailments while evaluating each individual patient impacted.

Primary Factors

Primary factors include otic parasites like *Otodectes cyanotis*, hypersensitivity diseases (food allergy, atopic dermatitis, contact hypersensitivity), endocrine diseases like hypothyroidism, otic neoplasia, and foreign bodies. These conditions can directly affect the external ear canal and result in otitis. The most frequent primary cause of otitis in dogs is underlying hypersensitivity illness [7].

Predisposing Factors

Predisposing factors are factors that alter the local ear canal environment and create an increased risk for development of otitis externa. Ears with excessive hair, stenotic ears, increased cerumen production in the canals, otic masses, frequent ear cleaning, as well as changes in external environmental temperature and humidity can all act as predisposing factors.

Factors that may predispose dogs to ear infections include:

• Moisture, which can create a prime growing environment for bacteria and yeast.
• Allergies, which lead to ear disease in about 50 percent of dogs with allergic skin disease and 80 percent of dogs with food sensitivities.
• Endocrine disorders, such as thyroid disease.
• Autoimmune disorders.
• Wax buildup.
• Foreign bodies.
• Injury to the ear canal.
• Excessive cleaning.

Perpetuating Factors

Perpetuating factors are factors that do not initiate inflammation but lead to exacerbation of the inflammatory process and maintain ear disease even if the primary factor has been identified and corrected. Bacteria such as *Staphylococcus* and *Pseudomonas,* and *Malassezia* yeast are common perpetuating factors. If infection travels to the tympanic bulla, presence of this infection in the middle ear can also act as a perpetuating factor, leading to recurrent external ear infections. Perpetuating factors are often the main reason for treatment failures in dogs affected with recurrent otitis externa [8].

DIAGNOSIS OF EAR DISEASES

If the dog is showing any of the common signs of ear infections, it's important to diagnose the root cause of it as soon as possible. Quick treatment is necessary not only for dog's comfort (these conditions can be painful!), but also to prevent the spread of infection to the middle and inner ear.

The veterinarian should take thorough history of the case. This is especially important for first-time infections. Some salient questions to be asked to owners must include:

- Duration of any symptoms, such as pain, swelling, discharge, and odor.
- If the dog has any allergies or other underlying medical conditions.
- Whether or not, the dog is on medication.
- What the dog has been eating.
- How often does the owner clean dog's ears and which dog ear cleaning products are used for that purpose.
- If the dog has undergone recent trimming or plucking of hair in dog's ears.
- Recent activities, such as baths, grooming, or swimming.
- If the dog has a history of ear infections, when they occurred, and how they were treated.

After obtaining history, the veterinarian should perform a physical examination. In severe cases, sedating the dog to facilitate examination deep within the ear canal is also recommended. Evaluation of both ears should be done simultaneously and it should include:

- Visual assessment to look for signs such as redness, swelling, and discharge.
- Examination with an otoscope, which allows evaluation of the ear canal and eardrum.
- Gentle palpation of the ear to assess level of pain.
- Microscopic examination of samples taken by swabbing the ear.
- Culture of samples from the ear.
- Biopsies or X-rays in severe or chronic cases.

Detecting ear diseases in dogs requires a combination of observation, examination, and, in some cases, specialized testing. When you notice any unusual signs or symptoms in dog's ears, it's essential to go for a proper diagnosis. Common diagnostic methods include:

Physical Examination

Inspecting dog's ears for redness, swelling, discharge, or signs of trauma. The veterinarian may also check for pain reactions during ear palpation.

Common Symptoms of Dog Ear Infections

Some dogs show no symptoms of ear infection aside from a buildup of wax and discharge in the ear canal. But ear infections often cause significant discomfort and affected dogs may show signs such as:

• Head shaking
• Scratching at the affected ear
• Dark discharge
• Odor
• Redness and swelling of the ear canal
• Itchiness

Crusting or scabs in the ears: Alopecia, excoriation, crusting, erythema, and hyperpigmentation are possible alterations of the ear pinna. Hyperemia, ulceration, ceruminous or suppurative discharge, tumors, stenosis, glandular alterations, or foreign bodies can all be seen in the external ear canal (Fig. **3**).

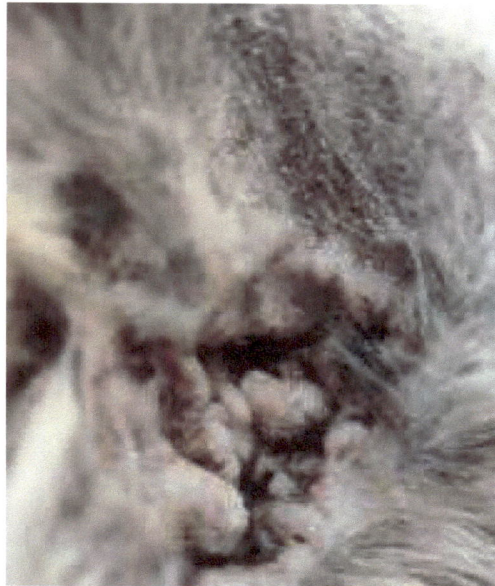

Fig. (3). Scab formation or crusting in ears.

In an afflicted ear, multiple aberrant findings are typically observed. An important aspect of the otoscopic examination is the assessment of the tympanic membrane, yet it can be challenging to do so in presence of otitis externa. It makes sense to postpone evaluating the tympanic membrane until after modifications linked to active otitis have been made [9].

Ear Cytology

This involves taking a sample from the ear canal to examine under a microscope. It helps identify the type of microorganisms present, such as yeast or bacteria, guiding treatment decisions.

Ear Culture and Sensitivity

In cases of chronic or recurring ear infections, a culture and sensitivity test may be performed to determine the specific bacteria involved and which antibiotics will be most effective.

Imaging

X-rays or advanced imaging like CT scans may be necessary if inner ear issues or tumors are suspected. It is possible to assess the ear canal and tympanic bulla radiographically, surgically, and otoscopically. Another imaging modality being considered for the diagnosis of otitis media is ultrasound, which is noninvasive and reasonably priced. Furthermore, there are sophisticated imaging methods available for imaging the ear, such as CT and MRI (Figs. **4a**, **4b**) . The ear canal and tympanic bulla can be examined noninvasively with these imaging techniques, although they require general anesthesia. To diagnose otic neoplasia, vestibular illness, otitis media, and congenital ear abnormalities, radiographs, CT scans, and MRIs may be used [10]. An infectious or inflammatory process as opposed to a neoplastic one, the degree of involvement in the middle or inner ear, peripheral as opposed to central vestibular disease, the chronicity of the disease process, involvement of nearby structures, and postsurgical complications are just a few of the important details about ear disease that can be obtained through imaging of the ear canal [11].

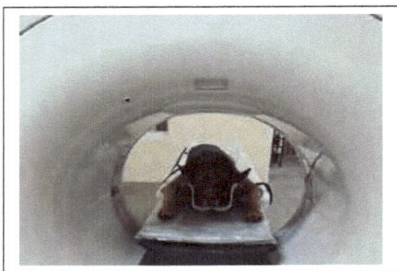
(a)

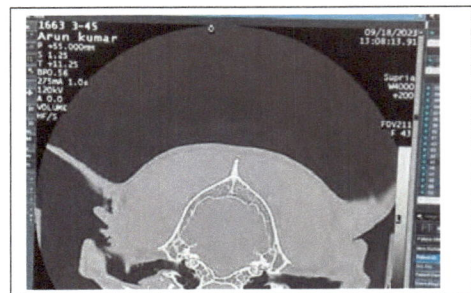
(b)

Fig. (4). Computed Tomographic examination (**a**) dorsoventral positioning of dog under general anesthesia (**b**) computed tomogram showing radiolucent right and left ear canal.

Biopsy

For suspected ear tumors, a biopsy may be needed to determine if they are benign or malignant [12]. The ear punch biopsy also provides a reliable method for sampling dogs with recurrent chronic ear disease irresponsive to treatment and proves useful for detecting benign and malignant growths of ear.

Treatment of Ear Diseases

The treatment approach for ear diseases in dogs depends on the underlying cause and the specific condition. Here are some common treatment methods:

Medications

Ear infections are often treated with topical or oral antibiotics or antifungal medications. Veterinarian must prescribe the appropriate medication based on the diagnosis.

Cleaning

Thorough ear cleaning is crucial for treating and preventing ear diseases. Veterinarian must demonstrate the proper technique for at-home cleanings or perform a deep cleaning under sedation if needed.

Surgery

In cases of severe ear hematomas or ear tumors, surgical intervention may be necessary. Surgery aims to drain blood from hematomas or remove tumors.

Lifestyle Adjustments

If allergies are the root cause, veterinarian may recommend dietary changes, environmental modifications, or allergy medications to manage the condition.

Long-Term Management

Chronic ear conditions may require ongoing management, including regular check-ups, ear cleaning, and medication to control symptoms and prevent recurrence.

Preventive Measures for Ear Diseases

Preventing ear diseases in dogs involves a combination of proactive measures. To help prevent majority of mentioned diseases in this chapter, following measures should be considered:

Regular Cleaning

Ear cleaning is recommended to prevent wax buildup and moisture retention.

Regular Veterinary Visits

Schedule regular check-ups to catch early signs of ear issues.

Allergen Management

If dog has allergies, the inflammatory triggers must be identified, and appropriate management strategies should be implemented.

Parasite Control

Maintain a year-round parasite control program to prevent ear mites and other parasites.

Prompt Treatment

Seek prompt treatment for any signs of ear discomfort, such as itching, redness, or discharge, to prevent conditions from worsening.

Gentle Handling

Handle dog's ears gently to avoid injury or discomfort.

Most uncomplicated ear infections resolve within 1–2 weeks, once appropriate treatment begins. But severe infections or those due to underlying conditions may take months to resolve or may become chronic problems. In cases of severe chronic disease where other treatments have failed, surgeries such as a Total Ear Canal Ablation (TECA) is recommended. A TECA surgery removes the ear canal, thus removing the diseased tissue and preventing the recurrence of infection [13]. TECA is often performed for the following reasons:

- Severe, incurable, or recurrent otitis externa (infection or inflammation of the ear canal), with little relief provided by medical treatment.
- Chronic ear disease-related ear canal constriction that makes it difficult to properly treat the ear canal.
- Unsuccessful ear canal disease management surgeries, such as Lateral Wall Resection (LWR) or Vertical Canal Ablation.
- Tumors limited to the canal of the ear.
- Otitis externa that is not improving with medication and has developed into otitis media, or middle ear inflammation or infection.
- Having trouble applying topical therapy for persistent otitis externa.

It is important to provide a detailed follow up to pet owners recommended recheck appointments. Lapses in treatment may lead to the recurrence of the infection. It is especially important to finish the full course of medication, even if dog appears to be getting better. Failure to finish the full course of treatment may lead to additional problems such as resistant infections.

CONCLUSION

In this chapter, we've laid the foundation for understanding the importance of ear health in dogs and introduced some common ear diseases. In the following chapters, we will delve deeper into each ear condition, exploring their diagnosis and treatment options. Remember that a proactive approach to ear health can significantly improve the quality of life for these furry companions.

Understanding the anatomy of a dog's ear, recognizing common ear diseases, and knowing how to diagnose and treat them are essential for responsible pet ownership. In the subsequent chapters, we will explore each ear condition in greater detail, providing comprehensive information to help you keep your canine companions ears healthy and free from disease. Remember that a proactive approach to ear care can lead to a happier and healthier life for these beloved pets.

REFERENCES

[1]   Huang HP, Little CJL, McNeil PE. Histological changes in the external ear canal of dogs with otitis externa. Vet Dermatol 2009; 20(5-6): 422-8.
[http://dx.doi.org/10.1111/j.1365-3164.2009.00853.x] [PMID: 20178479]

[2]   Zamankhan Malayeri H, Jamshidi S, Zahraei Salehi T. Identification and antimicrobial susceptibility patterns of bacteria causing otitis externa in dogs. Vet Res Commun 2010; 34(5): 435-44.
[http://dx.doi.org/10.1007/s11259-010-9417-y] [PMID: 20526674]

[3]   Saridomichelakis MN, Farmaki R, Leontides LS, Koutinas AF. Aetiology of canine otitis externa: a retrospective study of 100 cases. Vet Dermatol 2007; 18(5): 341-7.
[http://dx.doi.org/10.1111/j.1365-3164.2007.00619.x] [PMID: 17845622]

[4]   Morgan JL, Coulter DB, Marshall AE, Goetsch DD. Effects of neomycin on the waveform of auditory-evoked brain stem potentials in dogs. Am J Vet Res 1980; 41(7): 1077-81.
[PMID: 7436102]

[5]   Hewitt J, Bajwa J. Aural hematoma and it's treatment: A review. Can Vet J 2020; 61(3): 313-5.
[PMID: 32165757]

[6]   Little C, Pearson G, Lane J. Neoplasia involving the middle ear cavity of dogs. Vet Rec 1989; 124(3): 54-7.
[http://dx.doi.org/10.1136/vr.124.3.54] [PMID: 2919494]

[7]   Cole LK, Rajala-Schultz PJ, Lorch G. Conductive hearing loss in four dogs associated with the use of ointment-based otic medications. Vet Dermatol 2018; 29(4): 341-e120.
[http://dx.doi.org/10.1111/vde.12542] [PMID: 29664150]

[8]   Eger CE, Lindsay P. Effects of otitis on hearing in dogs characterised by brainstem auditory evoked response testing. J Small Anim Pract 1997; 38(9): 380-6.
[http://dx.doi.org/10.1111/j.1748-5827.1997.tb03490.x] [PMID: 9322176]

[9]   Griffiths LG, Sullivan M, O'Neill T, Reid SWJ. Ultrasonography *versus* radiography for detection of fluid in the canine tympanic bulla. Vet Radiol Ultrasound 2003; 44(2): 210-3.
[http://dx.doi.org/10.1111/j.1740-8261.2003.tb01273.x] [PMID: 12718358]

[10]   M.G. Bischoff, S.K. Kneller / Vet Clin Small Anim 34 (2004) 437–458.

[11]   Belmudes A, Pressanti C, Barthez PY, Castilla-Castaño E, Fabries L, Cadiergues MC. Computed tomographic findings in 205 dogs with clinical signs compatible with middle ear disease: a retrospective study. Vet Dermatol 2018; 29(1): 45-e20.
[http://dx.doi.org/10.1111/vde.12503] [PMID: 28994490]

[12]   Hnilica KA. Otitis externa small animal dermatology: a color atlas and therapeutic Guide. 3rd ed. St. Louis, Missouri: Elsevier Saunders 2011; pp. 395-8.

[13]   Cole LK, Kwochka KW, Kowalski JJ, Hillier A. Microbial flora and antimicrobial susceptibility patterns of isolated pathogens from the horizontal ear canal and middle ear in dogs with otitis media. J Am Vet Med Assoc 1998; 212(4): 534-8.
[http://dx.doi.org/10.2460/javma.1998.212.04.534] [PMID: 9491161]

CHAPTER 2

Normal Structure and Function of Ears

Jasvinder Singh Sasan[1,*], Shalini Suri[1] and Kamal Sarma[1]

[1] *Division of Veterinary Anatomy, Faculty of Veterinary Sciences and Animal Husbandry, Sher-E-Kashmir University of Agricultural Sciences and Technology of Jammu, Jammu and Kashmir, India*

Abstract: Hearing is one of the fundamental sense. Ear also known as the vestibulocochlear organ, is subdivided into three parts namely external, middle and inner ear. Auricle and external acoustic meatus comprise external ear. Sound waves are transmitted from the external ear to the middle ear. In dogs, breed-specific variances of external ear is noticeable. The auricle has a funnel-like shape which helps in sound collection. Auricle is divided into the proximal conchal cavity and distally located scapha. Anthelix divides the conchal cavity from the scapha and is located close to the conchal cavity. External acoustic meatus is made up of a proximal osseous portion and a distal cartilaginous portion. The cartilaginous portion of carnivores is relatively long and curved which hampers the passage of the straight otoscope for examination. The tympanic membrane consist of two parts, namely the pars flaccida and the pars tensa. The middle ear comprises the auditory ossicles (malleus, incus and stapes), muscles and auditory tube. Tympanic cavity is contained in the petrous temporal bone and has dorsal (epitympanicum), middle (mesotympanicum) and ventral (hypotympanicum) section. Auricular ossicles are located in the dorsal portion. The tympanic membrane is located on the lateral wall of the middle portion. The tympanic bulla is known as the ventral hypotympanicum. Internal ear has membranous and osseous labyrinth. The membrane labyrinth is filled with endolymph and includes the vestibular labyrinth which houses the receptor organ for balance and cochlear labyrinth containing the organ of hearing. The osseous labyrinth consists of vestibule, semicircular canals and cochlea. While defects in the inner ear may result in sensorineural hearing loss, defects in the outer, middle, and middle ear can cause conductive hearing loss. Therefore, it is crucial to research the anatomy and physiology of the ear. This chapter's main objective is to explore the fundamental anatomy and physiology of numerous components of the canine ear that plays a vital role in hearing.

Keywords: Auricle, Cochlea, Conchal cavity, Ear, Scapha, Tympanic membrane, Vestibule.

---

* **Corresponding author Jasvinder Singh Sasan:** Division of Veterinary Anatomy, Faculty of Veterinary Sciences and Animal Husbandry, Sher-E-Kashmir University of Agricultural Sciences and Technology of Jammu, Jammu and Kashmir, India; E-mail: jssasan216@gmail.com

Tanmoy Rana (Ed.)

INTRODUCTION

Ear houses both the hearing and the balancing organs thus known as the vestibulocochlear organ [1]. The cochlea receives and converts mechanical impulses from sound waves into electrical signals, and the vestibular organ provides animal a sense of position and movement in relation to gravity. The inner ear contains the receptors for both organs. The vestibulocochlear nerve is the physical and physiological relationship between the two organs. The ear can be divided into three subdivisions (Fig. **1**):

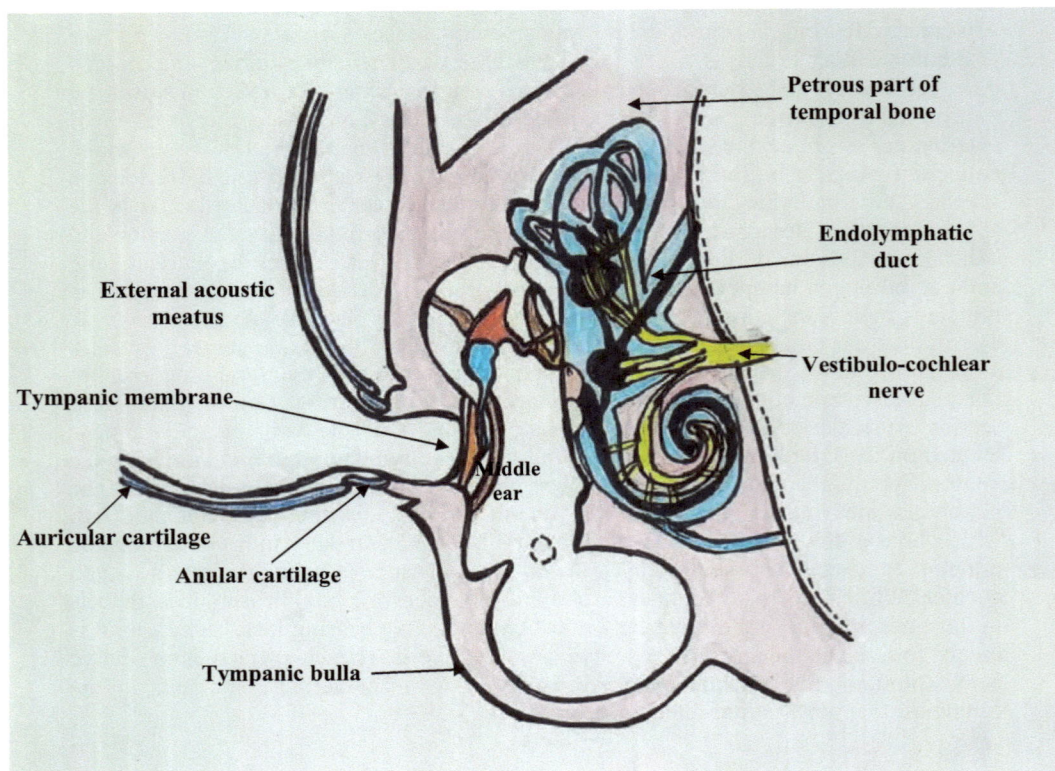

Fig. (1). Schematic diagram showing external acoustic meatus, middle ear and inner ear.

- External ear
- Middle ear
- Internal ear

The organ of balance (vestibular system) is restricted to the internal ear.

EXTERNAL EAR

The external ear consists of the following parts:

- Auricle along with the auricular cartilage.
- External acoustic meatus.
- Tympanic membrane.

When upright, the ears can be used independently to locate and gather sound. The tympanic membrane, located deep within the external acoustic meatus, receives sound waves *via* the external acoustic meatus.

Auricle

Auricle is also known as the ear leather to dog fanciers [2]. The size and shape of the external ear in domesticated animals varies widely between species and breeds (Fig. **2**). In dogs, breed-specific variances are particularly noticeable. Konig and Liebich [1] reported breed-specific ear forms as summarized in Table **1**.

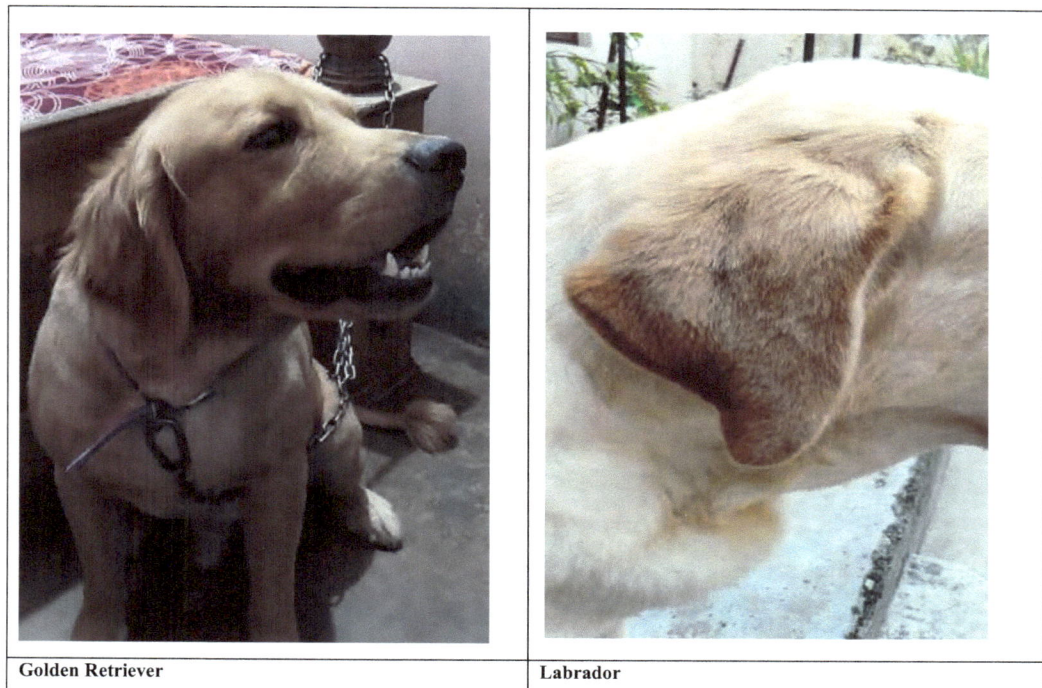

| Golden Retriever | Labrador |

(Fig. 2) contd.....

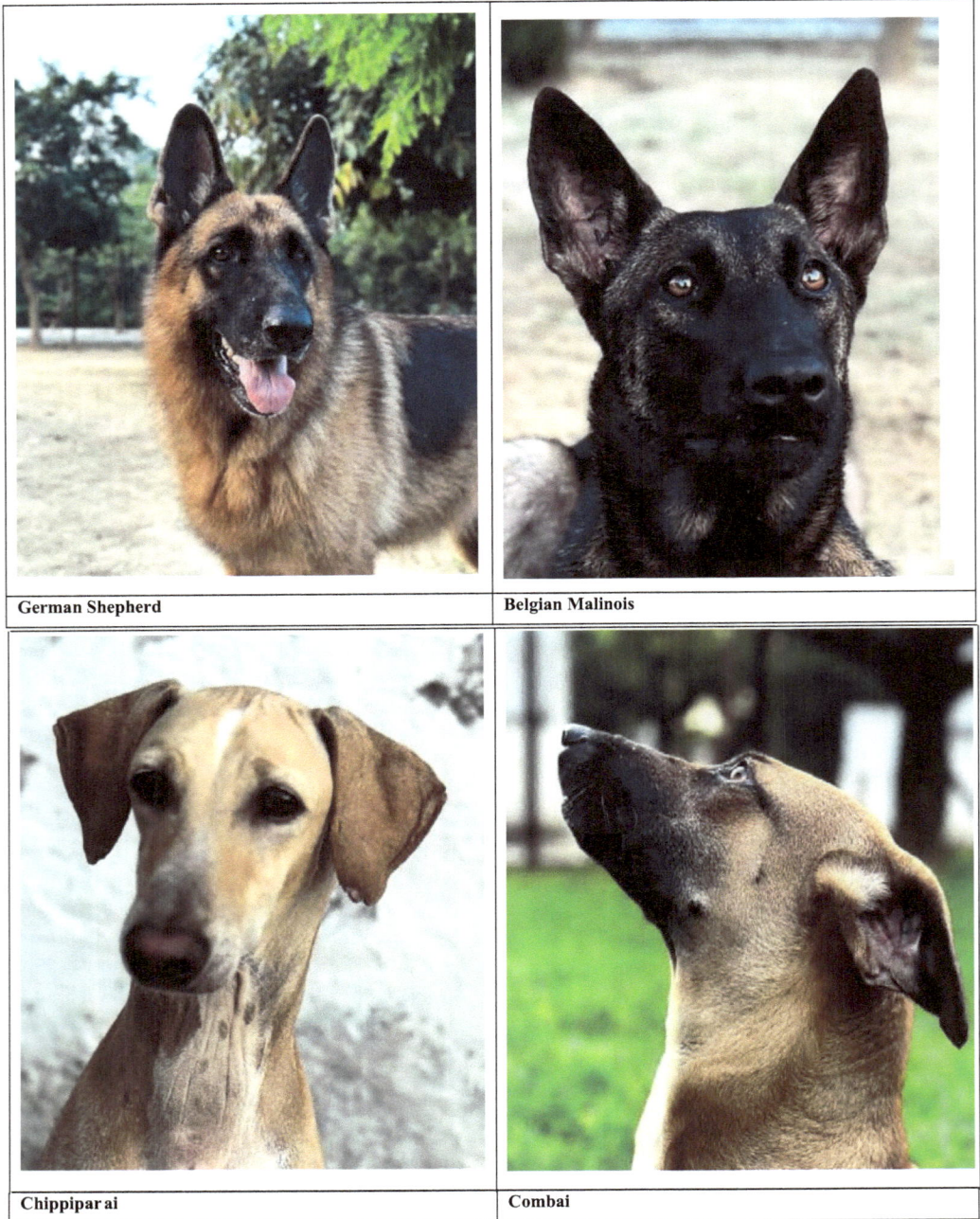

| German Shepherd | Belgian Malinois |
| Chippiparai | Combai |

Fig. (2). Showing shape of auricle in different breeds of dog.

Table 1. Ear shapes of various breeds of dogs.

Breed	Ear form
Spitz, northern sledge dog	Short erect ear
German shepherd	Long erect ear
French bulldog	Bat ear
Foxterrier, collie	Drop ear
Greyhounds	Rose ear with the ear tip lying close to the head
Great Dane, a few types of gun dogs	Lop-eared
Bloodhounds, a few hunting dogs	Lop-eared (long)

The auricle, which resembles a funnel, acts as a sound collecting structure. The auricular muscles move it to focus and gather sound. The muscles that move the auricle are coated in skin. The auricular muscles surround and insert onto the auricle. The external ear is turned and moved up and down.

The auricle's funnel-like distal opening narrows to form a tube at its proximal end. The skin-covered auricular cartilage determines the auricle's size and shape. Numerous foramina penetrate the auricular cartilage, allowing blood vessels and nerves to travel from the convex surface to the concave surface [3]. On the concave surface, the hairs are sparse and thin except few to guard the opening to the external auditory meatus. In dogs with pendulous ears in particular, the convex surface is covered in typical fur and has dense, long hairs.

The auricle on its concave surface is divided into two parts, namely proximal concha or conchal cavity and distally located flattened scapha (Fig. **3**).

The proximal part of the auricle, where it funnels into the external acoustic meatus, is known as the conchal cavity (cavum conchae). On the concave surface of the auricle, there is a transverse cartilage fold called the anthelix which divides the conchal cavity from the scapha and is located close to the distal section of the conchal cavity. The conchal tube's base is lined by an additional cartilaginous band called the anular cartilage (cartilago anularis), which connects to the osseous external acoustic meatus. The cutaneous marginal pouch (saccus cutaneus marginalis) is visible in the caudal edge of cats and dogs (Fig. **4**). In a dog of ordinary size, the anular cartilage is around 2 cm long. The conchal section of the auricular cartilage is rolled into a tube at the entry of the external auditory meatus, and there are several cartilaginous extensions there. A thick, blunt, quadrangular plate of cartilage called the tragus protrudes from the rostral edge of this opening. The antitragus, a thin, long cartilage projection next to the tragus on this rostral boundary, is present. The intertragic incisure (incisura intertragica), which divides the antitragus from the tragus, is present [4].

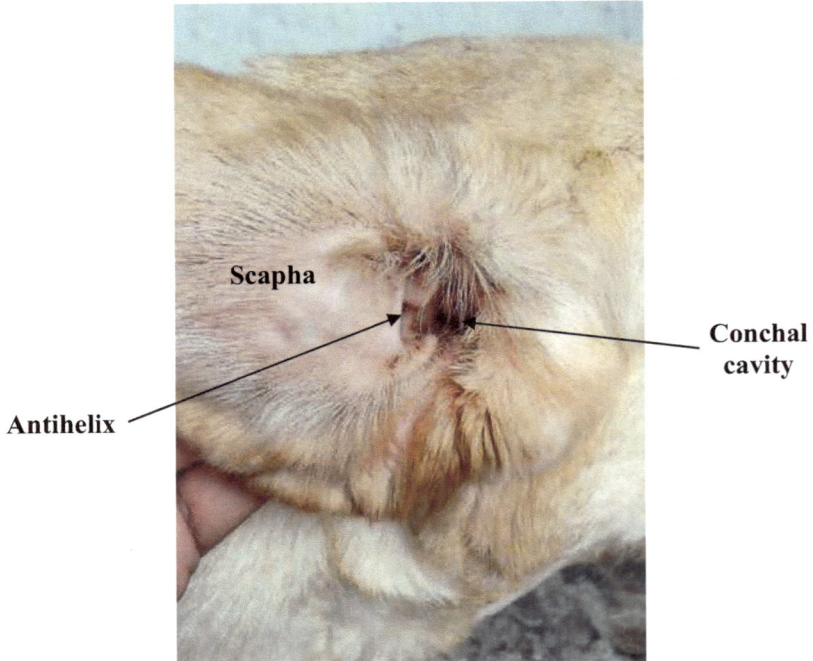

Fig. (3). Auricle of Labrador dog showing scapha and conchal cavity separated by antihelix.

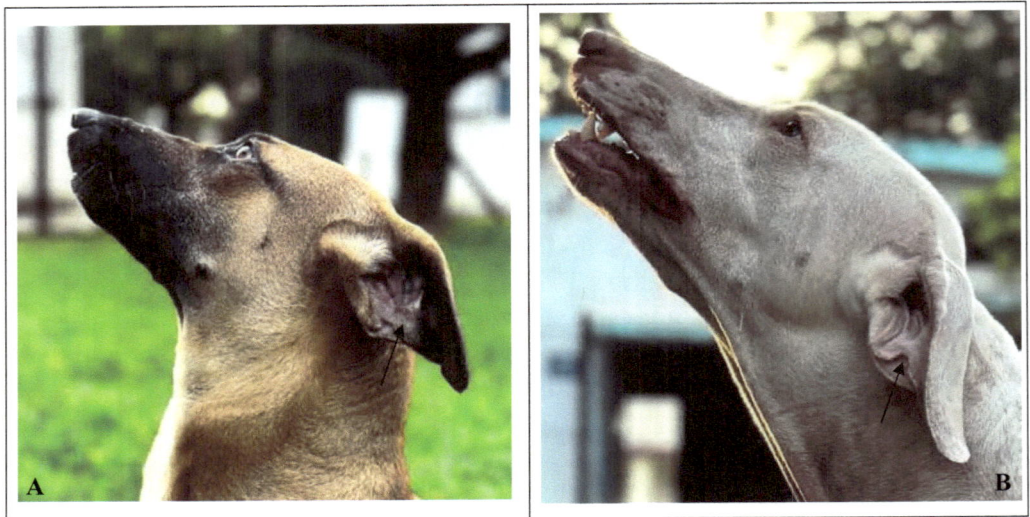

Fig. (4). Cutaneous marginal pouch (arrow) in Comboi (**A**) and Rajapalyam (**B**) breed of dog.

External Acoustic Meatus

It is the canal that runs from the base of the auricle to the tympanic membrane and is made up of a proximal osseous portion and a distal cartilaginous portion. The cartilaginous portion of carnivores is curved and relatively long, with its beginning portion oriented downward and its subsequent horizontal portion directed medially [1]. As it is curved, it hampers the passage of the straight otoscope for examination [2].

The anular cartilage connects the comparatively short osseous portion to the concha's basal region. The flexibility of external ear is due to configuration of a separate ring connecting the auricle and the external acoustic meatus. Stratified squamous epithelium contains sebaceous and tubular ceruminous glands. These glands secrete earwax (cerumen). These glands are located throughout the external acoustic meatus in carnivores [1].

Tympanic Membrane

The middle ear is separated from the external acoustic meatus by the tympanic membrane, commonly known as the eardrum. It transfers sound waves to the middle ear's auditory ossicles. It is a thin, oval-shaped sheet which is semi-transparent and is composed of three layers:

- Outer stratified squamous epidermis derived from ectoderm of first pharyngeal groove.
- Middle layer of fibrous connective tissue.
- Inner layer of mucosa which is of pharyngeal pouch origin.

The tympanic membrane can be divided into two parts: the pars flaccida and the pars tensa [1]. The malleus's short lateral process and the tympanic incisure's edges are separated by the pars flaccida, a small dorsal triangular area. The remaining portion of the membrane is known as the pars tensa. In the dog tympanum's connective tissue layer, Wakuri *et al.* [5] discovered outer radial and inner circular fibres in the pars tensa. The umbo membranae tympani is the name for the most depressed point, which is located opposite the distal end of the manubrium. The head of the malleus articulates with incus, body of neighbouring auditory ossicle, whereas the handle of the malleus is implanted in the tympanic membrane. Tympanic membrane converts incoming sound waves into mechanical impulses, which the auditory ossicles then transmit to inner ear. Sensory nerve fibres innervate richly vascularize the tympanic membrane.

To explore microangiology in relation to surgical procedures, Maher [6] removed the tympanic membranes and adnexa from neonatal dogs. He discovered that the canine tympanic membrane's anatomy and vascular supply are remarkably comparable to that of humans. There were two sources of vascular supply: intrinsic sources from the deep auricular and rostral tympanic branches of the maxillary artery, and extrinsic ones from the stylomastoid branch of the caudal auricular artery.

MIDDLE EAR

The middle ear comprises the:

- Air filled tympanic cavity (cavum tympani),
- Auditory ossicles (ossicula auditus) and
- Auditory tube (tuba auditiva, Eustachian tube).

Tympanic Cavity (Cavum Tympani)

The petrous temporal bone contains the tympanic cavity. It has a dorsal, middle, and ventral section. The auricular ossicles are located in the dorsal portion known as the epitympanicum [1]. The tympanic membrane is located on the lateral wall of the middle portion, or mesotympanicum, which enters *via* auditory tube into the nasopharynx rostrally. The tympanic bulla (bulla tympanica), also known as the ventral hypotympanicum, is an inflated, bulbous protrusion of temporal bone which in some species, is separated into a huge cell area [1]. The floor and a sizable portion of the lateral walls of the tympanic cavity are formed by the tympanic bulla. In canines, tympanic bulla is located medial to the muscular process of the mandible and great cornu of the hyoid bone [7]. The tympanic membrane is incorporated into the lateral wall of the tympanic cavity, and there are two windows on the medial side.

The base of the stapes occupies the oval vestibular window (fenestra vestibuli), which connects the tympanic cavity with the inner ear. It is situated rostrodorsally. The cochlear window (foramen cochleae), which is more caudally located and has a rounded form, connects to the cochlea cavity. The secondary tympanic membrane closes it. The promontorium, a bony protrusion from medial wall of tympanic cavity, houses cochlea. The tympanic cavity is lined by a single-layered epithelium that also covers the tympanic membrane and auricular ossicles.

The tympanic cavity's long axis measures around 15 mm in length and forms a caudolateral angle of roughly 45 degrees with the sagittal plane. The dimensions of the breadth and depth are roughly comparable, ranging from 8 to 10 mm. The tympanic membrane is slanted ventromedially [4].

The chorda tympani, which originates from the facial nerve and travels through the tympanic cavity medial to the malleus before joining the lingual nerve, is one of the nerves that can be seen running through the tympanic cavity. The tympanic plexus arising from the tympanic nerve (n. tympanicus) of the glossopharyngeal nerve lies on the promontory and supplies the tympanic mucosa and the minor petrosal nerve to the otic ganglion. This tympanic plexus also receives support from the internal carotid plexus' caroticotympanic nerves.

Auditory Ossicles

The three auditory ossicles transmit the vibrations that travel from the tympanic membrane through the tympanic cavity and into the inner ear (Fig. **5**):

- Hammer (malleus),
- Anvil (incus) and
- Stirrup (stapes).

These tiny bones, which stretch from the tympanic membrane to the vestibular window, are connected to one another by syndesmoses to form a chain.

The malleus, made up of the head, neck, and manubrium, is the most lateral of the auditory ossicles. The three-sided manubrium is embedded within the tympanic membrane. The neck, which extends above the tympanic membrane, connects it to the head. The head of the malleus articulates with the body of the incus. The muscular projection of the malleus, which extends medially and somewhat rostrally from the base of the manubrium, provided a little hook at its end for the attachment of the m. tensor tympani. The lengthy rostral process is deeply enmeshed in the tympanic membrane. Short lateral process is located opposite to the muscular process at an angle of approximately 90 degrees with the rostral process [4]. This is the most dorsal attachment of the manubrium to the tympanic membrane.

Incus is considerably smaller than malleolus. Its form is comparable to a bicuspid tooth with diverging roots in a human. Incus is made up of a body and two limbs, *i.e.* long and short limb. The short limb points caudally. Lenticular bone articulates with head of stapes.

The stapes is made up of a base, two limbs, a head, a neck, and a muscular process. It is horizontally positioned, with the base pointing medially. Through the lenticular process, the head articulates with the incus. The vestibular window's edge is covered by a fibrocartilaginous ring, which the base articulates with. The stapes, the smallest bone in the body with a length of about 2 mm, is the innermost ossicle [4]. The concave or opposing sides of the rostral and caudal limbs are hollowed out. A single crus shows as a narrow semicircle of bone when cut in half. The muscular process provides attachment site for stapedius muscle.

	Malleus 1. Head 2. Facet for incus 3. Neck 4. Manubrium 5. Lateral process 6. Anterior process
	Incus 1. Facet for malleus 2. Long crus 3. Short crus 4. Body 5. Lenticular process
	Stapes 1. Head 2. Neck 3. Crura 4. Base

Fig. (5). Schematic diagram showing auditory ossicles of dog.

Several ligaments attaches the ossicles to the wall of the tympanic cavity [8]. Lateral ligament of the malleus connects the lateral process of the malleus to the margins of the tympanic notch. Dorsal ligament of the malleus joins the head of the malleus to a small area on the roof of the epitympanic recess. Rostral ligament of the malleus attaches the rostral process of the malleus and the osseous tympanic ring just ventral to the canal by which the chorda tympani leave the tympanic cavity. Dorsal ligament of incus attaches the body of the incus to the roof of the epitympanic recess. The caudal ligament of the incus attaches the short limb to the fossa. An anular ligament attaches base of stapes to the cartilage that lines vestibular window.

The tympanic membrane's vibrations are not only transmitted but also at least 20 times magnified by the auditory ossicles. This is necessary to start waves in the inner ear's endolymph. The tensor tympani and stapedial muscles, two antagonistic muscles connected to the ossicles, play a significant part in the enhancement mechanism. The rostro-medial portion of the tympanic cavity is the origin of the tensor tympani muscle (m. tensor tympani), which inserts to the malleus. This muscle's contraction increases the transmission system's sensitivity by tensioning chain of auditory ossicles and tympanic membrane. The stapedius muscle (m. stapedius) inserts to the stapes from a tiny depression between the wall of the tympanic cavity and the facial canal. Transmission is attenuated when the stapedial muscle contracts, moving the stapes' base farther from the vestibular window. The facial nerve innervates the stapedial muscle, while pterygoid nerve, branch of the mandibular nerve, innervates tensor tympani muscle.

Auditory Tube (Eustachian Tube)

The auditory tube, which connects the tympanic cavity to the nasopharynx, is a tiny, slit-like tube, surrounded by a ventrally open trough which is cartilaginous near the throat and osseous close to the tympanic cavity (pars cartilaginea tubae auditivae). The ciliated epithelium that lines both portions contains goblet cells and is surrounded by a collagenous-elastic soft tissue that is populated by lymphoreticular cells. The medial wall is almost exactly twice as long as the lateral wall, which is around 8 mm long. The tube has an oval cross shape and a larger diameter of 1.5 mm. Auditory tubes open on the dorso-lateral wall of the naso-pharynx, levels with the landmark provided by the hamulus of the pterygoid bone, which is palpable through the mouth caudo-medial to the last tooth of the cheek [2].

INNER EAR

The membrane labyrinth, which makes up the internal ear, is a composite organ made up of a network of ducts and chambers filled with membranous fluid.

Endolymph, the fluid in this labyrinth, stimulates sensory cells in the membranous wall with its motions. The membranous labyrinth comprises of:

• Vestibular labyrinth containing the receptor organ for balance.
• Cochlear labyrinth with the organ of hearing.
• Ductus reuniens, through which both systems communicate.

The osseous labyrinth encircles the membrane labyrinth and is similar to the membranous labyrinth in terms of shape and partitions, but slightly bigger. The bony labyrinth consists of the following parts (Fig. **6**):

• Vestibule
• Semicircular canals
• Cochlea

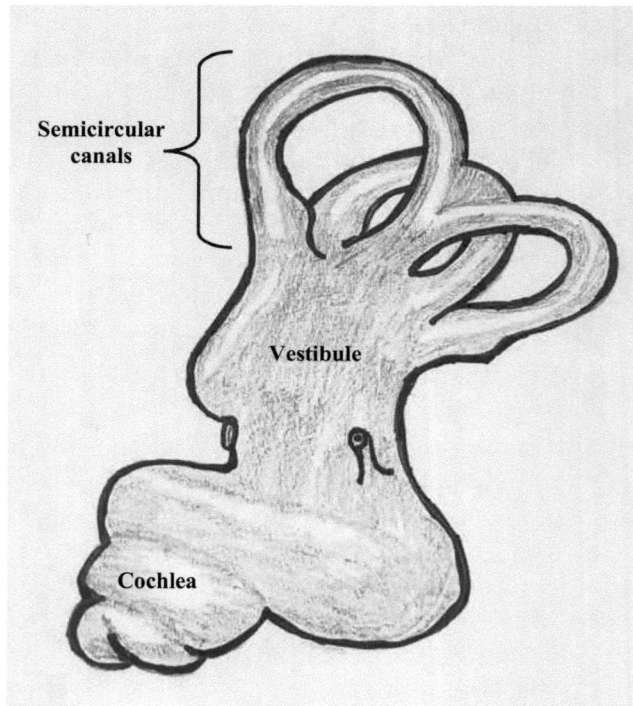

Fig. (6). Schematic diagram showing osseous labyrinth of inner ear which encloses membranous labyrinth.

The vestibule is the osseous labyrinth's primary chamber. It communicates caudally with the semicircular canals and rostrally with the cochlea. Two windows can be found on the vestibule's lateral wall: the vestibular window, which is blocked by the stapes, and the cochlear window, which is ventral to it and covered by secondary tympanic membrane. Vestibular labyrinth's semicircular duct is housed in the semicircular canals. The cochlea resembles a snail's shell in both size and form. It spirals around the modiolus, a hollow centre of the bone that houses the cochlear nerve. The spiral consists of three turns in carnivores [1]. The spiral lamina, an osseous shelf that extends into the spiral canal from the modiolus, partially divides the lumen into the scala tympani and scala vestibuli. The spiral lamina contains the spiral ganglion of the cochlear nerve. Three membranous channels in the cochlea encircle the modiolus. The vestibular and cochlear aqueducts connect the fluid-filled clefts (spatia perilymphatica) between the osseous and membranous labyrinths to the subarachnoid space of the meninges.

Vestibular Labyrinth

Saccule (sacculus), utricule (utriculus) and semicircular ducts (ductus semicirculares) make up the vestibular labyrinth (Fig. **7**). Each ampulla of the semicircular ducts has a sensory crista, while the sacculus and utriculus' walls both include sensory maculae. These use the vestibular nerve to sense and transmit balancing impulses.

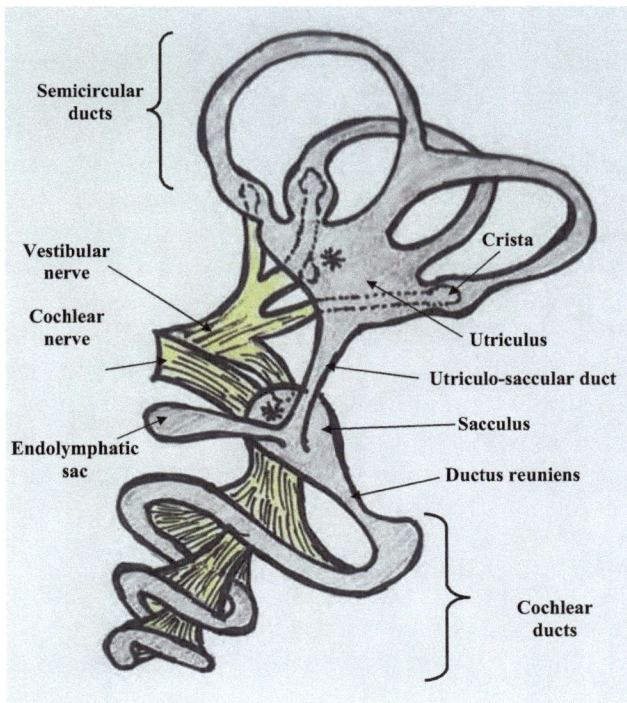

Fig. (7). Membranous labyrinth.

SACCULE (SACCULUS) AND UTRICLE (UTRICULUS)

Within osseous vestibule, there are two enlargements called saccule and utricle. The three semicircular ducts for balancing emerge from the utricle, and the spiral cochlear duct for hearing emerges from the saccule. Single-layered squamous epithelium with underlying loose connective tissue covers the wall of saccule and utricle. The elevated and oval-shaped saccule and utricle maculae (macula sacculi, macula utriculi) are formed by thickening of the medial wall. Modified epithelial cells function as receptors and are innervated by vestibular nerve fibres. These cells make up the sensory macula. A small network of non-myelinated nerve fibres surrounds the base of the epithelial cells before converging to create the vestibular nerve. These receptor cells' luminal region has a gelatinous layer that is encircled by sensory hairs. Otoliths, which are tiny calcium carbonate crystals, adhere to the gelatinous layer. The changes in the membrane's orientation causes pressure to be applied and the receptor cells to be stimulated. The vestibular nerve's efferent fibres subsequently carry the initiated impulse to the brain. Thus, changes in the vertical or horizontal plane are recorded by the maculae.

Semicircular Ducts (Ductus Semicirculares)

The osseous labyrinth's semicircular canals contain the three semicircular ducts. Each duct leaves the utricle and is semicircular having two crura. Near the point where one crus of each duct joins the utricule, there is a dilatation called an ampulla. Semicircular ducts stand roughly at right angles to each other. Orientation of anterior duct is transverse, posterior is sagittal, and lateral duct is horizontal. Structure of the wall of the ducts is comparable to those of the saccule and utricle. The sensory ampullary crest, also known as the crista ampullaris, protrudes from each ampulla. The receptor cells' sensory hairs are triggered by the movement of the glycoprotein layer (cupula) that surrounds them. Rotation causes the endolymph to move, causing the cupula to deform and the receptor cells to get stimulated. The vestibular component of the vestibulocochlear nerve supplies sensory nerves to the receptor cells of the vestibular labyrinth. The associated vestibular ganglion, which has direct branches to the vestibular receptor cells, is situated inside the internal acoustic meatus.

Cochlear Labyrinth (Pars Auditiva Labyrinthi)

The organ of hearing, which is made up of the organ of Corti (organum spirale) inside the cochlear duct (ductus cochlearis), is situated in the wall of the membranous cochlear labyrinth (Fig. **8**). Spiral canal of the cochlea is divided into three membranous ducts, which spiral around the modiolus to the apex of the cochlea:

- Scala vestibuli,
- Cochlear duct, also called the scala media, and
- Scala tympani.

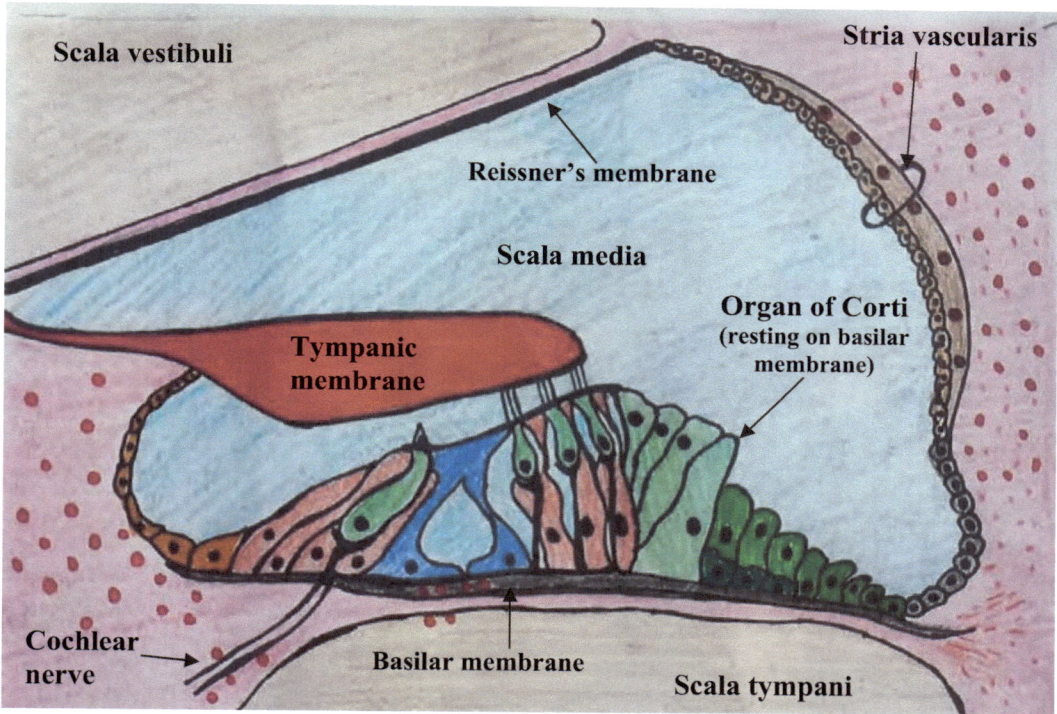

Fig. (8). Schematic diagram showing organ of corti.

Scala vestibuli, cochlear duct, and scala tympani make up the upper, middle, and lower channels, respectively. Around blind end of the cochlear duct, at the helicotrema of cochlea, the two scalae communicates. Scala vestibuli and scala tympani start at the vestibular window and secondary tympanic membrane, respectively, at the base of the cochlea, which covers the cochlear window. Both scalae contain perilymph and are bordered with a single layer of epithelium. The cochlear duct starts off blind, ascends *via* the osseous cochlea's spiral canal, and then terminates blind at the tip of the modiolus. It connects to the vestibular labyrinth *via* the ductus reuniens and contains endolymph.

Between the two scalae, the cochlear duct wraps around the modiolus. In cross section, it appears wedge-shaped, with the tip pointing in the direction of the modiolus. The Corti organ is located inside, submerged in endolymphatic fluid. The walls of the cochlear duct have three distinct segments: tympanic membrane, vestibular membrane and lateral membrane. The cochlear duct's roof, which separates it from the cochlea's scala vestibuli, is made up of the incredibly thin vestibular membrane. The spiral ligament (ligamentum spirale), which is securely attached to the spiral lamina's underlying periosteum, forms the lateral wall of the cochlear duct. It is highly vascularized and is charge of creating and secreting endolymph. The cochlear duct's floor is formed by the tympanic membrane, which also divides it from scala tympani. Organ of Corti is part of the tympanic membrane. Its connective tissue component is the basilar lamina, which is derived from the periosteum of the spiral lamina and continuous with spiral ligament of the lateral wall of the cochlear duct.

Organ of Corti (Organum Spirale)

The hearing receptor cells are part of the spiral organ, often known as the organ of Corti. It is located on the cochlear duct's tympanic membrane and follows the spirals throughout the cochlea. A gel-like membrane (membrana tectoria) covers the interior of the duct. Organ of Corti includes two different types of cells:

• sensory cells and
• supporting cells: columnar and phalangeal cells.

The columnar cells contact the basilar membrane with one end, while the other end is extended to form plates which provide stability to the receptor cells of the organ of Corti. The columnar cells are assisted by the phalangeal cells, which also support the receptor cells. Between the phalangeal cells are rows of receptor cells.

The auditory ossicles' chain carries mechanical vibrations of the tympanic membrane, which are caused by sound waves, from the external ear to the inner ear. The vestibular window and stapes come into direct touch, which causes the inner ear's perilymph to move. Due to the incompressibility of fluids, the movement of the perilymph is conveyed to the cochlear window through the scala tympani, helicotrema, and scala vestibuli, where it causes the secondary tympanic membrane to vibrate. The vestibular membrane transmits various frequencies to the endolymph of the cochlear duct. Pressure exerted by the endolymph on the tectorial membrane causes pressure on the sensory hairs, which in turn prompts impulses to be sent to the spiral ganglion by the receptor cells. The vestibulocochlear nerve's cochlear portion is made up of the combined axons of the spiral ganglion, and it travels to the appropriate nuclei of the medulla oblongata.

CONCLUDING REMARKS

Ear, one of the most advanced sense organs, is divided into three structural and functional sections. The tympanic membrane, which divides the outer ear from the middle ear, receives sound vibrations from the outer half, which includes the pinna and auditory canal. These vibrations are picked up by the middle ear, which houses the three ossicles (malleus, incus, and stapes) where they are amplified. The vibrations are transmitted from the middle ear to the inner ear, which houses the spiral-shaped cochlea as the sensing organ. The stereocilia found in the hair cells of the organ of Corti in the cochlea are responsible for opening the mechanotransduction channels, which allows the nerve signal to reach the brain. In this way, the vibrations are transformed into an audible sound.

REFERENCES

[1]   Konig HE, Liebich HG. Veterinary anatomy of domestic animals: Textbook and colour atlas. 7th ed. New York: George Thieme Verlag Stuttgart 2020; pp. 619-32.

[2]   Dyce KM, Sack WO, Wensing CJG. Textbook of Veterinary Anatomy. 3rd ed. Saunders Elsevier 2002; pp. 385-6.

[3]   Miller ME, Witter R. Applied anatomy of the external ear of the dog. Cornell Vet 1942; 32: 64-86.

[4]   Evans HE, de Lahunta A. Miller's anatomy of the dog. 4th ed. Elsvier Saunders 2013; pp. 731-45.

[5]   Wakuri H, Mori S, Mutoh K, Kataoka S, Watanabe S. Fiber arrangement in the canine tympanic membrane. Okajimas Folia Anat Jpn 1988; 65(1): 11-7.
[http://dx.doi.org/10.2535/ofaj1936.65.1_11] [PMID: 3405580]

[6]   Maher WP. Microvascular networks in tympanic membrane, malleus periosteum, and annulus perichondrium of neonatal mongrel dog: A vasculoanatomic model for surgical considerations. Am J Anat 1988; 183(4): 294-302.
[http://dx.doi.org/10.1002/aja.1001830403] [PMID: 3218619]

[7]   Done SH, Goody PC, Evans SA, *et al.* Color atlas of veterinary anatomy volume III Dog and Cat. 2nd ed. Mosby Elsvier 2009; 10.

[8]   Getty R, Foust HL, Presley ET, Miller ME. Macroscopic anatomy of the ear of the dog. Am J Vet Res 1956; 17(64): 364-75.
[PMID: 13340092]

CHAPTER 3

Physiology of Ear and Hearing

Archana Mahapatra[1,*], Satish Kumar Pathak[1], Prasanta Kumar Koustasa Mishra[2] and Thulasiraman Parkunan[3]

[1] *Department of Veterinary Anatomy, Faculty of Veterinary and Animal Sciences, Institute of Agricultural Sciences, Banaras Hindu University, Uttar Pradesh, India*

[2] *College of Veterinary Science and Animal Husbandry, OUAT, Odisha, India*

[3] *Department of Veterinary Physiology and Biochemistry, Faculty of Veterinary and Animal Sciences, Institute of Agricultural Sciences, Banaras Hindu University, Uttar Pradesh, India*

Abstract: Sense organs that is eye, ear, nose, tongue and skin provide a true sense to communicate with the outer world. Ear is the organ of hearing and balance. Ear is a complex organ consisting of three divisons, the outer, middle, and inner ear. The structures of the external ear are auricle, external auditory meatus and outer layers of the tympanic membrane. The middle ear is an air filled cavity (tympanum) consists of ear ossicles, auditory tube (Eustachian tube), middle ear muscles, inner layer of the tympanic membrane. The internal ear consists of the osseous labyrinth consisting of cochlea, vestibule and semicircular canals and membranous labyrinths and the vestibular and acoustic (spiral) ganglia associated with the eighth cranial nerve (vestibulocochlear nerve). The auditory system of ear convert sound waves into neural signals. The auricle acts as a condiut to collect the sound waves. The middle ear acts as a precochlear amplifier and impedance matching device. Transduction of sound occurs in the cochlea by spiral organs (formerly known as organs of Corti) resulting in an action potential that transmits along the auditory nerve to cochlear nucleus in the brainstem for hearing. The vestibular system plays an important role in maintaining the equilibrium and balance of the animal. It is a primary sensory organ consisting of vestibule and semicircular canals which orients with respect to the gravitational field of the earth and co-ordinates the movement of various sensory organs and thus the linear, rotatory, acceleration and deacceleration movements of the animal.

Keywords: Auricle, Balance, Basilar membrane, Cochlear duct, Crista ampullaris, Ear, Ear ossicles, External auditory meatus, Hair cells, Hearing, Impedance, Macula, Membranous sacculus, Membranous utriculus, Organ of Corti, Semicircular duct, Stereocilia, Tectorial membrane, Tympanic attenuation reflex, Tympanum.

* **Corresponding author Archana Mahapatra:** Department of Veterinary Anatomy, Faculty of Veterinary and Animal Sciences, Institute of Agricultural Sciences, Banaras Hindu University, Uttar Pradesh, India;
E-mail: archanamit88@gmail.com

Tanmoy Rana (Ed.)

INTRODUCTION

Human beings enjoy the companionship and benefit of dogs from the utility of many breeds. Domestication trained dogs communicate with humans in the best possible way that other animals cannot [1]. Ear is the organ of hearing and equilibrium. Hearing acuity in dogs is critically important for service, assistance, rescue, police and at military bases. Accurate hearing assessment is crucial as these dogs work on the auditory clues received in potentially life-threatening situations [2 - 4]. The form and function of ear will provide a deep insight for the hearing assessment.

STRUCTURAL COMPONENTS OF THE EAR

Ear is a complex organ consisting of three divisions, the outer, middle, and inner ear. The outer and middle ear are derived from the first and second pharyngeal arches, first pharyngeal cleft and pharyngeal pouch. The inner ear develops from the bilateral thickening of ectodermal otic placode placed lateral to the hindbrain. The principal structures of the ear are enclosed in the petrous temporal bones of the skull [5].

The structures of the external ear are auricle, external auditory meatus and outer layers of the tympanic membrane. The middle ear is an air filled cavity (tympanum) consists of ear ossicles, auditory tube (Eustachian tube), middle ear muscles, inner layer of the tympanic membrane. The internal ear consists of the osseous labyrinth consisting of cochlea, vestibule and semicircular canals and membranous labyrinths consisting of cochlear duct, membranous utriculus and sacculus, semicircular ducts and the vestibular and acoustic (spiral) ganglia associated with the eighth cranial nerve (vestibulocochlear nerve) [5].

PHYSIOLOGY OF HEARING

Energy waves produce the sound. These waves travel through a medium which causes movement of the molecules thereby increasing and decreasing the pressure waves (*i.e.*, alternating compression and rarefaction) of air within the environment [6].

The structures of ear convert sound waves into neural signals. The neural signals are sent directly to the brain *via* the auditory nerve (Fig. **1**). This transduction of sound occurs in the cochlea resulting in an action potential that transmits along the auditory nerve to cochlear nucleus in the brainstem. The external, middle and internal ear along with auditory nerve constitute peripheral auditory pathway. The brainstem and the brain constitute the central auditory pathway [7].

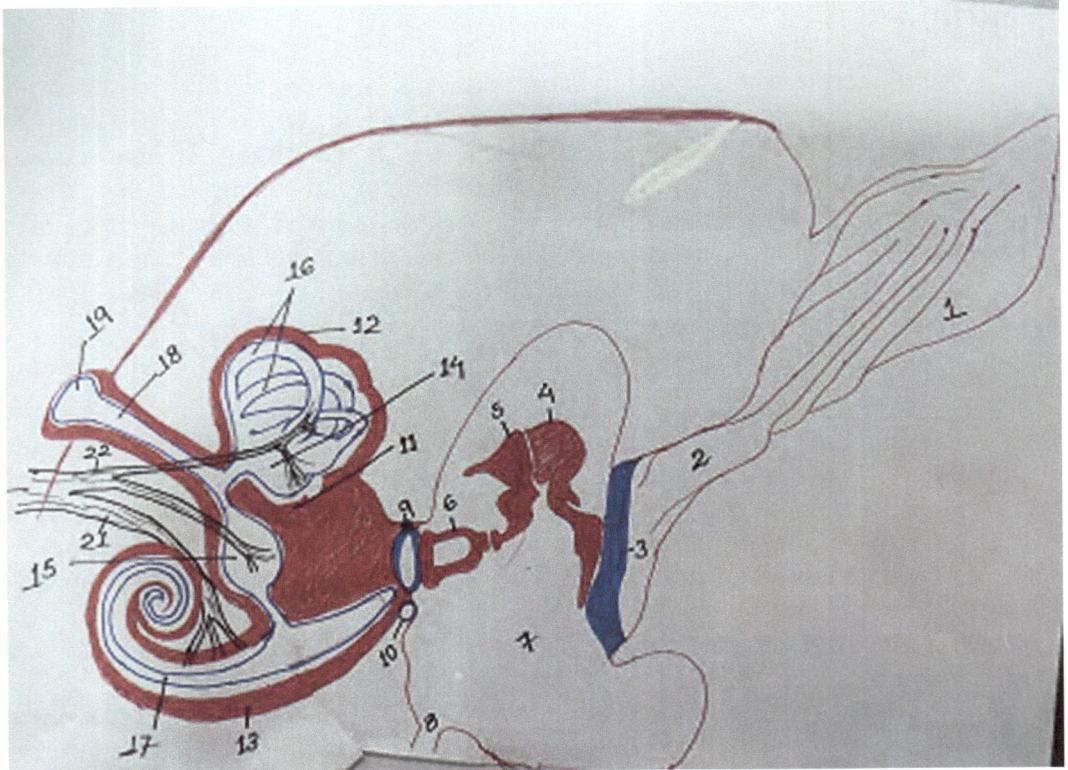

Fig. (1). Schematic diagram of canine ear exhibiting the structural component of outer, middle and inner ear. 1- Auricle, 2- External auditory meatus, 3-Tympanic membrane, 4-Malleus, 5-Incus, 6-Stapes, 7-Tympanic cavity, 8- Auditory tube, 9-Vestibular window, 10-Cochlear window, 11-Vestibule, 12-Semicircular canal, 13-Cochlea, 14-Utriculus, 15-Sacculus, 16-Semicircular duct, 17- Cochlear duct, 18- Endolymphatic duct, 19-Endolymphatic sac, 21-Cochlear branch of vestibulocochlear nerve, 22-Vestibular branch of vestibulocochlear nerve.

Function of the Outer Ear in Hearing

The auricle acts as a condiut to collect the sound waves. The well-developed muscles of the auricle of dog can direct it toward source of sound. There is variation in length of auricle in different breeds of dog. Dogs with large erect ears are good at localizing distant sounds. The ability to regulate the orientation of auricle improves hearing sensitivity up to 28 dB in dogs at higher frequencies [8, 9]. Many dogs are able to perceive the ultrasonic vocalization produced by mice and some insects [10]. The sound waves from the auricle are conveyed to auditory canal. The ear canal is long and L-shaped in dogs which helps to protect the tympanic membrane and amplify certain frequencies of sound. In the auditory canal these waves reach at the end of the external ear that is separated from the middle ear by tympanic membrane or ear drum (Fig. **2**).

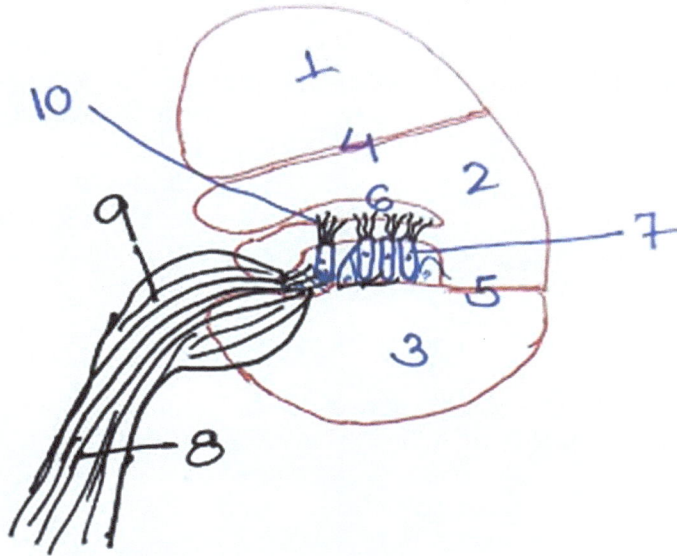

Fig. (2). Schematic diagram of cochlear duct (transverse section)
1- Scala vestibule, 2-Scala media, 3-Scala tympani, 4-Vestibular membrane, 5-Basilar membrane, 6-Tectorial membrane, 7- Hair cells, 8-Cochlear nerve, 9-Spiral ganglia, 10-Sterocilia.

Function of the Middle Ear in Hearing

In the middle ear the sound waves lead to the vibration of tympanic membrane, the outer boundary of tympanic cavity. Presence of collagen fibers in the tympanic membrane optimizes the sound transmission to the next level *i.e.* to the ear ossiccles [11]. The ear ossicles that is malleus, incus and stapes are attached with tympanic membrane and amplifies the sound waves. Sound-generated air pressure waves, vibrates the tympanic membrane. This membrane transfers and translates air pressure waves into fluid pressure waves within the labyrinth of internal ear. Air and fluid have different impedance (the tendency of a medium to oppose movement brought about by a pressure wave). The fluid has higher impedance than air thus a direct transfer of a pressure wave from air to water cannot bring the desired movement in the perilymph and endolypmh of the internal ear. This is known as "impedance mismatch" which is well managed by two efficient mechanism of the middle ear. First, by the extensive surface area of the tympanic membrane that is approximately 18-20 times larger than the surface area of the footplate of the stapes which is anchored to the vestibular or oval window. Secondarily, it is leveraged by the incus and malleus. These two phenomenal characteristics of the middle ear amplify the pressure wave and overcomes the impedance mismatch. This transfer of pressure within the middle ear is called as acoustic immitance (impedance *i.e.* restriction to the transfer of pressure + admittance *i.e.* transfer of pressure) [12 - 14]. Contraction of the middle ear muscles *i.e.* tensor tympani and stapedius blocks the loud or repetitive noises to enter into the middle ear and it also produces a transitory change in the impedance [15, 16]. This protective reflex mechanism known as tympanic attenuation reflex requires approximately 40-160 milliseconds to eventuate. Thus gun-shot like short loud noises causes hearing impairment among some haunting dogs [17]. So the middle ear acts as a precochlear amplifier and impedance matching device.

Function of the Inner Ear in Hearing

The internal ear portion of the auditory system consists of the cochlea, acoustic ganglia and the cochlear branch associated with vestibulocochlear nerve. It is separated from the middle ear by the vestibular (oval) and cochlear (round) windows. The highly coiled cochlea comprises of three separate fluid filled compartments *i.e.* scala vestibuli, scala media and scala tympani. Scala media is separated from the scala vestibule by vestibular membrane (Reissner's membrane) and from the scala tympani by the basilar membrane. Scala vestibuli and scala tympani both are filled by perilymph (similar to extracellular fluid) and scala media by endolymph (similar to intracellular fluid). Stapes of the middle ear is attached to the vestibular window through the foot plate. The sound waves from the stapes reach to the perilymph fluid of spiral shaped region of cochlea through oval window (fenestra vestibuli). Here it first passes through the fluid filled tube called the Scala vestibuli. The sound waves in this region are converted in to the same frequency fluid waves. These fluid waves reach to second fluid filled tube of cochlea called Scala tympani through the top of cochlea. These waves return to base of the cochlea that is round window (fenestra cochleae) as scala tympani attached to it by a membrane, but this time passes through cochlear duct. The waves of scala vestibuli and scala tympani are converted into neural signals by spiral organs (formerly known as organs of Corti) present in cochlear duct [18]. The hair cells are present in the spiral organs. Two types of hair cells are present, three rows of outer hair cells and one row of inner hair cells. The outer hair cells are the main part (over 75%) of the sensory cells within the cochlea. The microvilli like structures stereocilia extend from apical surface of hair cells to the overlying the tectorial membrane, a highly hydrated extracellular matrix. This membrane stimulates the hair cells. It is essential for cochlear sensitivity and frequency selectivity [19]. An influx of cations such as K^+ and Ca^{2+} into the cells, mediated by the mechanosenstive ion channels, depolarize the cells upon proper displacement of the sterocilia. The vibration of the basilar membrane drives the displacement of the stereocilia whilethe sound generates an electrical signal inside the cell. This results in further release of the chemical neurotransmitter at the cellular base and set off the action potentials in the cochlea-vestibular nerve [20] The afferent nerve fibers of cochlea-vestibular (eight cranial) nerve attached to these hair cells. These nerve fibers connect the inner ear with brain. In dogs, the hearing areas are located in the temporal poles of the brain [21]. The loudness of sound related with degree of bend in the hair cells. Higher amplitude of a propagating waves leads to the greater bend of the hair cells and more loudness of sound [22]. The interruption in pathway of sound waves or fluid waves can result in loss of hearing. Most of the times deafness in dog is related to disorders of the spiral organs. Dogs with erect and cropped ears are more prone to infection of ears. It is a common cause of hearing loss in dogs [23]. Brachycephalic dogs had significantly thicker tympanic bulla walls and smaller tympanic cavity volumes compared to nonbrachycephalic dogs predisposing them to subclinical middle ear lesions [24].

Function of Vestibular System in Maintenance of Equilibrium

The vestibular system plays an important role in maintaining the equilibrium and balance of the animal. It is a primary sensory organ which orients with respect to the gravitational field of the earth and co-ordinates the movement of various sensory organs and thus the linear, rotatory, acceleration and deacceleration movements of the animal. This sensory system of ectodermal origin is responsible for transmission of 'special proprioception" [25]. Any disturbance vestibular system may result in neurological incoordination. This system can be anatomically dissected into two components as peripheral and central. The peripheral component is housed in the temporal bone and consists of saccule, utricle and semi-circular canal and peripheral axons of the cranial nerve VIII. The cerebellar nuclei, vestibular nuclei in the medulla, spinal cord and rostral brainstem comprises the central component [26]. The localization of head is determined by the signal transmitted by the function of macula of saccule, utricle and crista ampullaris. This signal gets transmitted to the brain stem through VIII cranial nerve. The vestibular nuclei receive this signal and circulate among the different body parts. The signal reaches to the forebrain and creates perception of position. In cerebellum, the signal maintains an integration between movement of organs like eye, neck, body and limbs with respect to position of the head. It also reaches to the centre like reticular formation in brainstem which controls motion sickness and vomiting. It also regulates the eye ball movement through control of muscles. The eye movement can be classified into three categories as rotary, vertical and horizontal. Co-ordination between 12 muscles is important for the regulated response of eye movement. The rotary movement of the eye is controlled by the utricle and vertical semicircular canal. The horizontal eye movement is controlled by utricle and horizontal canal. Saccule and vertical semicircular control the vertical movement [27]. The manifestation of vestibular incoordination can be observed in the form of nystagmus, head tilt, strabismus, drooling, circling movement and ataxia *etc.* [25]. Idiopathic vestibular diseases are more common in aged dogs which is otherwise known as "old dog" vestibular disease [28].

CONCLUSION

The ear of dogs consists of the pinna, external ear canal, middle ear and inner ear. The external ear is made up of auricular as well as annular cartilage. The auricular cartilage of the pinna looks like a funnel-shaped at the starting point of the external ear canal. The middle ear is made up of an air-filled tympanic cavity with three auditory ossicles, and tympanic membrane. Interestingly, the tympanic membrane is a semitransparent membrane consists of different parts includingpars flaccida and pars tensa. The auditory ossicles play an important role in transmitting and amplifying air vibrations from the tympanic membrane towards the inner ear. The inner ear is housed within a bony labyrinth in the petrous portion of the temporal bone. Membranous labyrinth, a layer of covering with its sensory organs responsible for hearing as well as balance is sited within this bony labyrinth. The fluid-filled spiral-shaped cochlea known as the organ of hearing is present in the inner ear. The cochlea is, covered by a thin membrane. The vestibular (oval) window is located on the dorsolateral surface of the promontory, covered by a thin diaphragm over which the footplate of the stapes is attached. The vibration of the basilar membrane drives the displacement of the stereocilia of the hair cells and sound generates an electrical signal inside the cell. The vestibular system plays an important role in maintaining the equilibrium and balance of the animal by the function of crista ampullaris and macula of saccule, utricle. The auditory tube is a short canal that extends from the nasopharynx to the rostral portion of the tympanic cavity proper and equalizes the air pressure in between outer and middle ear and is efficacious in preventing damage to the tympanic membrane.

REFERENCES

[1]   Kaminski J, Waller BM, Diogo R, Hartstone-Rose A, Burrows AM. Evolution of facial muscle anatomy in dogs. Proc Natl Acad Sci USA 2019; 116(29): 14677-81.
[http://dx.doi.org/10.1073/pnas.1820653116] [PMID: 31209036]

[2]   Shiu JN, Munro KJ, Cox CL. Normative auditory brainstem response data for hearing threshold and neuro-otological diagnosis in the dog. J Small Anim Pract 1997; 38(3): 103-7.
[http://dx.doi.org/10.1111/j.1748-5827.1997.tb03328.x] [PMID: 9097241]

[3]   Wilson WJ, Mills PC. Brainstem auditory-evoked response in dogs. Am J Vet Res 2005; 66(12): 2177-87.

[http://dx.doi.org/10.2460/ajvr.2005.66.2177] [PMID: 16379665]

[4]   Munro KJ, Cox CL. Investigation of hearing impairment in Cavalier King Charles spaniels using auditory brainstem response audiometry. J Small Anim Pract 1997; 38(1): 2-5.
[http://dx.doi.org/10.1111/j.1748-5827.1997.tb02976.x] [PMID: 9121129]

[5]   Hyttel P, Sinowatz F, Vejlsted M, Eds. Keith Betteridge, Essentials of domestic animal embryology. 1ˢᵗ ed., Saunders Elsevier 2010.

[6]   Peterson DC, Reddy V, Hamel RN. Neuroanatomy, auditory pathway. StatPearls. Treasure Island, FL: StatPearls Publishing 2023.

[7]   Rowe DP, O'Leary SJ. (Eds): Michael J Aminoff, Robert B Daroff, Encyclopedia of the Neurological Sciences. 2ⁿᵈ ed. Academic Press 2014; pp. 329-34.
[http://dx.doi.org/10.1016/B978-0-12-385157-4.00121-4]

[8]   Nummela S. Hearing in aquatic mammals. In: Thewissen JGM, Nummela S, Eds. Sensory evolution on the threshold: Adaptationsin secondarily aquatic vertebrates. Berkeley: University of California Press 2008; pp. 211-24.

[9]   Phillips DP, Calford MB, Pettigrew JD, Aitkin LM, Semple MN. Directionality of sound pressure transformation at the cat's pinna. Hear Res 1982; 8(1): 13-28.
[http://dx.doi.org/10.1016/0378-5955(82)90031-4] [PMID: 7142030]

[10] Arriaga G, Jarvis ED. Mouse vocal communication system: Are ultrasounds learned or innate? Brain Lang 2013; 124(1): 96-116.
[http://dx.doi.org/10.1016/j.bandl.2012.10.002] [PMID: 23295209]

[11] O'Connor KN, Tam M, Blevins NH, Puria S. Tympanic membrane collagen fibers: a key to high-frequency sound conduction. Laryngoscope 2008; 118(3): 483-90.
[http://dx.doi.org/10.1097/MLG.0b013e31815b0d9f] [PMID: 18091335]

[12] National Research Council (US) Committee on Disability Determination for Individuals with Hearing Impairments. Hearing Loss: Determining Eligibility for Social Security Benefits. Dobie RA, Van Hemel S, editors. Washington (DC): National Academies Press (US); 2004.
[PMID: 25032316]

[13] Kumar, A. & Roman-Auerhahn, Margo. Anatomy of the Canine and Feline Ear. Small Animal Ear Diseases. (2005), 1-21.
[http://dx.doi.org/10.1016/B0-72-160137-5/50004-0]

[14] Connors BW. Sensory transduction. In: Boron WF, Boulpaep EL, Eds. Medical physiology updated edition. Philadelphia: Elsevier Saunders 2005; pp. 343-52.

[15] Heine PA. Anatomy of the ear. Vet Clin North Am Small Anim Pract 2004; 34(2): 379-95.
[http://dx.doi.org/10.1016/j.cvsm.2003.10.003] [PMID: 15062614]

[16] Sims MH. Electrodiagnostic evaluation of auditory function. Vet Clin North Am Small Anim Pract 1988; 18(4): 913-44.
[http://dx.doi.org/10.1016/S0195-5616(88)50090-6] [PMID: 3264964]

[17] Kumar MSA, clinically orientated anatomy of the dog and cat, 2ⁿᵈ edition Linus learnig, 2015, ISBN 10 1-60797-552-1.

[18] Echteler SM, Fay RR, Popper AN. Structure of the mammalian cochlea. In: Fay RR, Popper AN, Eds. Comparative Hearing: Mammals. New York: Springer-Verlag 1994; pp. 134-71.
[http://dx.doi.org/10.1007/978-1-4612-2700-7_5]

[19] Sellon JB, Ghaffari R, Freeman DM. The tectorial membrane: mechanical properties and functions. Cold Spring Harb Perspect Med 2019; 9(10): a033514.
[http://dx.doi.org/10.1101/cshperspect.a033514] [PMID: 30348837]

[20] Reichenbach T, Hudspeth AJ. The physics of hearing: fluid mechanics and the active process of the inner ear. Rep Prog Phys 2014; 77(7): 076601.

[http://dx.doi.org/10.1088/0034-4885/77/7/076601] [PMID: 25006839]

[21]   Andics A, Gábor A, Gácsi M, Faragó T, Szabó D, Miklósi Á. Neural mechanisms for lexical processing in dogs. Science 2016; 353(6303): 1030-2.
[http://dx.doi.org/10.1126/science.aaf3777] [PMID: 27576923]

[22]   Masaki K, Weiss TF, Freeman DM. Poroelastic bulk properties of the tectorial membrane measured with osmotic stress. Biophys J 2006; 91(6): 2356-70.
[http://dx.doi.org/10.1529/biophysj.105.078121] [PMID: 16815909]

[23]   Strain GM. Deafness in dogs and cats. Boston, MA: Cabi Publishing 2011.
[http://dx.doi.org/10.1079/9781845937645.0000]

[24]   Salgüero R, Herrtage M, Holmes M, Mannion P, Ladlow J. Comparison between computed tomographic characteristics of the middle ear in nonbrachycephalic and brachycephalic dogs with obstructive airway syndrome. Veterinary Radiology &Amp. Vet Radiol Ultrasound 2016; 57(2): 137-43.
[http://dx.doi.org/10.1111/vru.12337] [PMID: 26765680]

[25]   Garosi LS, Dennis R, Platt SR, Corletto F, de Lahunta A, Jakobs C. Thiamine deficiency in a dog: clinical, clinicopathologic, and magnetic resonance imaging findings. J Vet Intern Med 2003; 17(5): 719-23.
[http://dx.doi.org/10.1111/j.1939-1676.2003.tb02507.x] [PMID: 14529142]

[26]   Lowrie M, Vetmb M. Vestibular disease: anatomy, physiology, and clinical signs. Compend Contin Educ Vet 2012; 34(7): E1.
[PMID: 22847320]

[27]   Jenkins TW. The ear-hearing and equilibrium. Functional Mammalian Neuroanatomy. Philadelphia: Lea and Febiger 1978.

[28]   Blauch B, Martin CL. A vestibular syndrome in aged dogs. J Am Anim Hosp Assoc 1974; 10: 37-40.

CHAPTER 4

Microbiology of Ear

Anju Nayak[1,*], Vandana Gupta[1], Sanjay Shukla[1], Ajay Rai[1] and Poonam Shakya[1]

[1] *Department of Veterinary Microbiology, College of Veterinary Science & A.H., Jabalpur, Nanaji Deshmukh Veterinary Science University, Jabalpur, Madhya Pradesh, India*

Abstract: Otitis is an inflammation of ear in dogs, can be noted following primary, secondary, perpetuating and predisposing factors. Otitis externa is more frequent than otitis interna and otitis media. Globally the prevalence of otitis externa is 5-20% which reach up to 30-40% in tropical environment. Infections in otitis externa is generally secondary after inflammation. The mycotic microorganism reported from otitis are *Malassezia pachydermatis*, *Aspergillus* spp., *Candida* spp. While, the predominant bacteria belongs to *Staphylococcus* spp., *Enterococcus* spp., *Pseudomonas aeruginosa*, *Streptococcus* spp., *Corynebacterium* spp., *Proteus* spp., *Escherichia coli* and *Klebsiella* spp. In culture, the yeast *Malassezia pachydermatis* and bacteria *Staphylococcus pseudintermedius* predominates. With advent of metagenomics *Finegoldia magna*, *Peptostreptococcus canis* and *Porphyromonas cangingivalis* anaerobic bacteria were identified. Colonization of ears by antibiotic resistant microorganism makes the treatment challenging for the veterinarian. The bacterial culture along with antibiotic susceptibility test is recommended.

Keywords: Bacteria, *Malassezia pachydermatis*, Otitis, Otitis externa, *Staphylococcus pseudintermedius*, Yeast.

INTRODUCTION

Otitis is the inflammation of different parts of the ear. On the basis of location of inflammation it is classified as otitis externa, otitis media and otitis interna. Inflammation of epithelium and lining of the external auditory canal is termed as otitis externa. Otitis media is the inflammation of the middle ear. Otitis interna refers to a group of inflammatory conditions of the internal ear. The most common ear infection is otitis externa, it can be unilateral or bilateral. Globally the prevalence of otitis externa is 5-20% which reach up to 30-40% in tropical environment. Infections in otitis externa is generally secondary after inflammation. The main cause of otitis externa is Allergic dermatitis, which is

---
* **Corresponding author Anju Nayak:** Department of Veterinary Microbiology, College of Veterinary Science & A.H., Jabalpur, Nanaji Deshmukh Veterinary Science University, Jabalpur, Madhya Pradesh, India; E-mail: nayakanju1970@gmail.com

more than 60% [1]. *Malassezia pachydermatis* from the yeast and *Staphylococcus pseudintermedius* among the bacteria are prevalent microorganisms [2]. A large diversity of bacteria and fungi are habitat of the ear. Culture of bacteria and fungi are still gold standard tests, but it is time consuming. But only about 1% of all microorganisms are in fact culturable [3].

PCR-based methods are usually limited to a panel of only selected microbes. On the basis of metagenomics analysis, the three most predominant bacteria were *Cutibacterium acnes* (previously known as *Propionibacterium acnes*; 4.5%), *S. pseudintermedius* (3.8%) and *Streptococcus sp.* (1.1%). *M. pachydermatis* (6.1%), *Capnodiales* (3.7%) and *Pleosporales* (1.0%) were among the yeast [4] while, *Finegoldia magna, Peptostreptococcus canis,* and *Porphyromonas cangingivalis* are the anaerobic bacteria. Previously, in canine ear infections, these anaerobic microbes were not identified as pathogens. As in clinical laboratory, usually only aerobic bacteria are cultivated until and unless specified. Now a days molecular methods like next gen sequencing can be applied for identification of microbes from as single sample without culturing them. Multiple etiological agents can be identified leading to judicious use of antibiotics and antifungal agent.

Etiology and Classification of Otitis

Wide variety of causative agents leads to Otitis in dogs. The predisposing factors can be classified as primary, predisposing and perpetuating. Normal ears of the dogs can be affected by primary causes of otitis externa. Primary causes include causes such as, parasites, foreign bodies, hypersensitivity and allergic diseases, keratinization disorders, autoimmune diseases initiate otitis externa. Primary cause changes the environment in the ear, often allowing a secondary infection to develop (Fig. **1**). The predisposing factors such as anatomic and conformational factors, excessive moisture, iatrogenic factors and obstructive ear disease make the ear more susceptible to the development of otitis externa but do not cause it alone. Perpetuating factors of otitis are bacteria, yeast, otitis media, progressive pathologic changes which are responsible for aggravation of otitis and prevents normal healing [5, 6].

- Allergy (adverse food reaction, atopic dermatitis, contact).
- Parasites (*Otodectes, Demodex, Sarcoptes*).
- Autoimmune/immune-mediated (pemphigus foliaceus, vasculitis, others).
- Endocrine disease (hypothyroidism, hyperadrenocorticism).
- Epithelialization disorders (sebaceous adenitis, zinc-responsive dermatitis).
- Foreign bodies.
- Glandular disorders (sebaceous gland hyperplasia).
- Fungal (*Aspergillus*).

- Viral (Canine distemper).
- Miscellaneous (proliferative necrotizing otitis of cats, juvenile cellulitis).

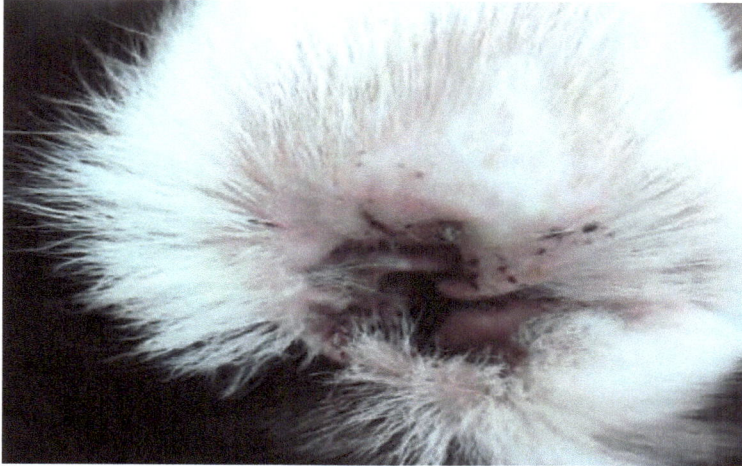

Fig. (1). Depicts ear infection of the ear of dogs.

Regardless of the primary ear lesion, the microbial contamination is the predominant cause of acute and suppurate otitis in case of dogs. *Staphylococcus intermedius* and *Malassezia pachydermatis* are the most common microorganisms isolated from canine otitis externa [7]. Otitis externa may occur irrespective of breed, gender or age of dog but predisposing factors are long pendulous ear, hairy pinna, higher density of compound hair follicles and ceruminous glands in the ear canal leading to heat retention and increase moisture.

Bacterial Etiology of Otitis

Among bacteria, 16 different bacterial species consisting of *Pseudomonas aeruginosa, Staphylococcus pseudintermedius/delphini, Proteus mirabilis, Streptococcus canis* were isolated by conventional method by conventional method. While, external ear canal 16S amplicon profiling resulted in 180 bacterial species from seven different phyla. The major species were *Pseudomonas aeruginosa, Corynebacterium auriscanis, Corynebacterium jeikeium/amycolatum, Porphyromonas cangingivalis* and *Staphylococcus delphini/pseudintermedius* [8].

Clinical Signs

The clinical signs of infected dogs include, anorexia, inflammation of mucosa and pain with violent head shaking, scratching and rubbing of ears, ceruminous or dark purulent discharge with foul odour.

Relationship between Otitis and Breed of Dogs

The medium and large ear breed dogs breeds like cocker spaniels and golden retrievers ear canal have more hairs in their ears, and have large and pendules ears. Therefore, we compared these pendules ear dogs with the dogs with vertical ear. In pendules ears dogs, it prevents the air circulation and heat dissipation, so the ear canal environment becomes moist. The moist, hot and humid environment of the ear canal is conducive for growth of microorganism. Their ear canal is rich in the cerumen glands. The presence and stimulation by the bacteria or parasites, leads to production of large quantity of substances from the cerumen glands. The exuberant hair prevents the secretions to move out of the ear canal, so that sufficient nutrients are available for growth of microorganisms. Although beagle dogs have drooping auricles but the incidence of ear diseases are less (Fig. **2**). Although, exceptionally higher incidence of ear diseases are recorded in huskies with vertical auricles. There is no direct relationship between structure of ears and otitis externa.

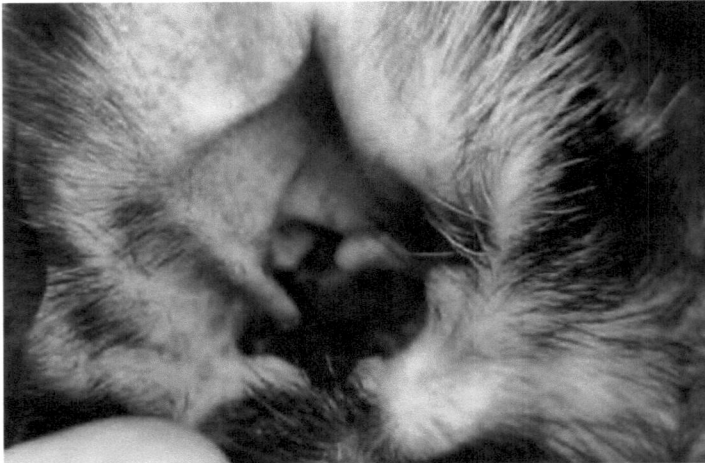

Fig. (2). Depicting ceruminoliths in the affected ear.

Further, the anatomy of ear in some breeds of dogs are different, which can lead to ear diseases. In certain breeds of dogs, namely sharkskin and bulldog, the structure of ear canal is genitally long and narrow and it has a certain angle to the horizontal plane. Which prevents normal discharging of the secretion, leading to higher incidence of ear diseases. Some conditions like ear canal edema, ear canal mass and ear canal hyperplasia can press the ear canal, leading to narrowing of the ear canal and thus causing ear diseases.

Relationship between Otitis and Gender of Dogs

There is no direct correlation between the gender of dogs and incidence of ear disease. In the male dogs, the secretion of sebaceous glands is affected by hormones and the androgen can results into hyperplasia and hypertrophy of sebaceous glands. In male dogs the exuberant sebum facilitates growth of microorganisms by providing nutritious environment. While, in case of females, there is degeneration of the sebaceous glands as the estrogen hormone declines their function, so females are less prone to the otitis. In some endocrine diseases there is excessive secretion of sebaceous glands, which may lead to ear disease. Now a days, due to improvement in living standards of human beings the diet provided to the dogs is also nutritious. The excessive intake of meat, which leads to the abnormal exuberant secretion of sebaceous glands, ultimately leading to pruritus and swelling [9].

Fungi and Yeast Etiology of Otitis

The yeast are present and can be normally isolated from the ear canal. Researchers indicated that if the environment inside the ear canal is favorable for the growth of yeast it can results in the otitis externa. The most common yeast isolated from otitis externa cases is *Malassezia pachydermitis* [10]. *Candida* spp., *Aspergillus* spp. may also be isolated from canine otitis externa. Although co existence of yeast *Malassezia* spp. with Gram positive cocci bacteria are very common.

CONCLUDING REMARKS

Most of the dogs presented with otitis to veterinary clinics usually suffer from otitis externa. The causative agent of otitis externa can be either bacterial, fungal or any other which must be identified first. The antibiotic sensitivity or if required anti fungal sensitivity must be performed for proper timely treatment of the dogs.

ACKNOWLEDGEMENTS

I acknowledge all the researchers, from whom I had quoted text or data to complete this manuscript.

REFERENCES

[1]   Saridomichelakis MN, Farmaki R, Leontides LS, Koutinas AF. Aetiology of canine otitis externa: a retrospective study of 100 cases. Vet Dermatol 2007; 18(5): 341-7.
[http://dx.doi.org/10.1111/j.1365-3164.2007.00619.x] [PMID: 17845622]

[2]   Graham-Mize CA, Rosser EJ Jr. Comparison of microbial isolates and susceptibility patterns from the external ear canal of dogs with otitis externa. J Am Anim Hosp Assoc 2004; 40(2): 102-8.
[http://dx.doi.org/10.5326/0400102] [PMID: 15007044]

[3]   Barcina I, Arana I. The viable but nonculturable phenotype: a crossroads in the life-cycle of non-

differentiating bacteria? Rev Environ Sci Biotechnol 2009; 8(3): 245-55.
[http://dx.doi.org/10.1007/s11157-009-9159-x]

[4]   Tang S, Prem A, Tjokrosurjo J, *et al.* The canine skin and ear microbiome: A comprehensive survey of pathogens implicated in canine skin and ear infections using a novel next-generation-sequencing-based assay. Vet Microbiol 2020; 247: 108764.
[http://dx.doi.org/10.1016/j.vetmic.2020.108764] [PMID: 32768216]

[5]   Rosser EJ. Causes of otitis externa. Vet Clin: Small animal practice, 2004; 34(2): 459-468.
[http://dx.doi.org/10.1016/j.cvsm.2003.10.006]

[6]   Lyskova P, Vydrzalova M, Mazurova J. Identification and antimicrobial susceptibility of bacteria and yeasts isolated from healthy dogs and dogs with otitis externa. J Vet Med A Physiol Pathol Clin Med 2007; 54(10): 559-63.
[http://dx.doi.org/10.1111/j.1439-0442.2007.00996.x] [PMID: 18045339]

[7]   Kiss G, Radványi S, Szigeti G. New combination for the therapy of canine otitis externa I Microbiology of otitis externa. J Small Anim Pract 1997; 38(2): 51-6.
[http://dx.doi.org/10.1111/j.1748-5827.1997.tb02987.x] [PMID: 9065882]

[8]   Leonard C, Thiry D, Taminiau B, Daube G, Fontaine J. External ear canal evaluation in dogs with chronic suppurative otitis externa: comparison of direct cytology, bacterial culture and 16s amplicon profiling. Vet Sci 2022; 9(7): 366.
[http://dx.doi.org/10.3390/vetsci9070366] [PMID: 35878383]

[9]   Di H. Evaluation of drug resistance to aminoglycosides in pathogenic microorganism of canine otitis externa. Beijing: China Agricultural University 2014.

[10]   Sarıerler M, Kırkan S. (2004). Microbiological diagnosis and therapy of canine otitis externa. Veterinercerrahi dergisi. 10(3- 4): 11-15.

CHAPTER 5

Cytology of Ear in Health and Diseases

Sirigireddy Sivajothi[1,*], **Bhavanam Sudhakara Reddy**[1] and **Dadireddy Narmada Raghavi**[1]

[1] *College of Veterinary Science-Proddatur, Sri Venkateswara Veterinary University, Andhra Pradesh, India*

Abstract: Ear diseases represent one of the most common clinical presentations in dogs seen by small animal practitioners. These conditions can arise from primary causes, secondary causes, and perpetuating factors, all of which are essential to identify for successful management. Cytology, the study of cells, offers a nonexpensive, readily available, and low cost diagnostic tool that can be utilized to screen dogs with ear diseases. The ear infection can be judged by the clinical examination, ear examination by otoscopy, imaging diagnostics, cytological intervention, and proper treatment should be undertaken based on the severity and duration of the infection in the ear. Cytology proves useful to clinicians for assessing the origin of types of infectious, such as yeast, mites, and bacteria; presence of types of leukocytes. In cases of recurrent or non-responsive ear diseases, cytology should be complemented with culture and susceptibility testing. Yeast, including *Malassezia* and *Candida*, can be identified on cytology by their specific morphology on cytology, which is crucial for selecting appropriate topical ear medications. Cytology also provides valuable information about mite infestations and the intensity of mite populations. It serves as a useful tool to assess the endpoint of therapy and ensure the resolution of infection. Additionally, cytology aids in decision-making by guiding the selection of antimicrobial medications and /or proceeding with further diagnostic methods, while also determining the endpoint of therapy. In cases where first-line therapy fails or bacilli are present, bacterial culture with an evaluation of antibiotic susceptibility is recommended. A comparison of healthy control dogs and clinical cases revealed significantly higher levels of organisms and inflammatory cells in the latter, with *Malassezia pachydermatis* isolated in both infected and healthy ears of dogs. Cytological examination of impression smears is a straightforward, readily applicable, and minimally cost-involved diagnostic method to provide the identification of etiological agents, which include bacteria, fungi, and mites. Processing and making the dermatological diagnostic cytological slide requires only professional skill without any special equipment, which can be evaluated in less time in routine clinical settings. Before receiving culture and sensitivity results, the immediate results of cytology are invaluable for making informed diagnostic decisions during consultations.

* **Corresponding author Sirigireddy Sivajothi:** College of Veterinary Science-Proddatur, Sri Venkateswara Veterinary University, Andhra Pradesh, India; E-mail: sivajothi579@gmail.com

Tanmoy Rana (Ed.)

Keywords: Bacteria, Cells, Cytology, Dog, Diagnosis, Ear diseases, Fungi, Mites.

INTRODUCTION

Ear diseases in dogs are often multifactorial and can pose significant challenges in management. Cytology, which involves the study of cells, is a crucial diagnostic tool in veterinary medicine. The term "cyto" originates from the Greek word "kytos," meaning "cell," and "logos" which means "science." Cytology enables quick, easy, and cost-effective diagnosis, making it one of the most important and commonly used diagnostic techniques in veterinary medicine. The presence of recurrent dermatological diseases, improper therapeutic regimens, treatment failures, and progressive loss of physical barriers in the ear canal can convert simple ear diseases into complicated ear diseases [1]. Ear diseases are a prevalent clinical presentation in dogs seen by small animal practitioners. These conditions can stem from primary, secondary, and perpetuating factors, all of which are crucial to diagnose, for successful management. Cytology, the study of cells, offers fast, low cost and immediate diagnostic facilities that can be utilized to screen dogs with ear diseases. When combined with clinical examination, ear examination by otoscopy, for assessing the primary infections, imaging diagnostic facilities and serial cytological procedures are useful in the assessment of secondary infections; along with the evaluation of therapeutic response to modify the appropriate managemental procedures. Cytological evaluations of ear swabs are vital for assessing and managing non-responsive or recurrent ear infections in small animal practice. It is recommended to perform cytology at each follow-up visit to assess therapeutic response or modify therapeutic protocols as needed [2]. The duration of cytological examination during revisits varies depending on the type of etiology for ear disease development and the treatment of affected patients. Many dermatological disorders share similar clinical signs and physical characteristics, making them challenging to differentiate from one another. Cytology serves as a crucial tool for evaluating ear diseases, enabling the assessment of the inflammatory response type and the identification of underlying causes. It aids in determining the presence of overgrowth and in guiding appropriate management strategies [3]. Cytology proves to be a reliable tool for rechecking examinations, assisting in the monitoring and adjustment of therapy as needed. *Malassezia* yeasts, characterized by their specific peanut shape, are normal commensals of canine skin. Ear diseases often have multifactorial etiologies and are classified into predisposing, primary, and perpetuating types. Predisposing factors include ear conformation, favorable environmental conditions, inappropriate treatment, and immunosuppressive diseases. Primary causes encompass foreign objects, parasites, hypersensitivity disorders, keratinization disorders, and immune-mediated diseases [4]. Effective management of ear diseases necessitates accurate diagnosis of primary diseases and perpetuating factors, followed by appropriate management strategies. Cytology provides a clear quantitative analysis of the organisms present, while microbiological analysis aids in identifying specific infectious organisms. Over time, various grading techniques have been employed in the cytological analysis of ear discharge to assess the severity of infection [5]. Cytological examination of ear discharges often reveals the presence of epithelial cells, bacterial organisms, *Malassezia* spp. Yeast organisms, and fungal hyphae [6, 7]. Persistent low-grade inflammation can increase the likelihood of developing neoplastic cells and ultimately result in permanent hearing loss [8, 9].

When to Perform the Cytology

Dogs exhibiting signs of ear diseases such as head shaking, ear scratching, erythema of the ears, pain upon palpation, foul odor from the ears, and ear discharges should undergo cytology. Ear cytology plays a crucial role in identifying primary, secondary, and perpetuating factors [10]. The primary pathogens identified in the literature are *Malassezia pachydermatis* and *Staphylococcus pseudintermedius*, which together account for over 70% of bacteria culture from ear discharges. Dogs with chronic ear infections, recurrent otitis, or non-responsive ear infections often present with suppurative otitis [11]. Common bacteria isolated from dogs with otitis include *Staphylococcus pseudintermedius, Enterococcus spp., Pseudomonas aeruginosa, Streptococcus spp., Corynebacterium spp.,* and *Escherichia coli* through bacterial isolation and culture. Initial treatment for most dogs with ear diseases typically involves first-line therapy, followed by assessing the response to treatment. If necessary, bacterial culture with the evaluation of antibiotic susceptibility is recommended [12]. In daily routine practice, discrepancies often arise between direct cytology and bacterial culture examinations. Differences exist between the examination of ears by cytology and the subsequent performance of sensitivity tests. This inconsistency may be attributed to the presence of uncultured bacteria or the emergence of rapidly growing bacterial strains [13, 14].

Indications of Ear Cytology

Indications for cytology in dogs with ear diseases include: assessing various cell types in the ears, distinguishing between inflammatory and neoplastic origins of cells, detecting underlying etiological causes such as parasites, bacteria, fungi, or allergies, differentiating clinical signs of ear diseases from systemic diseases, determining the extent of ear infections, evaluating the status of microbial populations, formulating effective therapeutic strategies, assessing the therapeutic efficacy of drugs against otitis, and monitoring therapeutic responses [13, 15].

Before cytology, it is crucial to visually inspect the discharge from the ears. Visual examination of ear discharge, including observing its color and odor, can provide valuable clues for preliminary diagnosis. Subsequently, cytology should be performed to further investigate the condition. Table **1** outlines the various colors and contents of ear discharges associated with different infectious processes. However, it is important to note that the proposed findings in the table are meant to aid in understanding and should not replace routine cytological examinations. Cytology serves as a preliminary examination to guide further investigation [16, 17]. Dry, grainy, and black discharges in dogs are commonly associated with *Otodectes cynotis* infestations. Waxy and brown exudate typically indicate *Malassezia* infection, while yellow-colored discharges are indicative of bacterial infection.

Table 1. Showing the type of ear discharge and type of ear infection.

Stage of Infection	Color of Ear Discharges	Clinical Signs
No infection	No discharge	Erythematous ear pinna and pruritic
Early infection	Dark brown ceruminous type	Wax-type material with no bacterial infection
Early infection	Pale brown ceruminous type	Wax-type material and the presence of *Malassezia*
Moderate infection	Pale brown–yellow ceruminous purulent type	Wax with inflammatory infiltrate. Presence of *Malassezia* and Gram-positive *cocci*
Moderate infection	Yellow–pale green purulent type	Wax with gram-positive and negative bacterial infection
Severe infection	Pale green mucopurulent type	Wax with mucus mixed contents Along with *Pseudomonas aeroginosa*

Samples Collection and Processing

The most commonly used instrument for the collection of ear samples was a cotton-tipped applicator (Fig. **1**). The location of sample collection varies depending on the anatomical location of ear discharges, such as the vertical and horizontal ear canals. The extent of swab insertion depends on factors like the presence of proliferative ear diseases, the degree of ear canal stenosis, and the intactness of the tympanic membranes. In cases of ruptured tympanic membranes, middle ear samples can be collected under general anesthesia. For cases where the tympanic membrane is intact, sampling requires a myringotomy using a spinal needle. Precautions during sample collection include obtaining samples at acute angles of both ear canals *i.e.* vertical and horizontal canals [18]. For optimal diagnostic slides, samples should be collected before the introduction of cleaning agents or other therapies. The swab should be rolled over the glass slide until the specimen is evenly distributed for drying (Fig. **2**). In cases of bilateral otitis in dogs, ear samples should be collected from both ears, with each sample marked as "R" for right and "L" for left on the slide to accurately document the infection status of each ear. Methylene blue stain is commonly used for simple and rapid staining. To reliably evaluate microorganisms, 5 to 10 high-power fields (magnification, 100×; with immersion oil) should be assessed, and the findings averaged and recorded. When ectoparasites are suspected, suspicious material should be placed on a microscopic slide with a few drops of mineral oil, followed by a cover slip [19]. Mites can be easily detected at low magnifications, typically 4× or 10×. Initially, microscopic examination of the slides can be carried out under the low magnification (x10 objective) which helps in wider area examination and selecting areas for further higher magnification (x40) or under oil immersion (x100) objective examination. The required instrumentation for sample collection was limited *i.e.* cotton sterile swabs, glass slides suitable for microscopic examination and suitable oil for mite identification, staining solutions such as Methylene blue or Romanowsky-type cytology stains, and a microscope equipped with 4x to 100x objective lenses. In the case of parasitic mites suspected in the ear swabs, ear exudates were collected with the help of ear swabs and mixed with the suitable mineral oil covered with a cover slip and examined under the lower and higher magnification to identify the type of mites [20, 21].

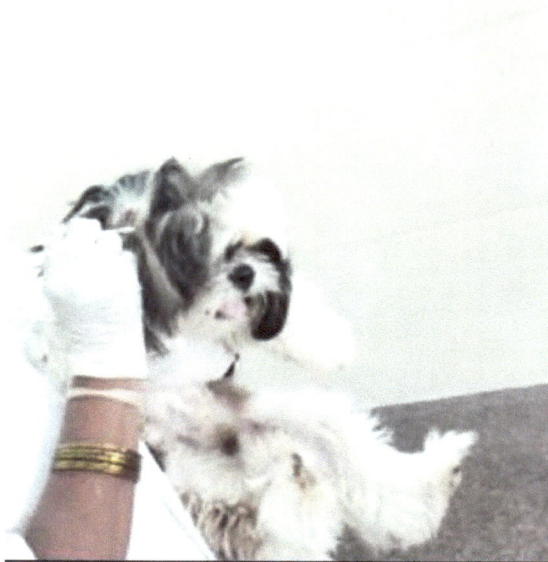

Fig. (1). Collection of swabs from the ears for cytology.

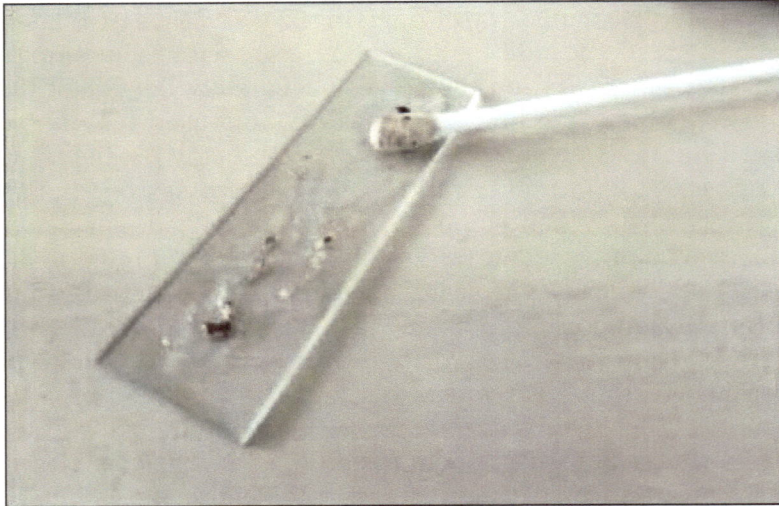

Fig. (2). Rolling the collected swab on the slides for examination.

Here are some key tips for cytology practice: 1. Label the frosted end of the slide with a pencil, noting the pet's name, case number, and examination date. 2. Avoid storing slides in formalin, as it can interfere with staining and cell identification. 3. Refrain from heat-fixing or refrigerating samples. Instead, allow smears to air dry and protect them from moisture by storing them in a slide container [22]. The suggested medical record for the documentation of the cytological findings in dogs is mentioned in Table **2**.

Table 2. Suggested format for documentation of ear cytology.

Left Ear Cytological Rxamination					
Yeast	Absence	Presence	Quantification	....	Number per field
Cocci	Absence	Presence	Quantification	....	Number per field
Rods	Absence	Presence	Quantification	....	Number per field
Neutrophils	Absence	Presence	Quantification	....	Number per field
Mites – Live	Absence	Presence	Quantification	....	Number per field
Mites- Dead	Absence	Presence	Quantification	....	Number per field
Phagocytosis	Absence	Presence	Quantification	....	Number per field
Right Ear Cytological Rxamination					
Yeast	Absence	Presence	Quantification	....	Number per field
Cocci	Absence	Presence	Quantification	....	Number per field
Rods	Absence	Presence	Quantification	....	Number per field

(Table 2) cont.....

Neutrophils	Absence	Presence	Quantification	....	Number per field
Mites – Live	Absence	Presence	Quantification	....	Number per field
Mites- Dead	Absence	Presence	Quantification	....	Number per field
Phagocytosis	Absence	Presence	Quantification	....	Number per field

Here are the guidelines for using a microscope: 1. Regularly clean and maintain the microscope to ensure optimal performance. 2. Use immersion oil sparingly and exclusively with the oil immersion objective. 3. Avoid leaving the oil immersion lens immersed in oil for extended periods, as it can cause irreparable damage. 4. Never submerge the 4X, 10X, or 40X objectives in immersion oil. If accidental immersion occurs, promptly clean the lens. 5. Immediately clean the lens with proper lens tissue after each use. 6. Keep the low-power objective in place when not in use and lower the stage. 7. Promptly clean away any spills of solvents or chemicals, including mineral oil, to prevent damage.

Results of the Ear Cytology

The initial microscopic examination of samples should be conducted at low magnification (4x), followed by higher magnification (100x). Key findings observed during microscopy examination of ear samples include inflammatory cells, fungi, bacteria, and parasitic mites. Classification of the different cells is mentioned in Tables **3** and **4**.

Table 3. Numeric scale for recording the number of organisms.

	Estimates The Number of Organisms Present As:
0	No organisms per HPF
1	1-3 organisms per HPF
2	4-10 organisms per HPF
3	11-30 organisms per HPF
4	Above 30 organisms per HPF

Table 4. Grading of ears based on the ear cytological examination.

Ear Grading	Type of Contents on Ear Cytology
0	No abnormal cells.
1	Very few bacteria, yeast, or inflammatory cells and difficult to find in the cytological examination.

(Table 4) cont.....

Ear Grading	Type of Contents on Ear Cytology
2	There are a few numbers of bacteria, yeast, or inflammatory cells and spotting is easy while cytological examination.
3	The presence of a huge number of bacteria, yeast, or inflammatory cells they were found easily through routine cytological examination.
4	The presence of a very huge number of bacteria, yeast, or inflammatory cells, and they were found easily without any difficulties.

Inflammatory Cells

The majority of cytological examinations conducted on slides derived from the ear canal revealed the presence of inflammatory cells. These cells aid in the assessment of various diseases, including pemphigus complex, cutaneous lupus, mucocutaneous pyoderma, and allergies [23 - 25].

Neutrophils

These cells are identified as acute inflammatory cells, tasked with combating infectious organisms. The presence of intracellular bacteria within these cells was noted. Bacterial overgrowth can be assessed by observing a higher quantity of bacteria, which may manifest as *cocci* or rod-shaped bacteria (Fig. 3).

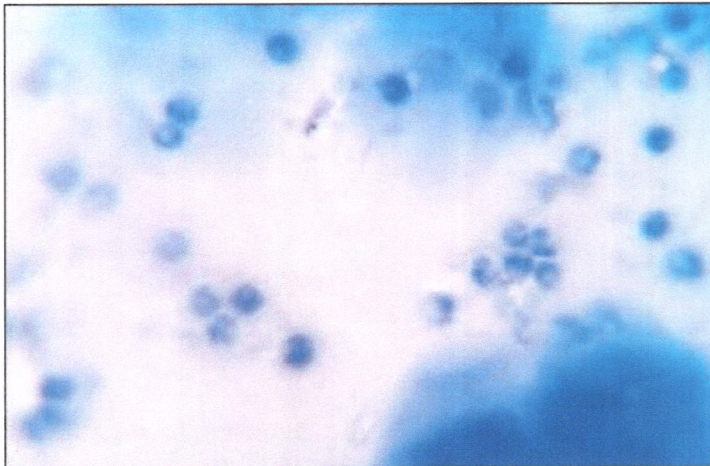

Fig. (3). Presence of neutrophils in stained smears (1000x magnification under oil immersion objective).

Eosinophils

In the inflammation process, eosinophils release a multitude of cytokines and mediators aimed at eliminating infectious organisms and recruiting other cells, such as mast cells. These eosinophils are also phagocytic and can engulf bacteria and fungi, indicating the presence of parasites, fungi, and food allergies.

Lymphocytes

Lymphocytes are very limited in ear cytology. These cells are direct results of the activities of neutrophils, eosinophils, and keratinocytes through releasing the cytokines.

Mast Cells

Mast cells are the cells responsible for the production of histamine, and are involved in ulcerated skin lesions in the ears.

Parasites

Demodex, Otodectes, and *Sarcoptes* are mites that may be visible on smears prepared from otic discharges. These mites can often lead to the development of dermatological signs in association with ear diseases. *Otodectes cynotis*, for instance, is commonly found in the ears of dogs with brownish wax. All these mites were photophobic in nature, and when they were examined with a light source they moved away from the light source and appeared as transparent to a reddish tinge based on the stages. *Demodex spp.* Mites are considered a normal inhabitant of the skin and called skin commensal in dogs and the presence of more numbers with different life stages in the cytological examination along with dermatological signs is considered as pathogenesis of the mites [26 - 28] (Figs. **4** and **5**).

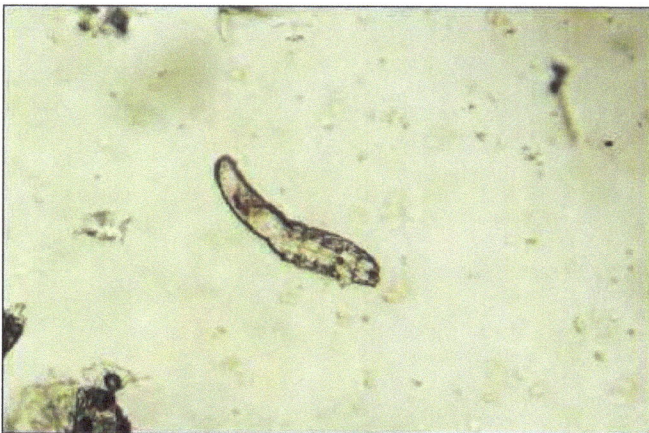

Fig. (4). Presence of *Demodex* mites in ear scrapings - direct visualization of ear discharges (400X magnification).

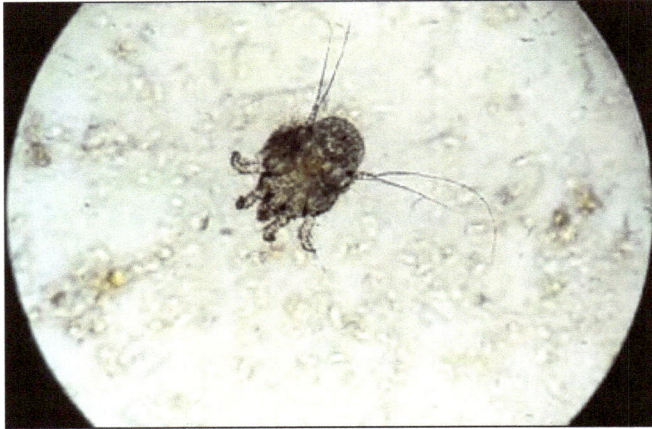

Fig. (5). Presence of *Otodectus* mites - direct visualization of ear discharges (400X magnification).

Fungi

Most fungal spores from dermatophytes are observed within neutrophils, occasionally appearing free between the neutrophils. Fungi typically appear as very small, round organisms with a clear halo and a basophilic center. In ear cytology, yeasts are generally larger than bacteria. *Malassezia pachydermatis* is the predominant yeast identified from the ears of dogs, presenting as dark blue/purple staining peanut-shaped organisms. In cases of dogs with a high infection of *Malassezia pachydermatis*, the ear discharges may appear very waxy, deviating from the typical inflammatory infiltrate, and improperly stained. In a few cases, *Candida spp.* may be found in the ears, appearing as more rounded shapes with a more defined waist, resembling a 'baker's bun' [29, 30] (Figs. **6** and 7).

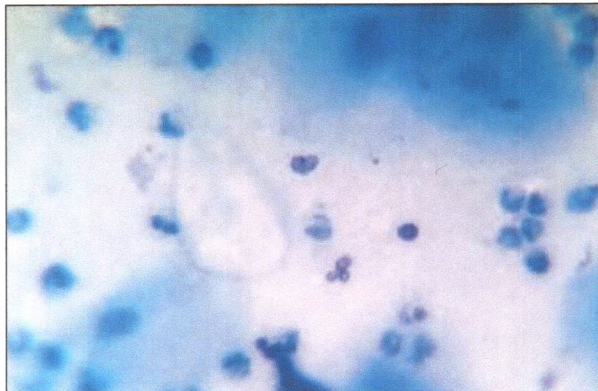

Fig. (6). Presence of *Candida* spp. organisms in stained smears (1000X magnification under oil immersion objective).

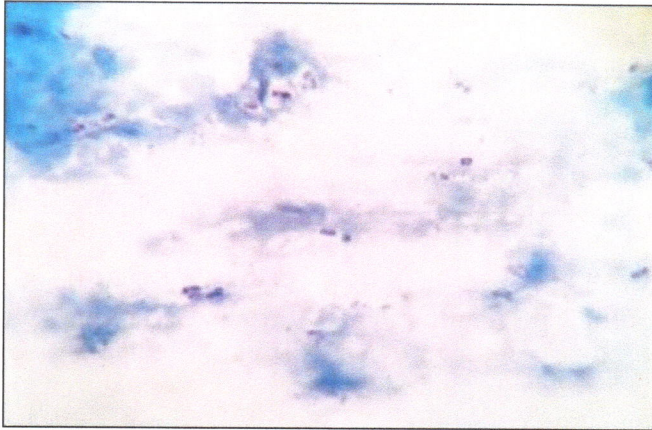

Fig. (7).   Stained smears examination of otic discharges - Peanut-shaped *Malassezia* spp. (1000X magnification under oil immersion objective).

Bacteria

Bacteria are the most common infectious organisms noticed in the cytology. Two types of bacteria are commonly noticed in the stained smears. *i.e. Cocci* and rods. *Cocci* are round in morphology, and appear individually or in clusters. Out of which cocci were found as intracellular *cocci,* which are indicative of true infection. *Cocci* are most often *Staphylococcus* or *Streptococcus* species. Further culture of the samples should be carried out for antibiotic sensitivity tests. Rods are often *Escherichia coli, Pseudomonas* species, or *Klebsiella* species [31, 32] (Fig. **8**).

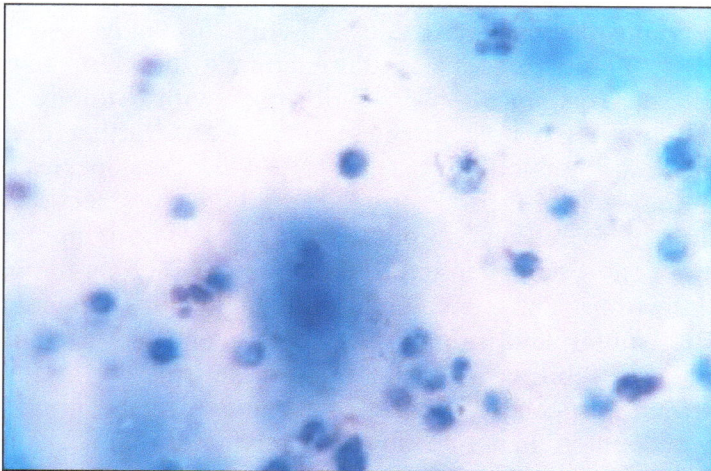

Fig. (8).   Presence of *Cocci* and rods in stained smears (1000X magnification under oil immersion objective).

Cytological Examinations

Based on the morphology and arrangements of bacteria in the cytological examination, bacteria are classified as rods *versus cocci*; arrangements in clusters, pairs, chains, and tetrads. The intensity of bacteria is classified on a scale of 1+, 2+, 3+, *etc.*, under 40× objective examination. Alternatively, methods may be used to denote increasing numbers. Various reporting schemes have been proposed based on the type and severity of lesions observed. Standardized criteria are used to report the severity of infection and the quantification of organisms found in the cytological examination [33 - 36]. Common organisms found in normal and diseased ears are mentioned in Table **5**. In healthy dogs, ear cytology analysis typically reveals a minimal number of organisms, with no rod-shaped bacteria or inflammatory cells present. Conversely, dogs with ear diseases exhibit a higher abundance of organisms, including *cocci*, rods, fungi, and parasites, along with various types of inflammatory cells. The otic microbiota isolated from control cases mainly consists of *Bacillus* spp. and *Staphylococcus* spp. In clinical cases, additional species such as *Pseudomonas spp., E. coli, Klebsiella spp.,* and *Alcaligenes spp.* may also be identified. Interestingly, the yeast *Malassezia pachydermatis* can be isolated from both infected and healthy ears of dogs [37]. Differences between the cytology and cultural tests in the determination of etiology for otitis in dogs are presented in Table **6**. Indications for culture and susceptibility testing in otitis: in certain dogs with ear diseases, along with cytology, antimicrobial sensitivity is advised. It is due to 1. In case of cytology findings rods and/or cocci seen. The most suitable antibiotic treatments can only be chosen if the organisms are known. 2. Marked purulent discharge without organisms being noted. 3. There is a possibility of finding a pathogen that is relevant, but organisms that are irrelevant clinically may also grow. 4. The presence of pyogranulomatous inflammation. In this uncommon ear inflammation, organisms are often difficult to see with cytology thus culture is obligatory. Culture should help direct secondary and further treatments when there is a suspicion of methicillin-resistant *Staphylococcus* species organisms [38 - 40]. Ear cytology plays a crucial role in guiding the selection of the initial antibiotic treatment for ear infections. However, determining the appropriate antibiotic therapy can be challenging due to factors such as the chronicity and recurrence of infections. The choice of antibiotic may vary depending on the type of bacteria, mites, fungi, and inflammatory cells identified in cytology samples. Assessing the susceptibility of these microorganisms to antibiotics can be particularly difficult, especially in cases of chronic or recurrent otitis. Therefore, clinicians may encounter challenges in accurately determining the most effective antibiotic regimen based solely on cytological findings. Additional diagnostic tests, such as culture and susceptibility testing, may be necessary to guide antibiotic selection and ensure successful treatment outcomes [41, 42]. Proper identification of the etiology of ear diseases in dogs relies on a comprehensive approach that considers past experiences, physical characteristics of discharges, odor, and cytological evidence from smears. Failure to thoroughly assess these factors may lead to misidentification of the primary pathogen and inappropriate selection of antimicrobial therapy, resulting in poor case management, prolonged treatment duration, treatment failures, and disease progression. In conclusion, cytology should be regarded as a fundamental preliminary diagnostic tool in the evaluation of every dog presenting with ear diseases in routine veterinary practice. Its role in guiding accurate diagnosis and treatment decisions cannot be overstated, contributing significantly to successful patient outcomes and effective management of ear conditions.

Table 5. Common organisms found in normal and diseased ears.

Microorganism Found In	
Normal Ears	**Ears with Otitis Externa**
Malassezia pachydermatis	*Malassezia* species
Lipid-dependent *Malassezia* species (*e.g., Malassezia furfur* and *Malassezia obtuse*)	*Staphylococcus pseudintermedius*
Staphylococcus pseudintermedius	*Pseudomonas aeruginosa*
Staphylococcus schleiferi subspecies coagulants	*Proteus mirabilis*
Coagulase-negative *Staphylococcus* species	*b-streptococci*
Bacillus species	*Corynebacterium* species
Corynebacterium species	*Enterococcus* species
Streptococci species	*Escherichia coli*
Micrococcus species	

Table 6. Comparison of cytology and cultural examination in dogs with otitis.

Factors	Cytology	Culture
Time to available results	Immediate	48–72 hours
Sensitivity for yeast	High	Low
Sensitivity for bacteria	High	Moderate to high
Sensitivity for leukocytes	High	None
Estimation of numbers	Semi quantitative	Categorical data
Rank significance in mixed infection.	Yes	No
Monitor response to therapy	Yes	No

(Table 6) cont.....

Factors	Cytology	Culture
Detection of antimicrobial resistance	No	Yes

CONCLUSION

Accurate diagnosis of the primary etiology and perpetuating factors is important for treating ear diseases. Cytological examination of ear samples serves as the most efficient, simple, practical, and rapid diagnostic tool that can be easily performed routinely for dogs with otitis. In addition to clinical examination, ear examination by otoscopy, assessing the primary infections, imaging diagnostic facilities, and serial cytological procedures are useful in the assessment of secondary infections; evaluation of therapeutic response, and making informed management decisions. Cytological evaluation focuses on characterizing three key features: yeast, bacteria, and leukocytes. Therapeutic interventions are based on the results of cytological tests. The abundance of leukocytes, including phagocytized bacteria, serves as a useful biomarker for distinguishing "true infection" from overgrowth. A combination of cytological examination, cultural studies, and antimicrobial sensitivity tests is the best method for identifying microbial growth and their susceptibility patterns. Culture testing provides valuable clues for selecting appropriate antibiotic therapy based on the specific pathogens identified.

REFERENCES

[1]   Angus JC. Otic cytology in health and disease. Vet Clin North Am Small Anim Pract 2004; 34(2): 411-24.
        [http://dx.doi.org/10.1016/j.cvsm.2003.10.005] [PMID: 15062616]

[2]   Bajwa J. Cutaneous cytology and the dermatology patient. Can Vet J 2017; 58(6): 625-7.
        [PMID: 28588342]

[3]   Shaw S. Pathogens in otitis externa: diagnostic techniques to identify secondary causes of ear disease. In Pract 2016; 38(S2): 12-6.
        [http://dx.doi.org/10.1136/inp.i461]

[4]   O'Neill DG, Volk AV, Soares T, Church DB, Brodbelt DC, Pegram C. Frequency and predisposing factors for canine otitis externa in the UK primary veterinary care epidemiological view. Canine Med Genet 2021; 8 (7).
        [http://dx.doi.org/10.1186/s40575-021-00106-1]

[5]   Ginel PJ, Lucena R, Rodriguez JC, Ortega J. A semiquantitative cytological evaluation of normal and pathological samples from the external ear canal of dogs and cats. Vet Dermatol 2002; 13(3): 151-6.
        [http://dx.doi.org/10.1046/j.1365-3164.2002.00288.x] [PMID: 12074704]

[6]   Saridomichelakis MN, Farmaki R, Leontides LS, Koutinas AF. Aetiology of canine otitis externa: a retrospective study of 100 cases. Vet Dermatol 2007; 18(5): 341-7.
        [http://dx.doi.org/10.1111/j.1365-3164.2007.00619.x] [PMID: 17845622]

[7]   Oliveira LC, Leite CA, Brilhante RS, Carvalho CB. Comparative study of the microbial profile from bilateral canine otitis externa. Can Vet J 2008; 49(8): 785-8.
        [PMID: 18978972]

[8]   Perry LR, MacLennan B, Korven R, Rawlings TA. Epidemiological study of dogs with otitis externa

in Cape Breton, Nova Scotia. Can Vet J 2017; 58(2): 168-74.
[PMID: 28216686]

[9]   Ghibaudo G, Peano A. Chronic monolateral otomycosis in a dog caused by *Aspergillus ochraceus*. Vet Dermatol 2010; 21(5): 522-6.
[http://dx.doi.org/10.1111/j.1365-3164.2010.00884.x] [PMID: 20409075]

[10]   Christopher MM, Hotz CS, Shelly SM, Pion PD. Use of cytology as a diagnostic method in veterinary practice and assessment of communication between veterinary practitioners and veterinary clinical pathologists. J Am Vet Med Assoc 2008; 232(5): 747-54.
[http://dx.doi.org/10.2460/javma.232.5.747] [PMID: 18312185]

[11]   Coatesworth J. Examination of the canine ear. Companion Anim 2011; 16(5): 31-5.
[http://dx.doi.org/10.1111/j.2044-3862.2011.00070.x]

[12]   Bugden DL. Identification and antibiotic susceptibility of bacterial isolates from dogs with otitis externa in Australia. Aust Vet J 2013; 91(1-2): 43-6.
[http://dx.doi.org/10.1111/avj.12007] [PMID: 23356371]

[13]   Bradley CW, Lee FF, Rankin SC, *et al.* The otic microbiota and mycobiota in a referral population of dogs in eastern USA with otitis externa. Vet Dermatol 2020; 31(3): 225-e49.
[http://dx.doi.org/10.1111/vde.12826] [PMID: 31960536]

[14]   Budach SC, Mueller RS. Reproducibility of a semiquantitative method to assess cutaneous cytology. Vet Dermatol 2012; 23(5): 426-e80.
[http://dx.doi.org/10.1111/j.1365-3164.2012.01075.x] [PMID: 22809453]

[15]   Girão MD, Prado MR, Brilhante RSN, *et al. Malassezia pachydermatis* isolated from normal and diseased external ear canals in dogs: A comparative analysis. Vet J 2006; 172(3): 544-8.
[http://dx.doi.org/10.1016/j.tvjl.2005.07.004] [PMID: 16154787]

[16]   Cole LK. Otoscopic evaluation of the ear canal. Vet Clin North Am Small Anim Pract 2004; 34(2): 397-410.
[http://dx.doi.org/10.1016/j.cvsm.2003.10.004] [PMID: 15062615]

[17]   Radlinsky MG. Advances in Otoscopy. Vet Clin North Am Small Anim Pract 2016; 46(1): 171-9.
[http://dx.doi.org/10.1016/j.cvsm.2015.08.006] [PMID: 26590676]

[18]   Miller WH, Griffin CE, Campbell KL. Muller and Kirk's Small Animal Dermatology. 7th ed. St Louis, MO, USA: Elsevier Health Sciences 2012; pp. 741-66.

[19]   Gotthelf LN. Factors that Predispose the Ear to Otitis Externa. Small Animal Ear Diseases: An Illustrated Guide. St Louis, MO: Saunders Elsevier 2005; pp. 142-55.
[http://dx.doi.org/10.1016/B0-72-160137-5/50010-6]

[20]   Lyskova P, Vydrzalova M, Mazurova J. Identification and antimicrobial susceptibility of bacteria and yeasts isolated from healthy dogs and dogs with otitis externa. J Vet Med A Physiol Pathol Clin Med 2007; 54(10): 559-63.
[http://dx.doi.org/10.1111/j.1439-0442.2007.00996.x] [PMID: 18045339]

[21]   Paterson S. Diagnostic approach to otitis in dogs. Todays Vet Pract 2011; 1(2): 27-32.

[22]   Kumar A, Singh K, Sharma A. Prevalence of *Malasezzia pachydermatis* and other organisms in healthy and infected dog ears. Isr J Vet Med 2002; 57: 145-8.

[23]   Favrot C, Steffan J, Seewald W, Picco F. A prospective study on the clinical features of chronic canine atopic dermatitis and its diagnosis. Vet Dermatol 2010; 21(1): 23-31.
[http://dx.doi.org/10.1111/j.1365-3164.2009.00758.x] [PMID: 20187911]

[24]   Tater KC, Scott DW, Miller WH Jr, Erb HN. The cytology of the external ear canal in the normal dog and cat. J Vet Med A Physiol Pathol Clin Med 2003; 50(7): 370-4.
[http://dx.doi.org/10.1046/j.1439-0442.2003.00548.x] [PMID: 14633232]

[25]   Wallace KA, DeHeer HL, Patel RT. The external ear canal. In: Valenciano AC, Cowell RL, Eds.

Diagnostic Cytology and Hematology of the Dog and Cat. 4th ed. St. Louis, MO: Elsevier Mosby 2013; pp. 171-9.

[26] Reddy BS, Kumari KN. Canine scabies - Its therapeutic management and zoonotic importance. Intas Polivet 2013; 14: 292-4.

[27] Reddy BS, Kumari KN. Demodicosis and its successful management in dogs. Ind J of Field Vet 2010; 6(2): 48-50.

[28] Reddy BS, Sivajothi S. Notoedric mange associated with *Malassezia* in cats. International Journal of Veterinary Health Science and Research 2014; 2: 101.

[29] Crespo MJ, Abarca ML, Cabañes FJ. Occurrence of *Malassezia* spp. in the external ear canals of dogs and cats with and without otitis externa. Med Mycol 2002; 40(2): 115-21.
[http://dx.doi.org/10.1080/mmy.40.2.115.121] [PMID: 12058723]

[30] DeBoer DJ, Moriello KA. Cutaneous Fungal Infections. In: Greene CE, Ed. Infectious Diseases of the Dog and Cat. St Louis, MO: Saunders Elsevier 2006; pp. 550-3.

[31] Fernandez GG, Barboza A, Villalobos O. Isolation and identification of microorganisms present in 53 dogs suffering otitis externa. Rev Cient Fac Cienc Vet Vet Uni Zulia 2006; 16: 23-30.

[32] Hariharan H, Coles M, Poole D, Lund L, Page R. Update on antimicrobial susceptibilities of bacterial isolates from canine and feline otitis externa. Can Vet J 2006; 47(3): 253-5.
[PMID: 16604982]

[33] Borriello G, Paradiso R, Catozzi C, *et al.* Cerumen microbial community shifts between healthy and otitis affected dogs. PLoS One 2020; 15(11): e0241447.
[http://dx.doi.org/10.1371/journal.pone.0241447] [PMID: 33237912]

[34] Bosznay J. Ear cytology in otitis externa: when, why, how? Vet Nurs 2014; 5(2): 70-5.
[http://dx.doi.org/10.12968/vetn.2014.5.2.70]

[35] Graham-Mize CA, Rosser EJ Jr. Comparison of microbial isolates and susceptibility patterns from the external ear canal of dogs with otitis externa. J Am Anim Hosp Assoc 2004; 40(2): 102-8.
[http://dx.doi.org/10.5326/0400102] [PMID: 15007044]

[36] Kasai T, Fukui Y, Aoki K, Ishii Y, Tateda K. Changes in the ear canal microbiota of dogs with otitis externa. J Appl Microbiol 2021; 130(4): 1084-91.
[http://dx.doi.org/10.1111/jam.14868] [PMID: 32979301]

[37] Korbelik J, Singh A, Rousseau J, Weese JS. Characterization of the otic bacterial microbiota in dogs with otitis externa compared to healthy individuals. Vet Dermatol 2019; 30(3): 228-e70.
[http://dx.doi.org/10.1111/vde.12734] [PMID: 30828896]

[38] Bellwood B, Andrasik-Catton M. Veterinary Technician's Handbook of Laboratory Procedures. Ames, IA: Wiley Blackwell 2014; pp. 144-5.

[39] Raskin RE. General categories of cytologic interpretation. In: Raskin RE, Meyer DJ, Eds. Canine and Feline Cytology. 3rd ed. St. Louis, MO: Elsevier Mosby 2016; pp. 16-33.
[http://dx.doi.org/10.1016/B978-1-4557-4083-3.00002-4]

[40] Tater KC, Scott DW, Miller WH Jr, Erb HN. The cytology of the external ear canal in the normal dog and cat. J Vet Med A Physiol Pathol Clin Med. 2003 Sep;50(7):370-4.

[41] Pierce-Hendry SA, Dennis J. Bacterial culture and antibiotic susceptibility testing. Compend Contin Educ Vet 2010; 32(7): E1-5.
[PMID: 20957608]

[42] Zamankhan Malayeri H, Jamshidi S, Zahraei Salehi T. Identification and antimicrobial susceptibility patterns of bacteria causing otitis externa in dogs. Vet Res Commun 2010; 34(5): 435-44.
[http://dx.doi.org/10.1007/s11259-010-9417-y] [PMID: 20526674]

CHAPTER 6

Procedure of Clearing of External Ear Canal

Alok Kumar Chaudhary[1,*]

[1] *Department of Veterinary Medicine, DUVASU, Mathura, India*

Abstract: The chapter underscores the vital role of ear health in dogs, covering various aspects of the subject. It highlights the importance of a dog's ears in maintaining overall health and well-being, focusing on sensory perception, communication, balance, and orientation. The anatomy of the external ear is detailed, explaining the functions of its components. The diagnostic approach for otitis externa is described, involving observations, external ear canal cytology, diagnostic imaging, and differential diagnosis. Basic principles of ear cleaning are outlined, including restraint and handling, observation, and the cleaning process itself, performed manually or using advanced techniques and solutions. Prevention strategies are provided, promoting routine ear care, proper drying after water exposure, regular inspections, allergy management, and collaboration with veterinarians. This abstract offers a comprehensive overview of canine ear health, serving as a valuable resource for veterinarians, and dog owners interested in this subject.

Keywords: Cytology, Ear cleaners, Pus in ear, Wax.

INTRODUCTION

Ears are the natural openings of the body that directly communicate with the environment and play crucial roles in sensory perception, communication, maintaining balance, orientation, and thermoregulation, ultimately contributing to overall health. Anatomically, it divided into three parts: the external ear, middle ear, and inner ear. The term "otitis" indicates inflammation of the ear and it can be otitis externa, otitis media or otitis interna depending upon involvement of parts of ear. Otitis externa is inflammation of the external ear canal and is the most frequently reported ear disorder in dogs, with a prevalence range of 8% to 30% [1]. Otitis externa may be acute or chronic (persistent or recurrent otitis lasting for 3 months or longer). It is caused by multiple etiological agents including bacteria, fungi, foreign objects, mites, allergens, or excessive moisture. Various factors contribute to ear infections in dogs, including ear shape, breed characteristics like

---

* **Corresponding author Alok Kumar Chaudhary:** Department of Veterinary Medicine, DUVASU, Mathura, India;
E-mail: dr.alokvet@gmail.com

Tanmoy Rana (Ed.)

long floppy ears, excess hair in the ear canals, swimming or bathing, and overproduction of earwax [2]. Common symptoms of otitis externa in dogs includes head shaking, scratching, bad odor, redness, swelling, discharge, severe pain and behavior changes. Cleaning the external ear of a dog is an essential aspect of routine grooming and hygiene maintenance [3]. Proper ear cleaning helps prevent ear infections, discomfort, and potential health issues.

UNDERSTANDING THE EXTERNAL EAR ANATOMY

Understanding the external ear anatomy of dogs is important for recognizing normal variations among breeds and for identifying any potential issues or conditions, such as infections (like otitis externa) or foreign bodies lodged in the ear canal. Regular inspection and care of the external ear can help maintain your dog's ear health and overall well-being. Anotomically, the external ear includes following structure:

Pinna (Auricle)

The pinna is the visible, outer part of the dog's ear. It is made of cartilage covered by skin and serves to capture and funnel sound waves into the ear canal. The shape and size of the pinna can vary widely among dog breeds.

Ear Canals (External Auditory Meatus)

This is a tube-like structure that extends from the pinna towards the middle ear. It's slightly curved and has a vertical orientation of about an inch before it turns horizontally towards the eardrum. It can be divided in to

Vertical Ear Canal

The initial part of the ear canal that runs vertically is important for funneling sound waves and protecting the middle ear.

Horizontal Ear Canal

After the vertical portion, the ear canal turns horizontally and leads to the tympanic membrane (eardrum). This part is important for protecting the inner structures of the ear.

Glands

The external ear canal contains sebaceous glands (which produce sebum, an oily substance) and ceruminous glands (which produce earwax or cerumen). These glands contribute to the health of the ear by moisturizing and protecting the ear canal.

Hair

Some dogs may have hair in and around the ear canal. Excessive hair in the ear canals can contribute to ear problems and should be regularly checked and, if necessary, trimmed.

Tympanic Membrane (Eardrum)

The eardrum separates the external ear from the middle ear. It vibrates in response to sound waves and transmits these vibrations to the middle ear's auditory ossicles (tiny bones), which then send the signals to the inner ear for processing.

IMPORTANCE OF EAR CLEANING

Cleaning your dog's ears is an integral part of pet care. Neglecting ear hygiene can lead to painful ear infections, discomfort for your dog, and even hearing loss. Regular cleaning helps remove debris, excess wax, and prevents the buildup of moisture, all of which contribute to a healthy ear environment.

Common Etiology and Predisposing Factors Associated with Ear Discharge in Dogs

The common etiology of ear discharge in dogs can be attributed to a variety of factors as described by Paterson, *et al.* [4], and Saridomichelakis [5].

Bacterial Agents

Various bacteria, including *Staphylococcus spp, Pseudomonas spp, Proteus spp, Enterococcus spp, Streptococcus spp, and Corynebacterium* spp, can lead to otitis externa in ear of dogs [6, 7]. These infections can cause inflammation, irritation, and discharge.

Parasites

Ear mite (*Otodectes cynotis*) is a common parasite that can infest a dog's ear canal, causing irritation, inflammation, and discharge. Other parasites like ticks, sarcoptic mange mites, demodex mites and ticks can also contribute to ear problems.

Dermatophytes

Fungal infections caused by dermatophytes like *Microsporum canis* and *Trichophyton mentagrophytes* can lead to ear issues and discharge in dogs. These fungi can cause skin and ear infections [8].

Hypersensitivity

Environmental allergies, food allergies, and flea allergies can cause inflammation and irritation in a dog's ears, leading to discharge. Allergic reactions can make the ear more susceptible to infections.

Endocrine Disorders

Conditions like hypothyroidism can impact the overall health of a dog's skin and ears, potentially leading to infections and discharge. Hormonal imbalances can affect the immune system's response to infections.

Foreign Bodies

Foreign objects, such as hair, plant materials, or debris, can become lodged in a dog's ear canal, causing irritation, inflammation, and a buildup of discharge.

Autoimmune Disorders

Autoimmune conditions like pemphigus complex and lupus erythematosus can affect the skin, including the skin lining the ears. These disorders can lead to inflammation, discharge, and secondary infections.

Glandular Disorders

Disorders of ceruminous, sebaceous, and apocrine glands can disrupt the normal production and composition of earwax, potentially leading to ear issues and discharge.

Benign and Malignant Tumors

Tumors, both benign and malignant, can develop in a dog's ear canal or surrounding tissues. These growths can cause various symptoms, including discharge, depending on their nature and location.

PREDISPOSING FACTORS

Several predisposing factors that can increase a dog's susceptibility to ear discharge and ear infections (otitis externa):

Anatomy

Dogs with floppy ears, such as Cocker Spaniels, Basset Hounds, and Poodles, have a greater risk of developing ear problems because their ear canals are often more closed off, creating a warm and moist environment that's conducive to bacterial and fungal growth.

Swimming or Bathing

Dogs that swim frequently or are bathed too often can end up with moisture trapped in their ear canals, promoting bacterial and fungal growth. It's important to thoroughly dry the ears after water exposure.

Poor Ear Cleaning

Over-cleaning or improper cleaning of a dog's ears can disrupt the natural balance of the ear canal, making it more susceptible to infections.

Previous Ear Infections

Dogs that have had ear infections in the past are more likely to experience recurring infections due to changes in the ear canal's environment or residual inflammation.

Excessive Hair in Ear Canals

Breeds with excessive hair growth in their ear canals, such as Poodles and Schnauzers, are at a higher risk of developing ear infections as the hair can trap debris and moisture.

Poor Air Circulation

Dogs that live in humid environments or have inadequate air circulation in their ears are more prone to fungal and bacterial growth.

Immunosuppression

Dogs with compromised immune systems due to illness, medications (*e.g.*, immunosuppressive drugs), or other factors are more susceptible to ear infections.

Behavioral Factors

Dogs that scratch or shake their heads excessively can traumatize the ear canal's lining, making it easier for bacteria and fungi to invade.

Age

Puppies and elderly dogs are generally more susceptible to ear infections due to their developing or weakened immune systems, respectively.

Poor Diet

Nutritional deficiencies can weaken a dog's immune system and overall health, making them more susceptible to infections, including ear infections.

PATHO-PHSIOLOGY OF EAR DISCHARGE IN DOGS

The patho-physiology of ear discharge in dogs can be understood by considering the normal anatomy and function of the ear, the production of earwax (cerumen), and how disruptions in this process can lead to various types of ear discharge External auditory canal ear canal contains sebaceous glands and ceruminous glands that normally produces cerumen or earwax. Cerumen, or ear wax, is a solid hydrophobic secretion of oily and waxy substances that coats. The primary functions of cerumen are to protect and to lubricate the skin lining the ear canal, prevent excessive moisture from entering the ear, and trap foreign particles (dust, debris, insects, *etc.*) to keep them from reaching the sensitive middle and inner ear. Under normal circumstances, cerumen is produced in a balanced manner and gradually migrates from the deeper parts of the ear canal toward the external ear, where it eventually dries up and falls out. However, various factors can disrupt this process:

Overproduction

Some dogs may produce excessive cerumen, leading to the rapid buildup of earwax in the ear canal.

Inadequate Drainage

Dogs with ear canal abnormalities, narrow ear canals, or ear conformation issues may not allow for proper drainage of earwax.

Foreign Bodies

Foreign objects, like grass seeds or debris, can become lodged in the ear canal, trapping cerumen and promoting bacterial or fungal growth.

Allergic Reactions and Inflammation

Allergies or infections can trigger an inflammatory response in the ear canal's skin, leading to increased cerumen production and disruption of normal earwax movement.

CLINICAL SYMPTOMS

The manifestations of clinical signs in dogs with otitis externa depend on the clinical condition. These signs can range from otalgia, which signifies mild ear discomfort or pruritus, to severe pain. Dogs affected by otalgia may exhibit symptoms such as head shaking, tilting their heads, imbalance, scratching, and chewing of the ears. In cases of otorrhea, there is a discharge either from or within the external auditory canal. Otorrhea is variable and can be characterized by the type of secretions, which may be thick, crusted, or adherent, and at times can occlude the ear canal. Additionally, the external auditory canal may become swollen and painful, accompanied by discharge and debris. Excesses accumulate of wax in the ear canal provide an ideal environment for bacteria and fungi to thrive (Figs. **1** and **2**). The presence of these microorganisms can lead to infection, further inflammation, and the development of various types of ear discharge [1].

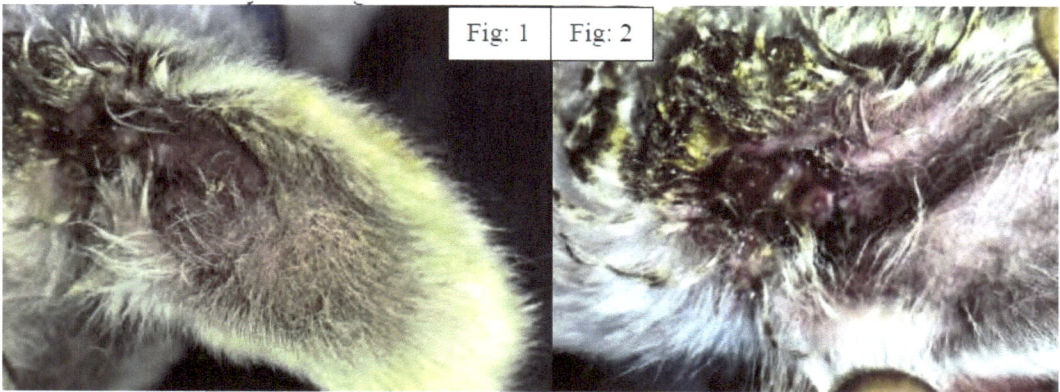

Fig: 1 | Fig: 2

Figs. (1 and 2). Shows the external canal of the ear with pus discharge.

Purulent Discharge

If bacteria are the primary culprits, a purulent (pus-like) discharge may result.

Foul Odor

Infections can produce a foul odor due to the breakdown of tissues and the presence of harmful microorganisms.

Waxy Discharge

In cases where the earwax itself becomes infected or inflamed, a waxy discharge may be observed.

Bloody Discharge

Severe infections or trauma to the ear canal can lead to a bloody discharge.

DIAGNOSTIC APPROACH

Diagnostic approach of otitis externa should be based on detailed history, ear canal examination, ear canal cytology and differential diagnosis [9, 10].

External Ear Canal Cytology

For the sample collection, carefully insert an applicator tip in the ear canal and, near the junction of the vertical and horizontal canals, collect material for cytologic examination. Transfer samples onto a glass slide directly and examine under microscope for mites and foreign body. for bacterial examination glass slide heat fix, and stain with Diff-Quik When examining samples under the microscope with oil immersion field (100X) for presence of bacteria, yeast and inflammatory cell. Sample should be testes in laboratory for culture & sensitivity [2].

Diagnostic Imaging of Ear Canal

Otoscopy

It clinically useful for assessment of canal proliferation, masses, foreign bodies, ruptured tympanic membrane and secretions. In advance tools, fiberoptic video-enhanced otoscopy is uses [11].

Computed tomography (CT)

Aids in differentiation of bony lesions in the bullae from soft tissue reactions.

Magnetic resonance imaging (MRI)

It is an expensive aids and useful in visualizing middle and inner ear and detects presence of fluids, such as endolymph within the cochlea and semicircular canals.

Ultrasound can be used for the detection of fluid within the tympanic bulla (Fig. 3).

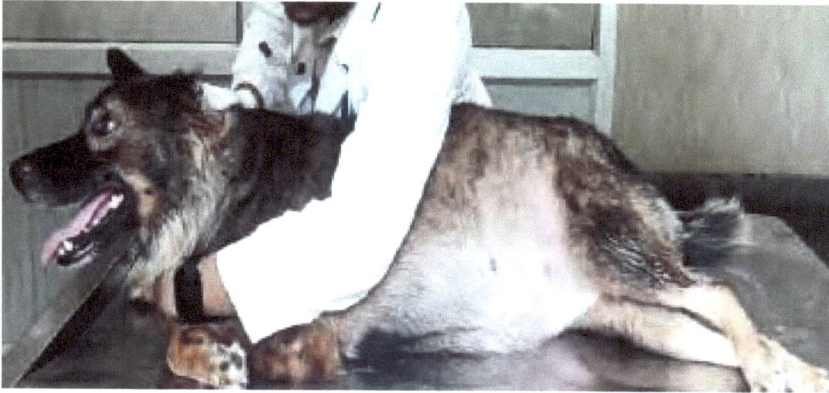

Fig. (3). Restraining of dog.

Radiograph

It can be applied for detects bony involvement of bullae; has limited value in soft tissue changes, especially in acute cases [3].

DIFFERENTIAL DIAGNOSIS

In the examination of the external ear, it's crucial to consider differential diagnoses to plan appropriate treatment. This includes distinguishing between acute or chronic bacterial infections, fungal infections, traumatic injuries, osteomyelitis, or cases presenting with otitis media and a perforated tympanic membrane. Noninfectious dermatologic causes of otitis externa should also be taken into account. Systemic diseases like atopic dermatitis, psoriasis, seborrheic dermatitis, acne, and lupus erythematosus can contribute to otitis externa. Additionally, local diseases such as contact dermatitis (irritant or allergic) may affect both the pinna and the external auditory canal. Understanding the specific condition and its underlying cause is vital for developing an effective treatment plan.

BASIC PRINCIPLE OF EXTERNAL EAR CLEANING

Ear cleaning in dogs is an important part of their overall grooming and health care routine. The basic principles of ear cleaning in dogs typically involves the following steps:

Restraint and Handling

Restraint and handling are crucial starting points for the proper cleaning of a dog's ear canal. This process should be undertaken in a calm and controlled environment to ensure the safety and comfort of the dog. When restraining the dog, it's essential to strike a balance, avoiding excessive tightness which could lead to stress or potential injury. This gentle and careful approach to restraint and handling sets the foundation for a successful and safe ear cleaning procedure, allowing both the dog and the owner to have a positive experience. Additionally, if a dog requires more extensive ear treatment or if the cleaning process becomes too uncomfortable for them, it may be necessary to consider general anesthesia as a means of ensuring the dog's well-being and the thoroughness of the cleaning procedure [4].

Observation

Observation is a critical first step in the ear cleaning process for dogs. Taking the time to thoroughly examine the dog's ear before proceeding allows you to gather important information about its condition. Look closely for any visible signs such as dirt, debris, redness, inflammation, discharge, or foul odor. These visual cues can serve as valuable indicators of the ear's health. Noticing any abnormalities or irregularities during this observation phase is crucial, as it can prompt you to seek veterinary advice if necessary. By carefully assessing the ear's appearance, you can tailor the cleaning process to address specific concerns and ensure your dog's ear health is properly maintained [5].

Cleaning

Cleaning process is a routine process for making healthy our pet because of proper ear cleaning of ear removes excessive wax and debris, bacterial by-products, degenerating cells, and free fatty acids that can be contribute to initiate inflammatory reaction in ear canal. In addition it also increases treatment efficacy through better penetration of topical medications. The cleaning phase in the process of caring for a dog's ears is a delicate but essential step. It usually performed by the several techniques based on clinical condition.

Manual Cleaning of Ear Canal

After restraining the dog carefully, lift the dog's ear flap to expose the visible parts of the ear canal. Apply the ear cleaning stick and gently wipe the dirt or debris (Fig. **4**). It's crucial to exercise caution during this process to avoid pushing any debris deeper into the ear canal, which could potentially worsen the issue. Using gentle, controlled movements is key to ensuring that the cleaning is effective while preventing any discomfort or harm to the dog. Repeat the process unit visual debris not clean [6].

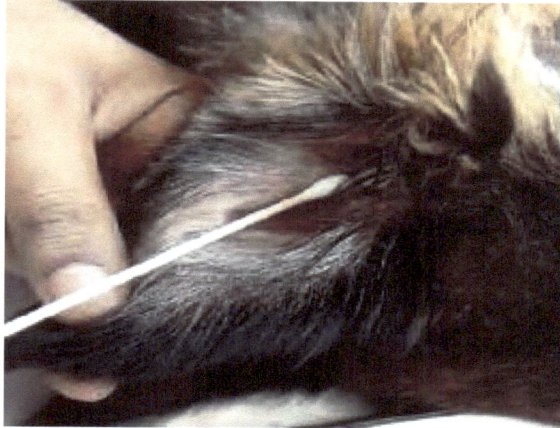

Fig. (4). Manuel cleaning of ear.

Cleaning of Ear Canal by Using Digital Otoscopy

Digital otoscopy is a modern and advanced method used for examining and cleaning the ear canal in both humans and animals, including dogs. This technique involves the use of a specialized tool called a digital otoscope, which provides a magnified and well-illuminated view of the ear canal on a digital screen (Fig. **5**).

Cleaning of Ear Canal by Suction Pump

Cleaning the ear canal using a suction pump, often referred to as ear lavage or ear irrigation, is a procedure commonly employed in medical settings to remove excess earwax (cerumen) or foreign objects from the ear canal (Fig. **6**).

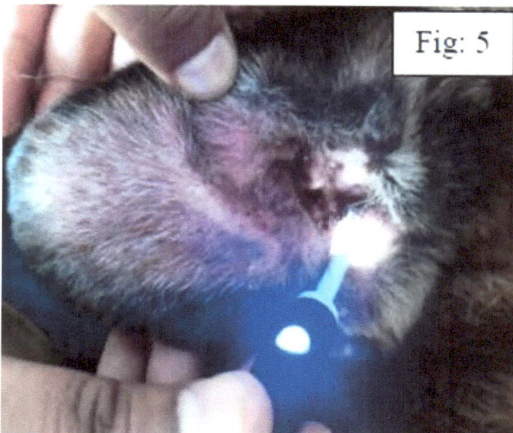

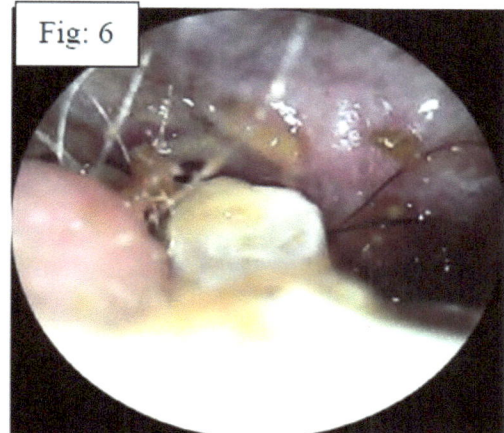

Figs. (5 and 6). Observation and cleaning of ear by using digital otoscopy.

Cleaning of Ear Canal by Using Solution or Agents

a) Normal saline: Normal saline is 0.9% saline, it means that there is 0.9g of salt (NaCl) per 100 ml of solution, or 9 g per liter. The salinity in the water is effective in breaking up the earwax and removing it with ease [7].

b) Cerumenolytic Agents: Cerumenolytic agents are substances designed to soften and break down earwax, making it easier to remove. These agents are typically in liquid or gel form and are applied directly into the ear canal. Common cerumenolytic agents includes:

Hydrogen Peroxide: Hydrogen peroxide is a mild antiseptic that can help to loosen and bubble away earwax. It can also have a mild antibacterial effect.

Dioctyl Sodium Sulfosuccinate: This is a surfactant that helps break down and disperse earwax and other debris. It acts as an emulsifying agent to make the wax easier to remove.

Urea and Carbamide Peroxide: These ingredients work as cerumenolytic agents by softening and dissolving earwax. They are often found in over-the-counter ear cleaning solutions.

Glycerin: Glycerin can help to moisturize and soften earwax, making it easier to remove.

Lanolin: Lanolin is a natural substance derived from sheep's wool, and it can help soften earwax. It also has moisturizing properties.

Propylene Glycol: Propylene glycol is a common ingredient in many ear cleaners. It can help to soften earwax and maintain moisture in the ear canal.

Phytosphingosine: Phytosphingosine is a lipid molecule with antiinflammatory properties. It may help soothe the ear canal while aiding in the breakdown of earwax.

Salicylic Acid: Salicylic acid is a beta-hydroxy acid that can help exfoliate and break down earwax. It is also known for its antiinflammatory properties [8].

c) Antibacterial agents: The most common indication of antibacterial agent is used to kill or inhibit the growth of bacterial agent in ear canal. It commonly recommended after cleaning of external auditory canal. Most commonly use antibacterial optic solution are:

i. Neomycin otic solutions and suspensions with polymyxin B–hydrocortisone

ii. Aminoglycoside ophthalmic solutions such as

1) Tobramycin sulfate 0.3%

2) Gentamicin sulfate 0.3%

iii. Quinolone ophthalmic solutions

1) Ofloxacin 0.3%

2) Ciprofloxacin 0.3%

3) Marbofloxacin

Some other solution are available with contain TrizEDTA (chelating agent), chlorhexidine, iodophors, boric acid, acetic acid

d) Anti fungal agent: Used for fungal infections, including Nystatin, Clotrimazole, Miconazole, and Ketoconazole.

Drying agents: Containing substances like isopropyl alcohol, acetic acid, or boric acid to help dry the ear canal.

e) Acidifying Agent: Maintain an acidic pH in the ear canal to prevent certain bacterial and yeast growth. Commonly used is 2% acetic acid.

f) Anti-inflammatory solution: 0.5% hydrocortisone is used as common ingredients in anti inflammatory solutions to reduce inflammation and provide relief from itching or discomfort caused by ear conditions [9].

DEEP EAR CLEANING

Deep ear cleaning, particularly when the tympanic membrane (eardrum) is not visible through routine diagnostics, is a specialized procedure that should be approached with care. Deep ear cleaning is typically indicated when routine diagnostics cannot visualize the tympanic membrane. This suggests that there may be a significant buildup of debris or other issues deeper in the ear canal that require attention. Deep ear cleaning should be performed with the patient under general anesthesia. This is because the procedure can be uncomfortable for the dog, and it allows for better control and thorough cleaning. Deep ear cleaning can be done using hand-held manual otoscopes or video-otoscopes. The latter is highly recommended as it provides improved visualization of the ear canal, making it easier to identify and address issues. Some specialized flushing devices have been developed for use with video-otoscopes. These devices combine suction and flushing capabilities and can be inserted through the channel on a video-otoscope or through the operating head of a manual otoscope. They are effective for ear cleaning. It is typically reserved for cases where routine diagnostics cannot visualize the eardrum, indicating the need for a more thorough examination and cleaning of the ear canal [10].

PREVENTION

1) Perform routine ear cleaning as needed to prevent the buildup of dirt, debris, and excess wax. Follow your veterinarian's recommendations for the frequency of cleaning.

2) When cleaning your dog's ears, use the appropriate cleaning solution and follow proper technique to avoid pushing debris deeper into the ear canal. Be gentle and cautious.

3) Make sure to thoroughly dry your dog's ears after bathing or swimming. Moisture in the ears can promote the growth of bacteria and yeast.

4) Minimize your dog's exposure to excessive moisture, such as heavy rain or prolonged water play, which can lead to ear problems.

5) Regularly inspect your dog's ears for signs of dirt, debris, redness, inflammation, discharge, or foul odor. Early detection of issues can prevent them from worsening.

6) Ensure your dog has a balanced diet to support overall health, including ear health.

7) If your dog has allergies, work with your veterinarian to manage them effectively. Allergies can contribute to ear problems [11].

CONCLUSION

In conclusion, maintaining the health of your dog's ears is an important aspect of responsible pet care. Proper ear care involves a combination of regular cleaning, preventive measures, and vigilance. By following the basic principles of external ear cleaning, such as gentle handling, observation, and the use of appropriate cleaning techniques and solutions, you can help keep your dog's ears clean and free from issues. Cerumenolytic agents, which soften and break down earwax, can be valuable tools in this process, and they are typically found in liquid or gel form applied directly into the ear canal. These agents, along with other cleaning solutions, can aid in the removal of dirt and debris, reducing the risk of infections and discomfort. To maintain good ear health in your dog, it's crucial to stay proactive with preventive measures. Regularly inspect your dog's ears, keep them dry after water exposure, and be attentive to signs of trouble. Consulting with your veterinarian for guidance and scheduling routine check-ups is essential for addressing specific ear health concerns and ensuring your dog's overall well-being.

REFERENCES

[1]   Sandeep K, Kafil H, Raman S, *et al.* Prevalence of canine otitis externa in jammu journal of animal research 2014; 4(1): 121-9.

[2]   Angus JC, Lichtensteiger C, Campbell KL, *et al.* Breed variations in histopathologic features of chronic severe otitis externa in dogs: 80 cases JAVMA 2002; 221:1000–1006.

[3]   Moog F, Mivielle J, Brun J, *et al.* Clinical and microbiological performances and effects on lipid and cytokine production of a ceruminolytic ear cleaner in canine erythemato-ceruminous otitis externa. Vet Sci 2022; 9(4): 185.
        [http://dx.doi.org/10.3390/vetsci9040185] [PMID: 35448682]

[4]   Paterson S, Matyskiewicz W. A study to evaluate the primary causes associated with *Pseudomonas otitis* in 60 dogs. J Small Anim Pract. 2018;59(4):238–242. 2.

[5]   Saridomichelakis MN, Farmaki R, Leontides LS, Koutinas AF. Aetiology of canine otitis externa: a retrospective study of 100 cases. Vet Dermatol 2007; 18(5): 341-7.
        [http://dx.doi.org/10.1111/j.1365-3164.2007.00619.x] [PMID: 17845622]

[6]   Zamankhan Malayeri H, Jamshidi S, Zahraei Salehi T. Identification and antimicrobial susceptibility patterns of bacteria causing otitis externa in dogs. Vet Res Commun 2010; 34(5): 435-44.
        [http://dx.doi.org/10.1007/s11259-010-9417-y] [PMID: 20526674]

[7]   Pye CC, Yu AA, Weese JS. Evaluation of biofilm production by *Pseudomonas aeruginosa* from canine ears and the impact of biofilm on antimicrobial susceptibility *in vitro*. Vet Dermatol 2013; 24(4): 446-449, e98-e99.
        [http://dx.doi.org/10.1111/vde.12040] [PMID: 23738965]

[8]   Chen T, Hill PB. The biology of *Malassezia* organisms and their ability to induce immune responses and skin disease. Vet Dermatol 2005; 16(1): 4-26.
        [http://dx.doi.org/10.1111/j.1365-3164.2005.00424.x] [PMID: 15725101]

[9]   Cole, L.K. Diagnostic tests and techniques for otitis. AVMA Convention Notes, 2003 AVMA, Denver, Colo.

[10]   Harvey R, Paterson S. Otitis Externa: An Essential Guide to Diagnosis and Treatment. Boca Raton, FL: CRC Press 2014.
        [http://dx.doi.org/10.1201/b16788]

[11]   Cole LK, Cole LK. Otoscopic evaluation of the ear canal. Vet Clin North Am Small Anim Pract 2004; 34(2): 397-410.
        [http://dx.doi.org/10.1016/j.cvsm.2003.10.004] [PMID: 15062615]

CHAPTER 7

Aural Haematoma and its Clinical Management

Ram Niwas[1,*], **Dinesh**[1] and **Sandeep Kumar**[1]

[1] *Department of Veterinary Surgery and Radiology, Lala Lajpat Rai University of Veterinary and Animal Sciences- Hisar, Haryana, India*

Abstract: Ear hematoma is collection of blood between skin and cartilage of ear, and it is one of common surgical condition. This occurs due to self-inflicted trauma or many other multiple reasons which leads to rupture of blood vessels and capillaries. Dog breeds with pendulous or heavy floppy ears are prone to ear hematoma. Both Surgical and non-surgical methods are adopted to treat this condition but surgical method have better treatment results as compare to later. Reoccurrence is one of the most common post operative complications irrespective of available treatment methods. However, control of inflammation, edema and drainage are important determinants for an effective treatment strategy.

Keywords: Cushing's disease, External ear, Hematoma, Hypothyroidism, Marshall putney's, Pendulous, S-shaped.

INTRODUCTION

An ear hematoma is also called an Ot, aural, or auricular hematoma. It is an abnormal accumulation of blood or serum and fibrin, usually between the cartilage and skin of the ear pinna [1]. More specifically, blood, serum, and fibrin clots are accumulated in between the cartilage and skin of the ear, usually involving the concave surface of the pinna, but less often may be present on the convex surface also [2]. It is one of the most common surgical conditions of the external ear [3]. Hematoma may appear as a focal, purplish, rounded, and hard area of swelling or may involve the whole surface of the pinna engorged with blood, leading to drooping of the affected pinna [2, 4, 5].

SURGICAL ANATOMY

The ear is composed of three parts: the internal, middle, and external ear. The internal ear consists of a bony labyrinth and a membranous labyrinth, which con-

---

*Corresponding author Ram Niwas: Department of Veterinary Surgery and Radiology, Lala Lajpat Rai University of Veterinary and Animal Sciences- Hisar, Haryana, India; E-mail: drsundariwal@luvas.edu.in

tain the cochlea, semicircular canals, and vestibule for hearing and balancing. The middle ear has ear ossicles, a tympanic membrane, and a tympanic cavity, which have connections with the pharynx *via* the eustachian tube (auditory tube). The external ear, which consists of the external acoustic meatus and pinna. Pinna again consists of skin, scutiform cartilage, annular cartilage, and auricular cartilage. Most aural hematomas occur in the auricular cartilage. The auricular cartilage is elastic in nature and is a thin, single-layered sheet that is pliable at the apex. On the convex side, the skin is relatively mobile, while on the concave side of the pinna, it is adherent to the cartilage tightly. The helix has medial and lateral borders, which are the free margins. Branches of the cranial auricular and the great posterior auricular arteries provide blood supply to the pinna. They provide branches to the margin of the auricle cartilage and pass through the foramina supplying the lateral surface. The venous drainage is provided by the maxillary vein [2].

ETIOLOGY

Generally, aural hematoma in dogs occurs due to self-inflicted trauma to the ear. Vigorous head shaking or scratching of the ear with paw causes rupture of blood vessels and capillaries, resulting in bleeding. The maxillary vein and the large posterior auricular artery are the main sources of the haemorrhage that arborizes over the pinna. This leads to the accumulation of blood and serosanguineous fluid in the space between skin and cartilage, leading to the formation of "haematoma". Due to this, the ear flap becomes initially soft and then thickens later on. The bleeding continues from the arteries until the pressure created by the accumulating blood equalizes with the pressure from the arteries themselves. Among other reasons, violent shaking of the head and pinna due to ear pain, otitis externa or media, neoplasia, hypersensitivity, and allergic dermatitis [6, 7]. In most allergic dermatitis cases, intradermal eosinophil and mast cell infiltrations have been described [8]. Water pouring in the ears during bathing can also result in violent head shaking, which can predispose the dog to hematoma formation. Parasites such as ear mites or ticks and foreign bodies (plant awns, grass seeds, or other debris) in or near the ear canal are also some predisposing factors for aural hematoma [9 - 12]. The association of otitis externa with aural hematoma and otodectic mange has been reported in most of the cases. Endocrine disorders such as hypothyroidism or Cushing's disease are also predisposing factors for hematoma. Hypothyroidism can lead to changes in the skin and coat quality due to which dogs may develop dry and itchy skin, which can contribute to ear scratching, while Cushing disease is associated with making the capillaries fragile, leading to early rupture and hematoma formation. In Cushing disease, the immune system of the dog is also compromised, which results in increased susceptibility to infection and irritation of the external ear canal. Some authors have proposed an immunological aetiology based on serological and immune histochemical examinations, which was supported by a successful response to corticosteroid therapy, but it is still a matter of debate and scientific validation [1, 13]. Certain haematological conditions, such as clotting disorders or immune-mediated thrombocytopenia, can increase the likelihood of spontaneous bleeding or poor clot formation. These underlying disorders can predispose dogs to ear hematomas. Although ear hematomas in dogs do not disturb other systemic functions.

BREED PREDISPOSITION AND OTHER RELATED FACTORS

Auricular hematoma is commonly associated with medium to large-sized canine breeds. Dog breeds with pendulous or heavy floppy ears, like the Cocker Spaniel, Labrador Retriever, Golden Retriever, German Shepherd, Basset Hound, Pit Bull, Boxer, and Spitz breeds, are more prone [14 - 16]. Dog breeds with long and droopy pinnas are more prone to bacterial infection as the droopy ear obscures the natural airing and drying of the ear canal. Droopy ears maintain darkness by blocking light, warmth, and a moist environment, which is suitable for yeast and bacterial infection. Middle to older-aged dogs are more likely to develop hematomas due to the association with cleavage of the cartilage plate because senility changes are associated with cartilage disruption that leads to hematoma [8, 17]. But sex-related predisposition associated with the occurrence of hematomas have not been recorded yet [15, 18, 19].

CLINICAL SIGNS AND DIAGNOSIS

The dog becomes restless and loses its pleasing looks due to pain. The dog frequently shakes his head and often scratches the affected ear. Clinical signs depend upon the duration of hematoma formation, the level of morphological changes in the ear, and the extent of the hematoma. Head tilting and circling towards the affected side are generally seen, which must be differentiated from otitis interna and media, encephalitis, and cerebellar ataxia. The diagnosis is based upon the history, clinical signs, symptoms, and clinical examination. On clinical examination, hematomas initially appear soft, fluctuating fluid-filled bulging mostly towards the concave side of the pinna, but gradually may become firmer and thicker due to fibrosis [2]. Confirmatory diagnosis of underlying otitis externa or media should be done with skull radiography in an appropriate radiographic view or by computed tomography. Other disease conditions like ear mites, hypersensitivity, Cushing's disease, and hypothyroidism must be considered to determine the aetiology of hematoma.

ANESTHETIC CONSIDERATION

The surgical procedure for the treatment of an aural hematoma is performed under general anaesthesia. After overnight fasting, a balanced anesthetic protocol should be followed to avoid any anesthetic emergencies. However, in this affection, systemic alterations in hemato-biochemical parameters are rarely observed. For conservative treatment, sedation might be necessary to keep the dog calm during the drainage process.

TREATMENT PROTOCOLS

The first concern before treating a hematoma is identifying and treating the root cause of irritation that stimulates the dog to scratch and shake his head violently. Always perform an otoscopic examination before starting the treatment to check for any foreign bodies or parasitic infestations. Both surgical and nonsurgical approaches have been described to treat this condition. But non-surgical procedures are either equal to or inferior to surgical procedures, depending on the size and site of hematoma formation. Early surgical intervention is necessary because, without treatment, the pinna is shrivelled and subsequent ossification of the cartilage mass causes continuous irritation. Shrivelling and scarring of the pinna may cause obstruction of the external auditory canal and thus induce chronic otitis externa [20]. Also, early treatment prevents permanent disfigurement of the ear pinna. If left untreated, fibrosis of the hematoma wall leads to folding and creasing of the cartilage, resulting in a permanent change in the contour and shape of the pinna. This curled-up appearance is termed as "Cauliflower ear" [21].

Non-surgical Procedure

Non-surgical methods are an alternative to surgical procedures. The most common conservative treatment is to relieve acute pain, and for this, fine needle aspiration is done. This procedure helps to relieve discomfort and pressure within the ear flap, but the chances of reoccurrence are very high. Fine needle aspiration in acute conditions with moderate swelling (less than 3cm) is an effective technique that may be performed with or without local infiltration of corticosteroids and antibiotics. Repeated aspiration and instillation of corticosteroids are more effective than single aspiration with pressure bandaging [17]. After hematoma drainage, a pressure bandage application around the ear helps minimize further accumulation of blood or fluid. The bandage should be snug but not too tight to impair circulation. It is important to monitor the bandage regularly for signs of excessive pressure or discomfort. Various types of cannulas, soft Penrose silicon drains, and other drains have been used to provide drainage for several weeks during the healing. Surgical treatment should be advocated after the organization of hematomas to prevent arterial bleeding postoperatively. To prevent the dog from scratching, after conservative or surgical treatment, an Elizabethan collar is usually recommended. This helps protect the ear and maintain the integrity of the bandage.

Surgical Procedure

The main objective of surgery is the drainage of hematomas, the removal of fibrin strands, and the promotion of granulation tissue formation that seals the skin incision. Irrespective of the surgical procedure adopted to treat it, failure to remove clots and fibrin strands inside the hematoma cavity results in contracture and subsequent disfigurement of the pinna even after surgery. All surgical procedures involve the incision of tissue overlying the hematoma, the removal of clotted blood and fibrin, the apposition of skin with sutures until a scar forms, recurrence prevention, and the retention of the normal anatomical appearance of the ear. A surgical procedure is preferred over conservative treatment if the hematoma is recurrent in nature or older than 7 days.

Various surgical techniques are available for the treatment of aural hematomas. These techniques include incisional drainage along with suturing of the concave and convex surface skin of the pinna together. After aseptic preparation of the pinna, an S-shaped or linear incision is made on the concave surface along the entire length of the hematoma (Figs. **1** and **2**). Before incision, the ear canal should be plugged with gauze to prevent the entry of blood into the auditory canal. The serosanguinous fluid, along with blood clots and fibrin strands, is drained out (Fig. **3**). The cartilage and internal lining of the integument are curetted and flushed with normal saline. The difference in various techniques lies in the methods of suturing to keep the inner and outer layers of the pinna in close approximation. Through and through, Horizontal interrupted mattress sutures with non-absorbable suture materials are applied parallel to the incision site without tension to obliterate the dead space. The first row of sutures is placed along the edges of the pinna, with each new row placed towards the skin incision. Knots are applied over the convex surface of the ear pinna (Fig. **4**). The staple technique using stainless steel sutures can be used for the obliteration of dead space created by hematoma; the use of staples again decreases the surgical time [22, 23]. However, metal staples induce severe inflammatory responses as compared to sutures [24].

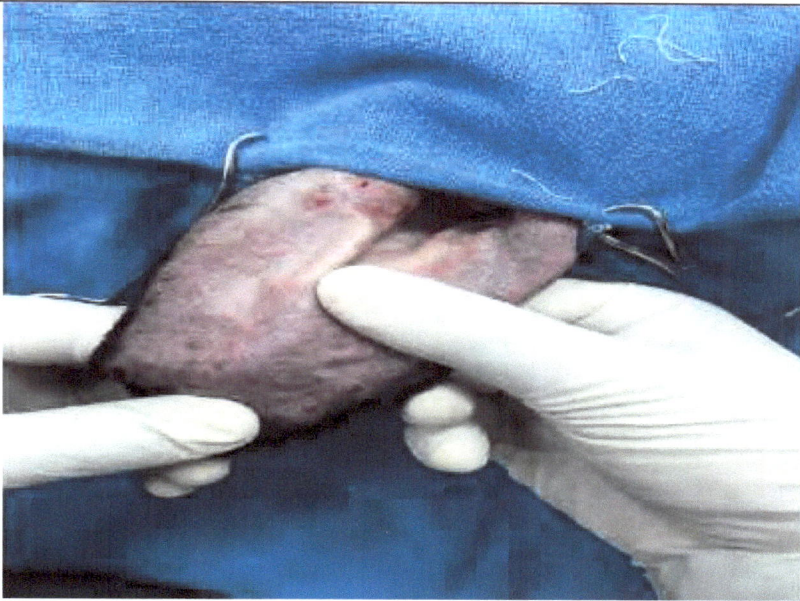

Fig. (1). Aseptic preparation and draping.

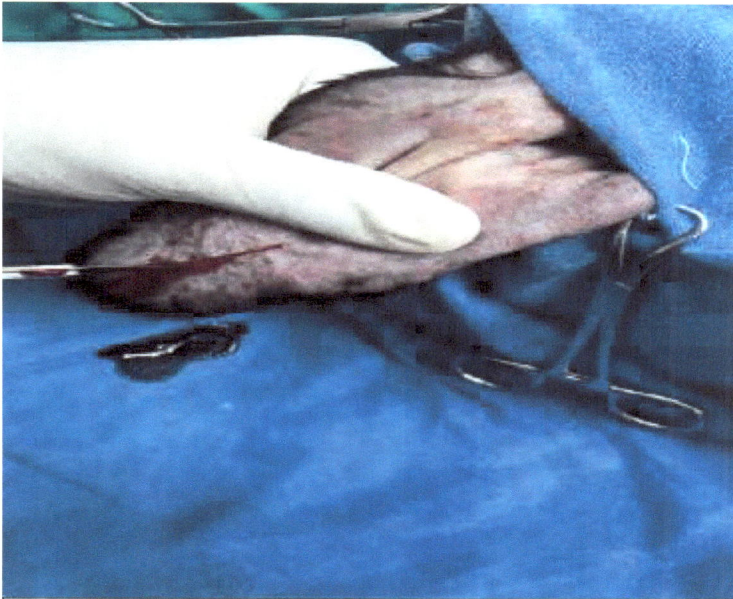

Fig. (2). Linear incision over hematoma.

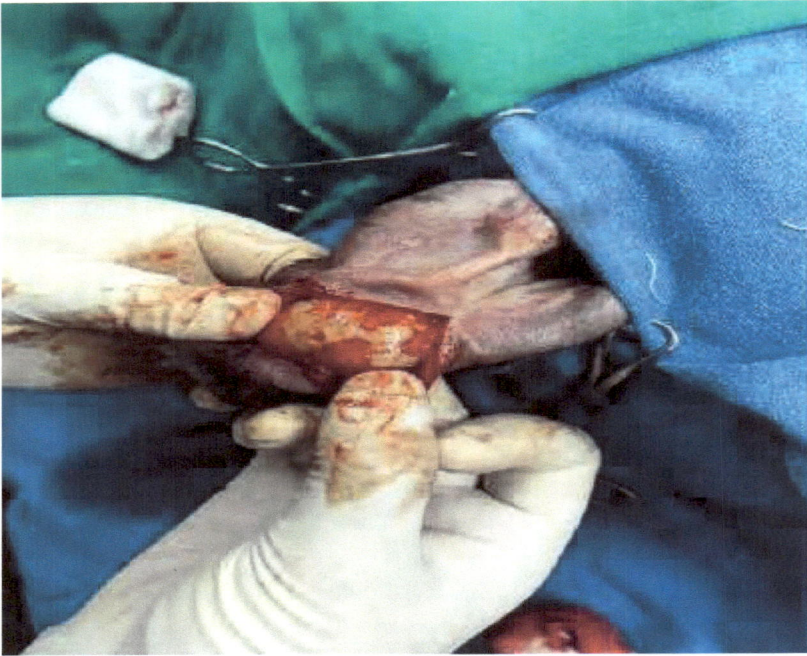

Fig. (3). Removal of sero-sanguinous fluid along with blood clots and fibrin.

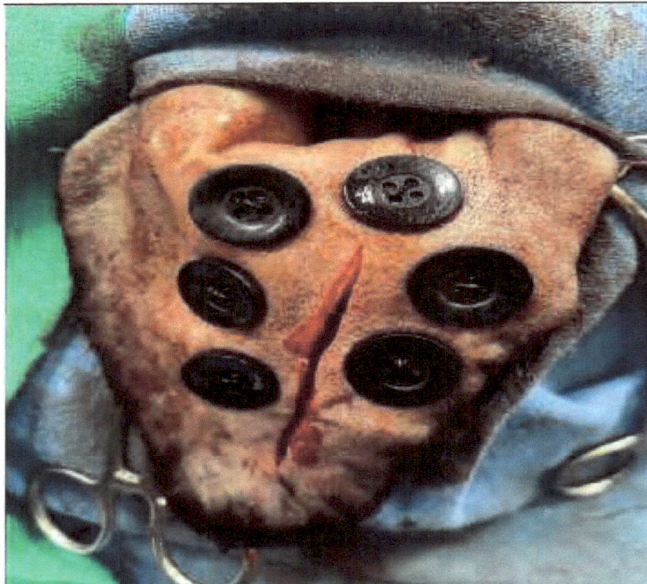

Fig. (4). Modified Marshall Putney's technique: Placement of sutures along with buttons on concave side of pinna.

In modified Marshall Putney's technique, or button suture technique, buttons are placed on both sides of the pinna during suturing, which leads to proper obliteration of dead space and, also prevents suture dehiscence (Fig. **5**). After suturing, a tight protective pressure bandage with an absorbent sterile gauge layer is applied over the ear, and the ear is placed on the dorsum of the head or neck. To prevent slipping of the bandage, adhesive tape is used to immobilise the ear pinna (Fig. **6**). Ear bandaging and antiseptic dressings should be done until suture removal. Healing in the pinna is slow, so sutures should be kept in place much longer than for other surgical wounds (typically four weeks or longer). Due to the length of time that the sutures must remain in place, non-absorbable suture materials without capillary action, like Polyamide or Nylon, are preferred over non absorbable Silk sutures.

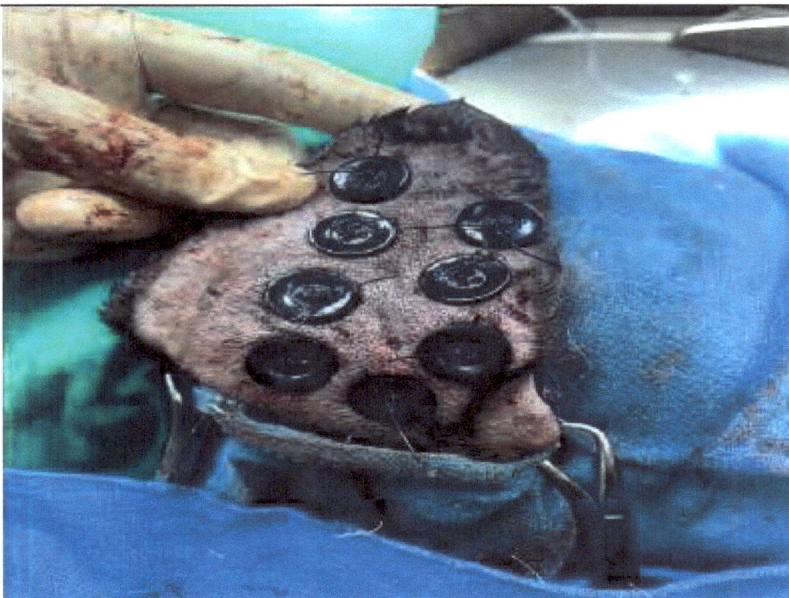

Fig. (5). Placement of sutures along with buttons on convex side of pinna.

Other surgical management involves a triangular-shaped incision made at the tip and base of the bulging, with subsequent drainage of hematoma, removal of fibrous adhesions, and passing of a flexible fenestrated sheath through the incisions [1, 15, 25]. In this technique, the fenestrated sheath is fixed by a stay suture with pinna for drainage. Lastly, the ear pinna is folded over a conical roll of sterile bandaging material kept on the concave side of the ear. The bandage is removed after 24 hours, and daily cleaning of the sheath using normal saline is recommended. The cavity should be infused with an antiseptic solution. In one of the suture-less techniques of repairing an aural hematoma, after incision and drainage, the pinna is fixed over the head with a cast of padding in between them. Hematomas can be treated with the minimum invasive technique of vacuum drainage through a lateral approach to the convex side of the pinna without compressive dressing [26]. The use of the carbon dioxide laser has also been reported for the treatment of aural hematomas. The laser is used to make multiple incisions in the hematoma to allow the evacuation of blood, and then multiple small incisions are made over the surface of the hematoma to stimulate adhesion formation. In this technique, sutures are not placed.

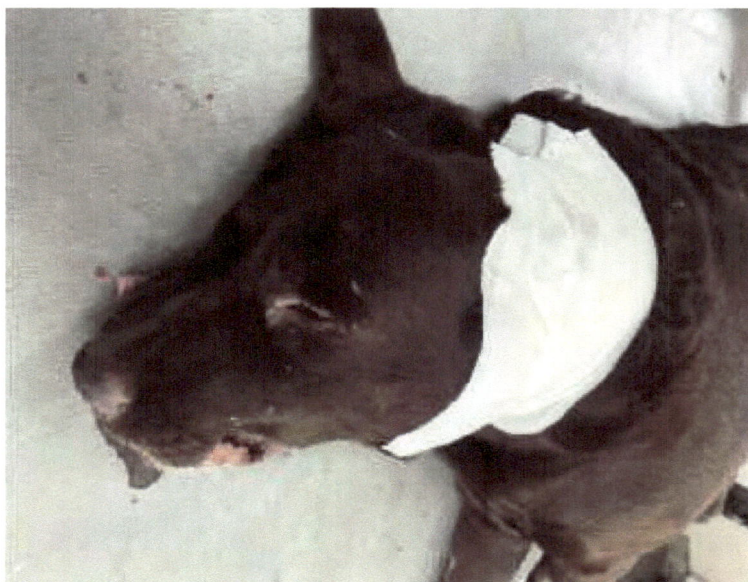

Fig. (6). Post operative dressing and bandaging.

COMPLICATIONS

Edema, discharge, inflammation, dehiscence and disturbances of the drainage sheath, pressure necrosis of the pinna, permanent scarring, and shrinkage are the main complications after surgical management [15, 27]. Abscess formation after use of local corticosteroid instillation during conservative treatment options is the most common complication reported [28]. Reoccurrence is one of the most common complications in both surgical and non-surgical treatment options [29, 30]. Partial erosions of auricular cartilage are the most consistent histopathological finding of the pinna surrounding the hematoma [13]. Control of edema, inflammation, and continuous drainage are important factors for an effective treatment strategy.

CONCLUSION

An aural hematoma, a blood-filled subcutaneous fluctuant swelling on the pinna formed when traumatic rupture of the capillaries and separation of the auricular cartilage and skin occurs. The prognosis for aural hematoma in dogs is good to excellent as long as the underlying etiological factors are addressed. Primary predisposing, and perpetuating factors are to be identified firstly for the detection/development of laural hematoma with a great resolution of the hematoma intervention. Always remembering to perform an otoscopic examination and otic cytology at initial presentation and at recheck examination will significantly aid in management of otitis.

REFERENCES

[1]   Kuwahara J. Canine and feline aural hematoma: clinical, experimental, and clinicopathologic observations. Am J Vet Res 1986; 47(10): 2300-8.
[PMID: 3490809]

[2]   Fossum TW. Aural hematoma and traumatic lesions of the pinna. In: Fossum TW, Ed. Small Animal Surgery. 4th ed. Mosby Elsevier Co 2007; pp. 307-12.

[3]   Ott RL. Ear in canine surgery, 2nd ed., Archibald, J., (eds). American Veterinary publications, Callifornia. 1974; 263-272.

[4]   Lanz OI, Wood BC. Surgery of the ear and pinna. Vet Clin North Am Small Anim Pract 2004; 34(2): 567-99.
[http://dx.doi.org/10.1016/j.cvsm.2003.10.011] [PMID: 15062625]

[5]   Brown C. Surgical management of canine aural hematoma. Lab Anim (NY) 2010; 39(4): 104-5.
[http://dx.doi.org/10.1038/laban0410-104] [PMID: 20305632]

[6]   Blättler U, Harlin O, Mattison RG, Rampelberg F. Fibrin sealant as a treatment for canine aural haematoma: A case history. Vet J 2007; 173(3): 697-700.
[http://dx.doi.org/10.1016/j.tvjl.2006.02.009] [PMID: 16624600]

[7]   Ahirwar V, Chandrapuria VP, Bhargava MK, Swamy M, Shahi A, Jawre S. A comparative study on the surgical management of canine aural haematoma. Indian J Vet Surg 2007; 28: 98-100.

[8]   Cynthia MK. Disease of the Pinna. The Merck Veterinary Manual. 9th ed. Merck Co. Inc 2005; c: 419-20.

[9]   Mayer K. The Ear in canine Surgery, 4th ed.. Santa Barbara American Veterinary Publications 1957; pp. 291-6.

[10]   Archibald J. Ears in canine surgery, 2nd ed.. Santa Barbara American Veterinary Publications 1974; pp. 263-90.

[11]   Slatter D. The pinna. T. B. of Small Animal Surgery 2nd ed.. Philadelphia: W.B. Saunder 1993; pp. 1545-l549.

[12]   Henderson RA, Horne R. Pinna. Slatter Douglas, Textbook of small animal surgery. 3rd ed.. Philadelphia: Saunders W.B. Publishers 2003; pp. 1737-41.

[13]   Joyce JA, Day MJ. Immunopathogenesis of canine aural haematoma. J Small Anim Pract 1997; 38(4): 152-8.
[http://dx.doi.org/10.1111/j.1748-5827.1997.tb03453.x] [PMID: 9127283]

[14]   Judith J. Canine aural Haematoma. Wattnam Focus 2000; 10: 4.

[15] Hassan AZ, Yila AS, Adeyanju JB, Hassan FB, Adawa DAY, Jahun BM. Aural haematoma in dogs: a review of 55 cases. Niger J Surg Res 2002; 4(1): 50-6.
[http://dx.doi.org/10.4314/njsr.v4i1.12169]

[16] Győrffy A, Szijártó A. A new operative technique for aural haematoma in dogs: A retrospective clinical study. Acta Vet Hung 2014; 62(3): 340-7.
[http://dx.doi.org/10.1556/avet.2014.016] [PMID: 25038951]

[17] Mikawa K, Itoh T, Ishikawa K, Kushima K, Uchida K, Shii H. Epidemiological and etiological studies on 59 aural hematomas in 49 dogs. Nihon Jui Masui Gekagaku Zasshi 2005; 36(4): 87-91.
[http://dx.doi.org/10.2327/jvas.36.87]

[18] Mohsin AJF. Surgical treatment of ear haematoma in dogs. Bas. J Vet Res (Pulawy) 2010; 9: 65-70.

[19] Feyisa A, Regassa F, Abebe F. Aural hematoma in dog: Surgical drainage followed by loose interrupted vertical mattress stitch. Int. J Case. Rep Clin Image 2020; 2: 128.

[20] Sherding RG. Diseases & Surgery of ear. 1994.

[21] Medleau L, Hnilica KA. Small animal dermatology: A color atlas and therapeutic guide. 2nd ed.. Philadelphia: Saunders W.B. Publishers 2006.

[22] Mattoo S, Mohindroo J, Sangwan V. Modified use of stainless-steel skin staplers for treatment of ear haematoma in dogs. XXXI Annual congress of Indian society for Veterinary Surgery and National symposium patients. 49-50.

[23] Manisha ND, Dhakate MS, Upadhye SV, Kamble M, Akhare SB. Comparative evaluation of surgical techniques for management of aural haematoma's in canine. Intas Polivet 2016; 17: 258-9.

[24] Fick JL, Novo RE, Kirchhof N. Comparison of gross and histologic tissue responses of skin incisions closed by use of absorbable subcuticular staples, cutaneous metal staples, and polyglactin 910 suture in pigs. Am J Vet Res 2005; 66(11): 1975-84.
[http://dx.doi.org/10.2460/ajvr.2005.66.1975] [PMID: 16334959]

[25] Giles WC, Iverson KC, King JD, Hill FC, Woody EA, Bouknight AL. Incision and drainage followed by mattress suture repair of auricular hematoma. Laryngoscope 2007; 117(12): 2097-9.
[http://dx.doi.org/10.1097/MLG.0b013e318145386c] [PMID: 17921905]

[26] Lahiani J, Niebauer GW. On the nature of canine aural haematoma and its treatment with continuous vacuum drainage. J Small Anim Pract 2020; 61(3): 195-201.
[http://dx.doi.org/10.1111/jsap.13107] [PMID: 31975442]

[27] Balagoplan TP, Arul Jothi N, Rameshkumar B. Needle aspiration and drain tube techniques for management of aural haematoma in dogs. Indian Vet J 2013; 90: 26-7.

[28] Seibert R, Tobias KM. Surgical treatment for aural haematoma. North American Veterinary Conference Clinicians Brief. 29-32.

[29] Joyce JA. Treatment of canine aural haernatorna using an indwelling drain and corticosteroids. J Small Anim Pract 1994; 35(7): 341-4.
[http://dx.doi.org/10.1111/j.1748-5827.1994.tb01711.x]

[30] Hall J, Weir S, Ladlow J. Treatment of canine aural haematoma by UK veterinarians. J Small Anim Pract 2016; 57(7): 360-4.
[http://dx.doi.org/10.1111/jsap.12524] [PMID: 27385623]

CHAPTER 8

Traumatic Injuries and its Clinical Management

Apoorva Mishra[1,*], Apra Shahi[1], Randhir Singh[1] and **Diva Dhingra[1]**

[1] *Department of Veterinary Surgery and Radiology, College of Veterinary Science and A.H., N.D.V.S.U, Jabalpur (M.P.), India*

Abstract: Traumatic ear injuries in dogs are relatively common due to their propensity to play, fight, scratch, and explore. Trauma to the ears can result from an external source or it could also be self-inflicted. Ear injuries can happen as a result of vehicular accidents, dog bites, ear burns, exposure to cold temperatures, faulty ear cropping techniques, and sharp objects. Mite and tick infestation, insect bite dermatitis, food allergies, and fly bites lead to intense pruritus and discomfort. Intense itching associated with such conditions can lead to excessive scratching and head shaking-associated traumas. Such trauma can lead to conditions like an aural hematoma, ear lacerations, broken ear cartilages, separation of auricular and annular cartilages, avulsion injuries, ear tip injuries, fractures of the tympanic bulla, tympanic membrane rupture *etc.* Medicinal treatment helps in management of ear infections but surgical intervention is required to deal with traumatic injuries.

Keywords: Aural hematomas, Avulsion injuries, Accidents, Broken cartilages, Bulla fracture, Ear burn, Frostbite, Lacerations, Tympanic membrane rupture.

INTRODUCTION

Trauma to the pinna is frequent in dogs. It can occur as a result of various accidents or incidents which may range from mild to severe. Traumatic injuries include hematomas, lacerations, burns, frostbite, fractures, torn ear tips, otitis externa. When trauma is left untreated, as might occur in some cases, it may lead to complications. Though with critical care and suitable treatment, most dogs recover fully. Head shaking leads to more pinnal trauma than fighting. Fight wounds may cause tearing of pinna, often with profuse bleeding. Trauma to pinna, particularly to the periphery may also be caused by Otodectic mange, otic foreign bodies, otitis media and facial pruritus.

---

[*] **Corresponding author Apoorva Mishra:** Department of Veterinary Surgery and Radiology, College of Veterinary Science and A.H., N.D.V.S.U, Jabalpur (M.P.), India; E-mail: mishra.ap07@gmail.com

Aural Hematoma

Aural hematoma most commonly occurs as a result of traumatic injury of ear in dogs [1]. Inflicted trauma from the ipsilateral rear foot or from vigorous head shaking due to underlying otitis externa may be there. Trauma may also result from ectoparasite infestations, allergy, and otic foreign bodies [2]. Otitis externa is not often associated with aural hematoma [3]. Lesion develops at the base of concave aspect of the ear initially which progresses towards the apex causing acute pain and discomfort to the dog. Aural hematomas present as warm, tense, rounded, occasionally bluish-purple fluid filled lesions and require surgical intervention. Surgical preparation of pinna is followed by a single, straight incision along the long axis of the ear. Drainage of the cavity is done, fibrin is curetted out, and then sterile saline is used for further flushing of the cavity. Longitudinal placement of full-thickness sutures minimizes the risk of blood vessel damage. Sutures are removed after a period of 2-3 weeks. Inadequate post-operative management of pain leads to violent head shaking and self-inflicted trauma which results in hemorrhage (Figs. **1a, b, & c**).

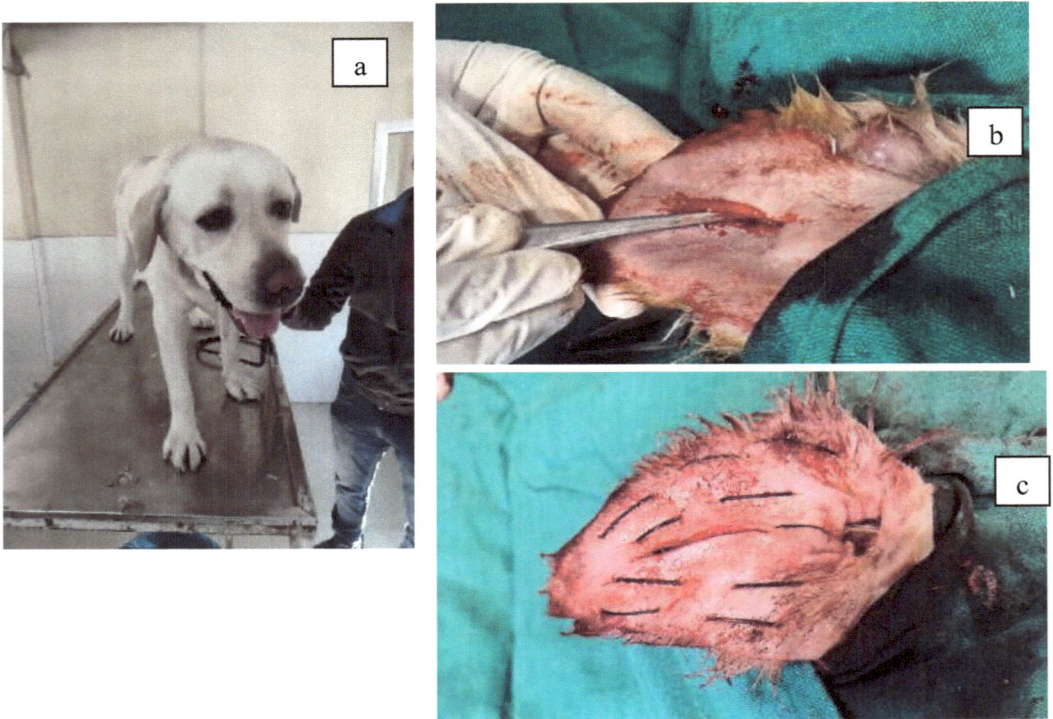

Figs. (1a, b, & c). Typical appearance of an aural hematoma, its operative procedure including curation and placement of horizontal mattress sutures.

Ear Laceration

Ear laceration may occur as a result of fighting or other trauma associated with sharp objects and invariably results in wound infection. Such wounds may involve only one skin surface and are superficial while others may perforate cartilage involving both skin surfaces. They may have more aesthetic appearance when sutures are placed or maybe left to heal by secondary intention. Cleaning, debridement, tissue apposition, protection, and prevention of secondary infection are the general principles of treatment [4]. Conservative treatment by simply clipping and cleaning can be done for small lacerated wounds. Small lacerations are managed by the use of adhesive, hydroactive dressings. Although in an ideal circumstances, where general anesthesia is not indicated, not much efficient can be achieved with careful surgical apposition and suturing. 1 cm overlap of margin should at least be there when dressing is cut to shape and applied over clean dried wound. Gentle handling of the dressing for few minutes should be done until it gets adhered. These dressings are considered to be advantageous since they are light weighted and are also tolerated well by the patient. Also, epithelialization is encouraged as there is suppression of bacterial infection, if any. When hydro active dressings breaks down, there is often presence of a discharge beneath them. Gentle peeling off the remains of these dressings after a period of two weeks is recommended. Large lacerations require early surgical intervention [4]. Surgical preparation and careful debridement of pinna is done and first sutures are placed at margins of the pinna ensuring better alignment. Closure of full-thickness lacerations is done either with rows of simple interrupted sutures on both aspects or with simple interrupted sutures on one face and vertical mattress sutures on the other face (Fig. **2**).

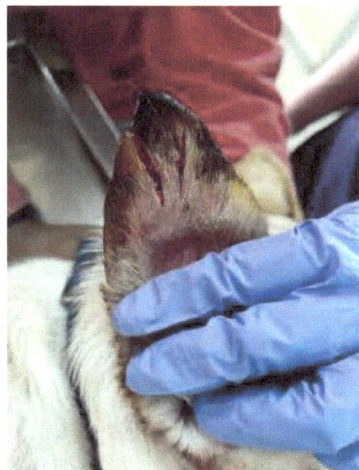

Fig. (2). Ear laceration in dog.

Foreign Body

Plant material (*e.g.,* grass seeds, foxtails) can work their way deep into the ear canal, causing pain, inflammation, and infection. Foxtails, in particular, can be quite dangerous due to their barbed structure. While playing or digging, a dog may get dirt or sand in its ears which can cause irritation and, if not removed, potential infection. Especially in puppies, tiny toys or parts of toys when lodged in the ear can sometimes end up causing trauma. Various other objects, such as small pieces of trash or household items or splinters or burrs, can potentially get stuck in a dog's ear, particularly if they're curious and like to rummage. Lodgement of foreign body in the ear causes irritation, pain, head shaking and ear scratching at or near the ear. Also, violent head shaking and scratching are common clinical signs of parasitic infection and acute bacterial infection. This leads to self-inflicted trauma which progresses to ear canal inflammation or infection (otitis externa) requiring prompt veterinary attention. Dogs that have long, pendulous ears (*e.g.,* Basset Hounds, Spaniels) and those with abundant hair present in the ear canal (*e.g.,* Poodles) are more susceptible to developing this condition. German Shephards are most frequently affected breed of dogs among erect-eared. When medical management of the condition fails or when cases involve stenotic ear canals due to proliferative growth, surgical intervention is considered. When cases do not have middle ear involvement, a lateral ear canal resection or a vertical ear canal ablation or a TECA can be performed. In order to avoid contamination as well as trauma to the site of operation, proper bandaging of the ear is advocated. Excessive head shaking, pawing or scratching at the bandage site is often seen. Post-operative complications include persistent infection (dissecting cellulitis, prolonged wound drainage, periauricular abscess formation), nystagmus, head tilt, postural abnormalities, and loss of hearing (Fig. **3**). The patient should be closely monitored post-operatively and usage of an Elizabethan collar is highly recommended.

Otitis

Otitis media typically develops from otitis externa that extends through the tympanum [5]. One-sided otitis media has several specific causes, including foreign body penetration into the tympanum, the presence of inflammatory polyps, and neoplasms like squamous cell carcinomas and fibromas [6]. Along with other clinical indications including ataxia, head tilt, nystagmus, Horner's syndrome, or facial nerve paralysis, there may be a strong head shaking that could injure the ear [7, 8]. A lateral ear canal resection with a ventral bulla osteotomy and a lateral bulla osteotomy, or a TECA with a lateral bulla osteotomy, can be done in cases where otitis externa is present concurrently. The purpose of treatment for these individuals is alleviation of otitis externa with establishment of drainage and flushing of the bulla. While cases without any evidence of otitis externa, a ventral bulla osteotomy is preferred [9].

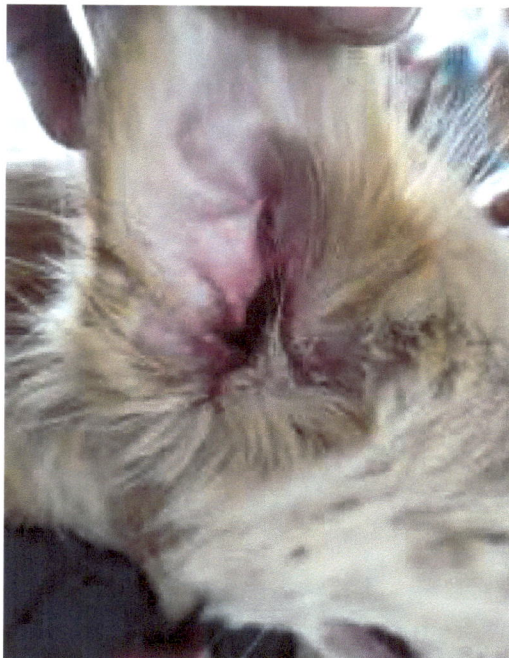

Fig. (3). Otitis externa with erythema in a dog with history of allergy due to wild grass.

Otodectes cynotis mites in dogs, which are a common cause of otitis externa, are usually seen in the horizontal and vertical canals of ear. Vigorous head shaking and constant ear scratching are common clinical signs that cause traumatic injuries. Ear drooping and pruritus may also be present. Severe cases show suppurative otitis externa and possible perforation of the tympanic membrane with accumulation of dark brown cerumen in ear. Application of a suitable ceruminolytic agent for ear cleansing is recommended along with any therapy. Outer ear may also be affected by another parasitic mite *Sarcoptes scabiei* that burrows into the top layers of skin and forms small, red, round bumps on the skin initially. These later become irritated open sores on outer edges of ear. Clinical signs such as head shaking and ear scratching put stress to the ear resulting in trauma. Dips, injections, spot-on and oral medications are useful treatment options. The dog's environment including the bedding, brushes and other objects need to be thoroughly cleaned as these mites can survive off the host for a considerable amount of time. Arthropod bite pinnal dermatitis occurs either through direct damage from an arthropod bite or as a result of a hypersensitivity reaction. Ticks are commonly found on the pinna or in the ear canal that cause severe irritation at the site of their attachment. A soft-shelled tick, *Otobius megnini*, also known as the spinous ear tick is known to parasitize the external ear canal of dogs. Vigorous and constant head rubbing and shaking leads to traumatic injuries to the ear. Treatment options are mechanical removal and use of acaricides (Fig. **4**).

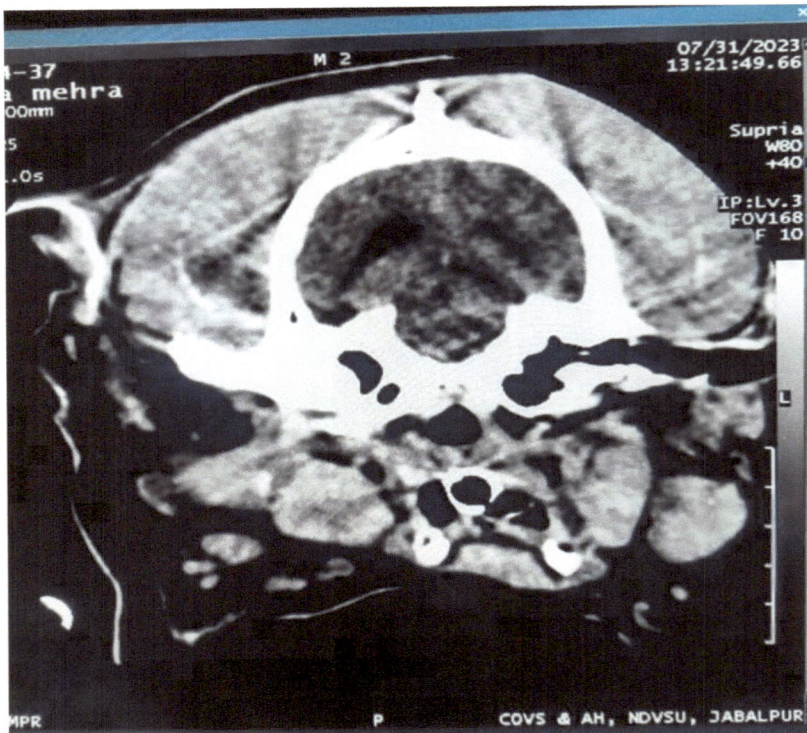

Fig. (4). Computed Tomographic image of ossified right ear canal of dog in case of chronic otitis media.

Frostbite

Frostbite occurs when the body's tissues freeze, which can happen when a dog is exposed to very low temperatures for a prolonged period. It's a serious condition, and the extremities, like the ears, are most susceptible due to their distance from the core of the body. Dogs that are poorly adapted to cold climates, breeds with floppy ears, very young animals and those that are undernourished are more susceptible. This condition is most commonly seen in wet or windy weather mainly affecting poorly insulated body regions such as ear tips. There may be temporary chilling of tissues or there may be necrosis and freezing of some portion of tissue which depends upon the degree of severity of frostbite. In mild cases, the ear appears pale initially and might also be bloodless. Intense redness, acute pain, heat and swelling follows thereafter. Falling off of the hair, with peeling off of the epidermis, may also be noticed. Whereas in severe cases of frost bite, the affected portion becomes swollen and painful, which later undergoes necrosis. There appears to be a demarcating line between healthy tissues and any necrosed area. A raw surface is left after the dead skin is sloughed off. There may also be occurrence of blisters or skin ulcers few days after the freezing event happens. Rapid, gentle warming and supportive care are treatment options. The affected area is warmed using lukewarm water (not hot). Use of direct heat like a heating pad should be avoided, as this can cause burns, especially when the skin can't feel the heat. Massaging or rubbing the frostbitten area should also be refrained from, as this can cause more damage. Once the tissue has been thawed out, refreezing should be avoided as it leads to more trauma to the ear. Mild antiseptics are recommended for use over such lesions. Turpentine, ammonia and chloroform preparation having one part each in six parts of a bland oily base is applied over the lesion. Amputation of the affected part may be required in severe cases when such frostbitten tissue becomes necrotic and there is shedding of the tips of the outer ears.

Broken Ear Cartilage

Sometimes there may be loss of integrity of the ear cartilage in dogs. Minor injuries resulting from play or accidents is one of the most important cause of a broken ear cartilage. Puppies are more susceptible to suffer from minor ear injuries. Ear mites and ticks do not directly harm the ear cartilage but cause severe discomfort and irritation. In an attempt to get relief from pain, this leads to continuous pawing and scratching by the dog which might cause damage to the cartilage. Another cause of a broken ear cartilage is excruciating pain from chronic ear infections which makes the dog scratch to extreme extent. Moreover, dogs with floppy ears tend to have naturally weak and flexible cartilage that makes them predisposed to suffering from a broken ear cartilage. While breeds of dogs which have a rigid ear cartilage (*e.g.,* German Shephard) also tend to have more prominent injuries from broken cartilages. Healthy cartilage formation in dogs require nutrients like magnesium, sulfur and collagen in adequate amounts. Deprivation of such nutrients, particularly in the early formative stages, leads to weaker cartilage and higher chances of ear injury. Severely irritated and itchy skin due to skin infections compels the dog to scratch incessantly which again leads to cartilage damage. Lastly, an improper ear cleaning technique opted by an inexperienced professional or an ignorant owner may lead to severe trauma and a broken cartilage. Broken ear cartilages are not much of an issue but harm the aesthetic appearance of the dog which may be of some concern to the owner. Although dogs with floppy ears tend to suffer from some hearing loss due to the shape of their ears. Treatment must be done for the underlying cause before proceeding for repair of broken cartilage. This is followed by placement of sutures to reattach the cartilage. Surgical intervention restores the original hearing abilities and aesthetic appearance of the dog but fails to restore the normal mobility of the ear.

Tympanic Membrane Rupture

The tympanic membrane or eardrum is a thin membrane separating the outer ear canal from the middle and inner ear. It is responsible for the transmission of sound from the environment to the middle ear bones, progressing to the labyrinth. Tympanic membrane rupture may also occur as a result of trauma since it is extremely delicate and easily gets damaged during cleaning of ear or any ear disease. A dog's ability to hearing is significantly impaired due to an infection or perforation that compromises the integrity and structure of the tympanic membrane. Perforation of the ruptured eardrum results into entry of tears, bacteria or fungi. This progresses to otitis media or the infection of the middle ear. Thick and pus like or bloody discharge from ear, sudden hearing loss, red and inflamed ear canal, pain on touching the ear, and head tilt are commonly observed clinical signs of a ruptured eardrum. Otoscopy can be performed after gentle flushing of the ear canal to remove the debris in order to diagnose a perforated eardrum. Other diagnostic tests such as a CT scan may also be used for an eardrum rupture and possible infection of the inner ear. A thorough ear flushing is advised in mild cases but surgical intervention may be needed in severe, irreparable changes of the outer ear. Healing occurs in most cases without any significant complications with ruptured eardrums being healed in less than three to five weeks without undergoing any surgical procedure. Oral medications for up to four to six weeks, frequent examinations and follow-up care are mandatory to ensure proper healing of the eardrum.

Injury to Ear Tip

Dogs with long, floppy ears are susceptible to tearing or injury to the ear tips, which may bleed and require medical attention. An ear infection that induces a dog to shake the head vigorously causes a tear on the ear or may form a blood blister. Ear tip injuries are difficult to heal as dogs constantly move around and the scabs easily come off when there is shaking of the head. This disrupts the healing process making such ear injuries more prone to trauma. Keeping the ear tips clean, dry and immobile with the help of wrap around bandages serves the purpose of healing.

Auricular Avulsion Injuries

Traumatic separation of all or a part of the ear causes damage to the auricular blood vessels [10]. Auricular avulsion injuries most commonly results from motor vehicle accidents, falls and incidents of assault [11, 12]. Management of such injuries becomes complex and difficult owing to the delicate auricular skin, intricate vasculature and cartilaginous boundaries. The unique ear positioning on either side of the head and their outward projection make them more vulnerable to trauma. Composite graft method for reattachment is mostly beneficial for smaller segments and have more chances of survival. This also generates good aesthetic results. Segments larger than one-third the size of the ear generally have a poor outcome because they undergo necrosis leaving large residual defect [13]. For a successful microvascular repair, identification and tagging of suitable arteries under the bench microdissection method is done. Vein grafts helps in simplification of microsurgical access and prevention of anastomotic tension in order to allow resection of damaged blood vessels. Under ideal conditions, the avulsed segment is anastomosed with the vein grafts. This is followed by reattachment of ear segment and arterial anastomosis [14]. In the Baudet method, a posturicular flap is created after excision of the posterior skin from the severed part. Large fenestrations are created by the perforation of the cartilage of the amputed ear [15]. Tissue survival is improved by this technique as contact between the graft and underlying vascular bed is allowed by such perforations. Suturing of the amputed part to the anterior stump of the ear and postauricular flap helps in reattachment followed by elevation of the ear with application of a full thickness skin graft [16, 17]. Major complication associated with microvascular repair of the ear is venous congestion. This can be managed with leech therapy or the surgical perforation of the reattached segment [18-22]. Another "sandwich" technique is employed where an auricular cartilage of an avulsed ear segment is inserted under a thin platysma muscle. Vascularization of the cartilage from both the anterior and posterior surfaces makes this Platysma myocutaneous flap method advantageous [23]. The TPF (Temporo Parietal Fascia) flap method is demonstrated useful in the repair of congenital deformities of the ear and provides vascular support for the repair of traumatically avulsed auricles. The method involves degloving the skin of the amputed ear, suturing of the amputed part to its original position, application of a TPF flap and covering the area with a full thickness skin graft [24 - 26]. Pocket principle involves minimal debridement of the skin edges with dermabrasion of the skin of the avulsed segment. Creation of a subcutaneous postauricular pocket is done followed by reattachment of the ear. This reattached portion of the ear is inserted into the pocket [27]. Microvascular repair and composite graft reattachment are considered best treatment options for an auricular avulsion repair. Other repair techniques such as the Baudet method, the pocket principle, and the techniques that involve periauricular skin flaps and TPF flaps should not be considered for management of auricular avulsion injuries in acute cases. TPF flap method causes cartilage resorption and fibrosis which leads to shrinkage and distortion of the ear.

The avulsed ear segment is often denuded of skin with the remaining cartilage being placed under post auricular skin. This practice reaps poor outcome and should strictly be discouraged as the ear cartilage becomes unusable and has difficulty withstanding the forces of contraction that occur following the secondary reconstruction. In pocket principle method, there is loss of cartilage stability and complexity [28].

Fly Bites and Maggot Wounds

Dogs, especially those with floppy ears or those who spend a lot of time outside, are most commonly afflicted by fly bites. Flies are attracted to ears because they often have small amounts of moisture and minor wounds, making them an appealing site for feeding and breeding. Unclean kennel areas exacerbate the problem. Sometimes an underlying ear infection or another condition can make the ears more attractive to flies. Clinical signs include red and inflamed patches which are often round and can be found especially on the tips and edges of the ears, bleeding or scabbing as repeated biting can cause the skin to break, incessant ear scratching and head shaking as the bites can be very itchy, dark crusts which might form from dried blood or scabs and presence of flies in their fur. Over abundance of flies may also lead to secondary infection. The bitten areas are gently cleaned with a mild antiseptic solution or saline which helps to reduce the risk of infection. There are topical ointments specifically designed to help soothe and heal fly bites on dogs that often contain ingredients that repel flies and prevent further bites. Application of a pet-safe fly repellent should be considered to deter the flies. When treatment is delayed, it may lead to a maggot-infested wound which may cause severe tissue damage. Visible white or yellowish larvae are seen moving within the wound which emanates a foul odor, there is presence of fluid discharge, and swelling around the affected area. The dog may be in obvious distress, constantly shaking its head, or scratching at the wound. The wound area is gently cleaned with saline solution for an easy visibility and accessibility of the maggots. Forceps are used to pick out as many maggots as possible because it's essential to remove all of them, as leaving even a few behind can lead to continued tissue destruction and infection. After manual removal of maggots present superficially, a chloroform, turpentine or camphor-in-oil dipped gauze is left inside the wound for a period of 24 hours (Fig. **5a & b**). The majority of the maggots have been killed by the time the gauze piece is removed. The wound has to be treated like an open wound thereafter. Application of fly repellants such as neem oil is advised. Loraxane ICI having the composition of insecticide loraxane and proflavin as an antiseptic can be used. Fresh Annona leaves which are a good fly repellant and antiseptic can also be tried by grinding it well followed by its application over the wound area.

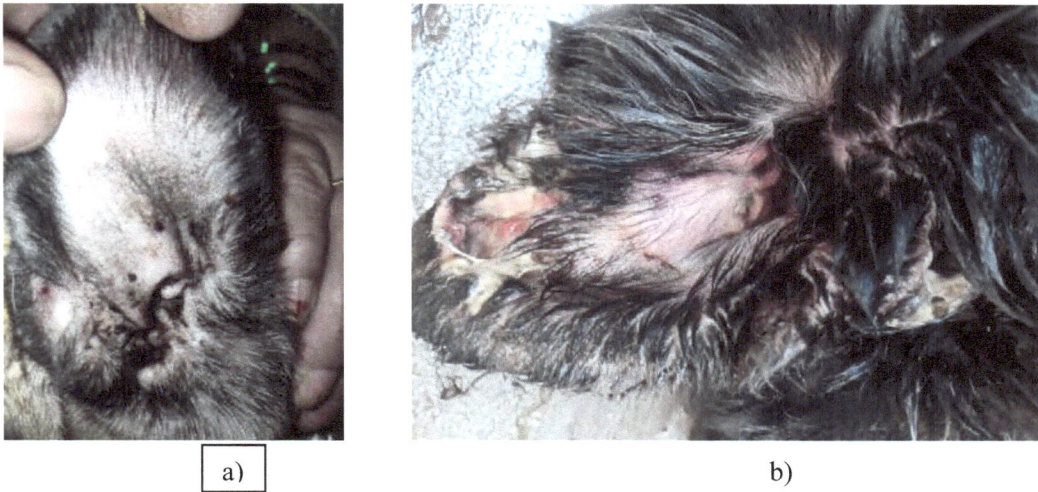

a)   b)

Fig. (5). Distribution of skin lesions on the ear pinna in dogs with tick infestation in semi-erected ears (**a**) and maggot wound due to flies in pendulous ears (**b**).

Separation of traumatic and annular cartilage

The ear of a dog is a complex structure comprising of skin, cartilage, blood vessels, and connective tissues. The auricular and annular cartilages are parts of the external ear and play a role in its shape and flexibility. A traumatic separation between these cartilages can be a significant concern, although rare, for dogs and requires prompt veterinary attention. Direct physical trauma, such as being hit by a car, a fall, or an altercation with another animal, can lead to a separation of the auricular and annular cartilages. Dogs that are dealing with ear infections or infestations might scratch their ears violently, leading to such injuries. Playing roughly with other dogs or humans can result in unintentional injuries. Improper handling which is seen especially in grooming sessions where aggressive handling or pulling of the ear might occur. Symptoms include an altered shape of the ear. A significant change in the shape or position of the ear is often the first sign. The dog might show signs of pain, like whining or being sensitive to touch. The injured area may become swollen or red. The ear might not move or flex as it usually does. Sometimes, there might be a crackling sound when the ear is touched, indicating air or fluid between the layers. A thorough physical examination needs to be conducted, with gentle palpation of the ear to ascertain the extent of the separation. Radiographs or ultrasound may be necessary to visualize the separation and check for any associated injuries. In some cases, surgical intervention, that is, TECA and lateral bulla osteotomy or vertical canal ablation might be necessary to realign the separated cartilages and ensure proper healing. The dog should be prevented from scratching the ear, and activities should be limited during the recovery phase. For many dogs, traumatic separation of the auricular and annular cartilages, if addressed promptly, may not have long-term implications. However, in some cases, it's important to consider the potential for recurrence, especially in dogs that have experienced severe trauma. Such dogs may need to be closely monitored, especially during activities that might strain the ear. Post-surgical healing might lead to scar tissue formation. While generally harmless, scar tissue may alter the appearance or flexibility of the ear.

The ear is a significant sensory organ for dogs, and injuries might make them more sensitive to sounds or touch. Some dogs might react more strongly to loud noises or avoid situations where their ears might be touched. When a dog exhibits symptoms of discomfort or pain in the ear, it can be quite distressing for both the pet and the owner.

Ear Burn

Just as humans can get sunburned, dogs too can suffer from burns on areas that are exposed, including their ears. Causes of ear burn in dogs are prolonged exposure to the sun especially in dogs with white or light-colored coats, hairless breeds, or breeds with thin fur on the ears; harsh chemicals found in certain grooming products or household cleaners can cause chemical burns if they come in contact with the dog's ears; contact with hot objects. Symptoms of ear burn include redness which is the most obvious sign, and can be quite pronounced in lighter-skinned breeds; the ear may become swollen or appear thicker than usual; in severe cases, the skin might start peeling or flaking off; the ear might feel warm to the touch, indicative of inflammation, the dog might scratch its ears frequently, whine, or shake its head; in the worst cases, blisters might form which can be painful and, if broken, can lead to infections. If an ear burn is suspected, the first step is to remove the causative agent from the environment. If sun exposure is the culprit, the dog is brought into a shaded area. Application of Aloe vera can soothe and heal sunburned skin. If a chemical is the cause, it may be neutralized by a suitable acid or alkaline solution. When burns are due to some acidic chemical, then alkalies such as sodium bicarbonate and soap solution are recommended. Use of acidic solutions is recommended when burns result from an alkaline chemical. Washing of the burn wound with plenty of plain water can also be resorted to, if suitable acid or alkaline solutions are not available. If the burn is due to exposure of some hot object and is recent, cool (not cold) water should be used to gently rinse the area for several minutes. Direct application of ice is not recommended. Also, indiscriminate ointment usage should be avoided as some substances can trap heat or cause further irritation. If left untreated or not addressed promptly, ear burns in dogs can lead to further complications such as secondary infections where broken skin or blisters provide an entry point for bacteria. Infected ears may ooze pus, exude a foul odor, or show increased redness. There may be chronic ear inflammation as repeated burns can cause the ear tissue to become chronically inflamed, leading to persistent discomfort and potential hearing impairment. Persistent pain and discomfort might cause behavioral changes as they may become more irritable, less active, or show signs of depression. Severe or recurrent burns can result in scar tissue formation, which may alter the appearance of the ear or affect its flexibility. Burnt skin of the ear being highly sensitive should not be touched or scratched as it might introduce bacteria and cause delay in the wound healing process. This necessitates the use of an Elizabethan collar.

Dog Bites

Dog bites can be painful and can lead to infections, and when it comes to the ears, which have a significant blood supply, they can bleed profusely. When a dog suffers a bite on its ear, whether during play or due to aggression, it's essential to address it promptly to prevent complications. Plenty of soap and water should be used for washing the wound properly. Alcohol or hydrogen peroxide are not directly used as they can be too harsh and cause further trauma. Also, the use of carbolic acid for cauterization is unnecessary. A clean cloth to be applied with gentle pressure to achieve hemostasis. The depth and severity of the bite wound are to be assessed. The dog might want to scratch or shake its head, which can interfere with wound healing. Swelling, excessive redness, discharge, foul odor, or increased pain might be indicative of a secondary bacterial infection. There is chance of contracting rabies following a dog bite if bitten by a rabid animal. Wherever possible, the dog should be kept under vigilant observation for a period of ten days to rule out any possibility of rabies.

Ear Cropping or Ear Trimming or Cosmetic Otoplasty

It is a controversial surgical procedure that involves removing a portion of a dog's ears to make them stand erect. The procedure is otherwise indicated when there is any irreparable injury or gangrene present. While traditionally done for certain breeds such as Affenpinscher, American Staffordshire Terrier, Boston Terrier, Bouvier des Flandres, Boxer, Briard, Brussels Griffon, Doberman Pinscher, German Pinscher, Giant Schnauzer, Great Dane, Manchester Terrier, Miniature Pinscher, Miniature Schnauzer, Neapolitan Mastiff, and Standard Schnauzer in order to achieve a specific aesthetic look, many animal welfare organizations, veterinarians, and pet owners, view it as a cosmetic procedure that offers no medical benefit to the dog. The ear has to be trimmed to the desired shape. Continuous sutures are applied to suture the skin over the cartilage, after the cartilage is trimmed short of the skin edges. When performed by inexperienced professionals, or due to the intricate vasculature and delicate structure of the ear, there are chances of causing a traumatic injury to the ear during the surgical procedure leaving the dog in excruciating pain. Post surgery, this causes more discomfort to the dog and a delayed wound healing process. A traumatic injury further increases the risk of secondary bacterial infection necessitating additional treatments. Scarring can occur as well, potentially affecting the dog's appearance. The dog becomes stressed and frustrated, and scratches or rubs its ear to relieve pain causing more trauma.

Insect Bites

Dogs' ears, particularly if they are floppy, provide a warm, protected space that can be attractive to various insects. Bites from these insects can be irritating and occasionally lead to more severe complications such as traumatic injuries caused as a result of pawing or violent head shaking. Identifying, treating, and preventing these bites are crucial for the comfort and health of the dog. Inflammatory mediators or toxic substances are present in the saliva of various hematophagous insects and cause insect bite dermatitis. Common culprits include mosquitoes for whom the thin skin of the ears is a particularly easy target; fleas are tiny pests that can bite anywhere but often favor areas with thin skin, like the ears. The rabbit flea (*Spilopsyllus cuniculi*), which is an important vector of diseases including myxomatosis, can affect dogs, and it adheres tightly to the skin of the tip and edges of the pinna, where it may cause dermatitis. The bite site is typically red and may swell. Small papules and wheals are present with central hemorrhagic crusts that can progress to multiple small ulcers. The apexes of the pinnae of dogs with erect ears or on the folded surfaces of the pinnae of dogs with floppy ears have got the lesions. The dog may scratch its ears excessively or shake its head. The bitten or affected area is gently washed with mild soap and water. In order to alleviate inflammation and pruritus in severe cases, use of topical or oral glucocorticoids preferably short acting may be recommended. Therapeutic face masks with ears can be use to decrease insect exposure. Insects like bees, wasps, and hornets can sting dogs. Due to the relatively thin skin and accessibility, a dog's ears are a common area to receive such stings. A sting can be painful for the dog and, in some cases, can lead to more severe reactions. The site of the sting usually becomes red and swollen; the dog might yelp at the moment of the sting and show signs of discomfort afterward; it may scratch its ears excessively or rub its head against objects leading to traumatic injury to the ear; the affected area might feel warm to the touch; in reaction to the pain or discomfort, some dogs might drool or paw at their face and ears. Bees, in paticular, can leave a stinger behind which should gently be scraped instead of using tweezers as squeezing can release more venom. A cold compress to the affected area should be applied to reduce swelling and provide relief. Use of anti-histamines and painkillers are advocated (Fig. **6**). A mix of baking soda and water can be applied to the sting site to neutralize the acidity and reduce pain.

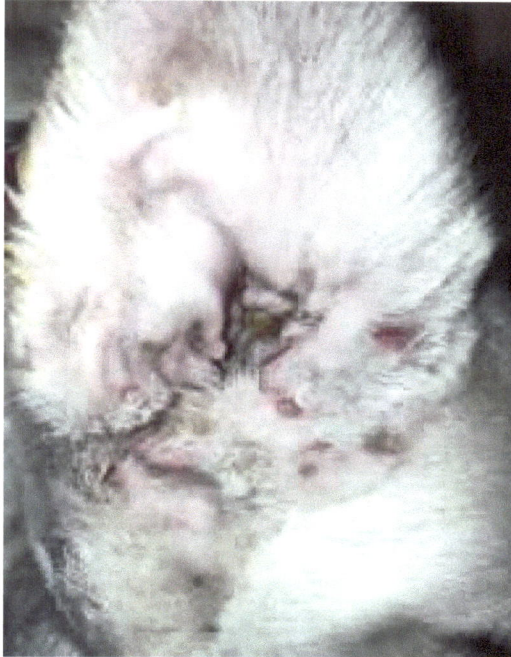

Fig. (6). Suspected case of insect bite in dog with multiple small lesions.

Tympanic Bullae Fractures

There are rare occurrences of traumatic tympanic bullae fractures in the ear of dogs [29]. These occurrences are the result of severe head trauma injuries and are also associated with neurological deficits. Facial nerve paralysis and Horner's syndrome can occur due to the damage caused to the structures associated with tympanic bulla [30]. As a result of extensive trauma to the region of the middle ear, there is facial nerve deficits on the ipsilateral side. Neurological examination is indicative of reduced movement of ipsilateral facial muscles, nostril & ear. Slight facial asymmetry may be observed with drooping lip and ear of ipsilateral side [31]. CT is more sensitive than plain radiography for the identification of skull fractures in dogs due to the complex anatomy of the skull [32]. The only realistic options for the management of traumatic tympanic bulla fractures include surgical exploration, facial nerve decompression if needed and bulla fragment removal. These type of injuries in small animals are commonly associated with neoplastic or infectious causes, or secondary to known surgical intervention such as ventral bulla osteotomy, or lateral bulla osteotomy [33].

Vehicular Accidents

Vehicular accidents involving dogs can lead to a range of injuries, some of which can directly or indirectly affect the ears. The ears, due to their exposed and delicate nature, can be especially susceptible to various forms of trauma during such accidents. Direct trauma to the ears include lacerations and abrasions where sharp objects or broken glass from the vehicle can cause cuts or scrapes on the dog's ears; bruising and hematomas as blunt trauma can cause blood vessels in the ear flap to rupture, leading to swelling or aural hematomas where the ear may appear puffy and fluid-filled. In severe crashes, explosions or fires can result in burns to exposed areas, including the ears. Indirect trauma affecting the ears include head trauma where a significant blow to the head can affect the inner structures of the ear, potentially leading to hearing loss, balance issues, or tinnitus (ringing in the ears); the sheer trauma of the accident can cause extreme stress or anxiety in dogs, leading them to excessively scratch or shake their head, which can subsequently cause more injury to the ears. There may also be some post-accident concerns. If lacerations or abrasions are not cleaned and treated promptly, they can become infected, leading to increased discomfort, redness, swelling, and discharge. Severe trauma can result in damage to the inner ear structures responsible for hearing, potentially leading to permanent hearing loss. Untreated or improperly treated ear injuries can also lead to chronic problems, such as persistent infections or the development of scar tissue. Until fully recovered, vigorous activities that might exacerbate ear injuries should be restricted. An Elizabethan collar (or cone) can prevent the dog from scratching or rubbing its injured ears, while allowing them to heal.

Facial Pruritus

It refers to itching or an uncomfortable sensation that prompts a dog to scratch, rub, lick, or chew the affected area. When a dog experiences facial pruritus, it often results in them scratching or rubbing their face and ears, potentially causing trauma to these areas. The potential causes are varied, including environmental allergens (pollens, mold, dust mites), food allergies, or flea bite hypersensitivity; mites (like Demodex or Sarcoptes), fleas, or ticks can cause itching; bacterial or fungal infections; conditions like seborrhea, autoimmune disorders, or certain tumors. The incessant scratching, rubbing, or shaking caused by pruritus can result in aural hematomas, cuts and abrasions, and secondary infections. The cause has to be first identified with skin scrapings, culture, allergy testing and dietary trials. This is followed by its management with the help of antiparasitic medications, antibiotics, antifungals, or allergen specific therapies. Soothing shampoos, creams, or sprays can provide relief. Short term steroids or anti-itch medications might be used to reduce inflammation and itching. Aural hematoma may require surgical drainage. Use of an Elizabethan collar is advocated to prevent further trauma to the affected ear.

Exposure to Allergens

Coal tar is a byproduct of coal processing. It has been used in various dermatological treatments, primarily for conditions like psoriasis, dandruff, and eczema because of its anti inflammatory and anti scaling properties. However, when used in or around the sensitive ear area of dogs, there can be some concerns. The skin inside a dog's ears is thin and sensitive and coal tar can lead to irritation, causing redness and discomfort. This might result in constant pawing and trauma. It might also dry out the skin inside the ears, leading to flakiness or scaling. An inflammatory response might occur, leading to swelling and further discomfort. This can also exacerbate ear infections if present. With repeated exposure, some dogs might develop an allergy or sensitivity to coal tar, leading to more severe reactions in the future. In rare cases, especially with prolonged contact or use of highly concentrated products, coal tar can cause chemical burns, leading to severe damage. The hair is to be shaved off from the affected and surrounding areas. Warm vegetable oil or coconut oil helps to soften the tar. The area should gently be massaged to remove the tar. Cold water helps to cool down the effect of burning skin area. Neosporin powder may also be helpful as it dissolves the tar. The thick, sticky nature of coal tar products can lead to residue buildup inside the ear, potentially leading to blockages that may require surgical intervention.

It is unknown how dogs get common food allergies. 28 excellent manuscripts from a recent literature analysis revealed that the reported prevalence of food allergies differed based on the particular demographic studied. For instance, food allergies were discovered in 1%–2% of dogs seeking any type of veterinarian care [34]. This percentage significantly increased in animals that presented with pruritus (9%–40% of dogs) or any kind of dermatitis (0%–24% of dogs) [35]. The most frequent food sources also tend to have the most common food allergies. Common food allergens include chicken, beef, lamb, wheat, dairy products while less common food allergens are soy, corn, egg, pork, fish and rice. Animals may exhibit multiple food source hypersensitivity. Food allergies can develop at a very young age or later in life. The age of onset has been documented to range from 6 months to 13 years, despite the fact that dogs with food allergies often also show clinical symptoms when they are young adults (1-4 years old) [36]. Food allergy may therefore be a differential diagnosis that is especially likely to be made in patients who initially arrive with skin illness at either a very early or very advanced age. A definite sex inclination does not seem to exist. Breed predispositions differ slightly based on the predominance of each breed locally. German Shepherds, Labrador Retrievers, French bulldogs, and West Highland

White Terriers, on the other hand, seem to be overrepresented in the majority of western nations. Food allergies can cause a wide range of clinical symptoms. The most frequently mentioned cutaneous clinical symptom in dogs is itching. Generalized or focused/multifocal pruritus can occur. In addition to other places, the pinnae are frequently impacted. When it comes to severity, canine scabies and the pruritis linked with food allergies are comparable. Otitis externa (with or without secondary infection) and recurrent infections with *Staphylococcus* spp. or *Malassezia* are other common symptoms of food allergies in dogs. Patients with food allergies who have no pruritus but have secondary infections can still develop them if the first infection is managed. Pyotraumatic dermatitis, angioedema, and urticaria are less frequent cutaneous symptoms [37]. A dietary elimination experiment is the only effective procedure for diagnosing food allergies as of now. This involves feeding the dog a limited ingredient or hypoallergenic diet for a set period (often 8-12 weeks) and observing for an improvement in symptoms [38]. If symptoms improve, ingredients are gradually reintroduced to identify the specific allergen. Food allergies can cause intense itching and discomfort, which can cause serious self-trauma on the ears. This traumatic event might trigger an inflammatory reaction and prolong pruritus on its own. Due to this, patients may use any antipruritic medicine required to manage their symptoms during the diet experiment.

Traumatic experiences can lead to behavioral changes as well. A dog that has experienced significant pain associated with its ears might become more wary or fearful, especially around other dogs or when being handled. Rehabilitation and behavioral therapy are advocated. Depending on the severity of the injury and subsequent treatment, some dogs might benefit from physical rehabilitation. This could include gentle massage to promote blood flow, increase flexibility, and reduce scar tissue buildup.

CONCLUSION

Ear remains a common structure that is routinely damaged due to its delicate anatomical as well as prominent position. The external ear injuries include simple and complex lacerations, hematoma formation, as well as varying avulsive injuries. The treatment has been done according to clinical history. Surgical intervention can also be performed as per severity of the case.

REFERENCES

[1]   Joyce JA. Treatment of canine aural haernatorna using an indwelling drain and corticosteroids. J Small Anim Pract 1994; 35(7): 341-4.
       [http://dx.doi.org/10.1111/j.1748-5827.1994.tb01711.x]

[2]   Henderson RA, Horne RD. The pinna. In: Slatter D, Ed. Textbook of Small Animal Surgery. 2nd ed. Philadelphia: WB Saunders 1993; pp. 1545-59.

[3]   Evans EK, Fernandez AL. Current trends in the management of canine traumatic brain injury: An Internet-based survey. Can Vet J. 2019; 60(1): 73-79.

[4]   Horne RD, Henderson RA. Pinna. In: Slatter D, Ed. Textbook of Small Animal Surgery. 3rd ed. Philadelphia: WB Saunders 2003; pp. 1737-45.

[5]   Cole LK, Kwochka KW, Kowalski JJ, Hillier A. Microbial flora and antimicrobial susceptibility patterns of isolated pathogens from the horizontal ear canal and middle ear in dogs with otitis media. J Am Vet Med Assoc 1998; 212(4): 534-8.
[http://dx.doi.org/10.2460/javma.1998.212.04.534] [PMID: 9491161]

[6]   Adams GL, McCoid G, Weisbeski D. Cerebrospinal fluid otorrhea presenting as serous otitis media. Minn Med 1982; 65(7): 410-7.
[PMID: 7202112]

[7]   Little C, Lane J, Gibbs C, Pearson G. Inflammatory middle ear disease of the dog: the clinical and pathological features of cholesteatoma, a complication of otitis media. Vet Rec 1991; 128(14): 319-22.
[http://dx.doi.org/10.1136/vr.128.14.319] [PMID: 2063523]

[8]   Bruyette DS, Lorenz MD. Otitis externa and otitis media: diagnostic and medical aspects. Semin Vet Med Surg (Small Anim) 1993; 8(1): 3-9.
[PMID: 8456201]

[9]   Parker AJ, Chrisman CL. How do I treat? Otitis media-interna in dogs and cats. Prog Veter Neur 1995; 6: 139-41.

[10]   Elsahy NI. Ear replanation. Clin Plast Surg 2002; 29(2): 221-31.
[http://dx.doi.org/10.1016/S0094-1298(01)00005-0] [PMID: 12120679]

[11]   Bardsley AF, Mercer DM. The injured ear: a review of 50 cases. Br J Plast Surg 1983; 36(4): 466-9.
[http://dx.doi.org/10.1016/0007-1226(83)90131-5] [PMID: 6626828]

[12]   Gault D. Post traumatic ear reconstruction. J Plast Reconstr Aesthet Surg 2008; 61 (Suppl. 1): S5-S12.
[http://dx.doi.org/10.1016/j.bjps.2008.09.015] [PMID: 18996782]

[13]   Pennington DG, Lai MF, Pelly AD, Pennington DG. Successful replantation of a completely avulsed ear by microvascular anastomosis. Plast Reconstr Surg 1980; 65(6): 820-3.
[http://dx.doi.org/10.1097/00006534-198006000-00017] [PMID: 7384284]

[14]   Kyrmizakis DE, Karatzanis AD, Bourolias CA, Hadjiioannou JK, Velegrakis GA. Nonmicrosurgical reconstruction of the auricle after traumatic amputation due to human bite. Head Face Med 2006; 2(1): 45.
[http://dx.doi.org/10.1186/1746-160X-2-45] [PMID: 17140448]

[15]   Norman ZI, Cracchiolo JR, Allen SH, Soliman AMS. Auricular reconstruction after human bite amputation using the Baudet technique. Ann Otol Rhinol Laryngol 2015; 124(1): 45-8.
[http://dx.doi.org/10.1177/0003489414542090] [PMID: 25024463]

[16]   Horta R, Costa-Ferreira A, Costa J, et al. Ear replantation after human bite avulsion injury. J Craniofac Surg 2011; 22(4): 1457-9.
[http://dx.doi.org/10.1097/SCS.0b013e31821d1879] [PMID: 21772155]

[17]   Mutimer KL, Banis JC, Upton J, Upton J. Microsurgical reattachment of totally amputated ears. Plast Reconstr Surg 1987; 79(4): 535-41.
[http://dx.doi.org/10.1097/00006534-198704000-00003] [PMID: 3823244]

[18]   Katsaros J, Tan E, Sheen R. Microvascular ear replantation. Br J Plast Surg 1988; 41(5): 496-9.
[http://dx.doi.org/10.1016/0007-1226(88)90006-9] [PMID: 3179595]

[19]   Akyürek M, Safak T, Keçik A. Microsurgical ear replantation without venous repair: failure of development of venous channels despite patency of arterial anastomosis for 14 days. Ann Plast Surg 2001; 46(4): 439-42.
[http://dx.doi.org/10.1097/00000637-200104000-00016] [PMID: 11324890]

[20]   Anthony JP, Lineaweaver WC, Davis JW Jr, Buncke HJ. Quantitative fluorimetric effects of leeching on a replanted ear. Microsurgery 1989; 10(3): 167-9.
[http://dx.doi.org/10.1002/micr.1920100304] [PMID: 2796712]

[21]   Sadove RC. Successful replantation of a totally amputated ear. Ann Plast Surg 1990; 24(4): 366-70.
[http://dx.doi.org/10.1097/00000637-199004000-00012] [PMID: 2353788]

[22]   Mello-Filho FV, Mamede RCM, Koury AP. Use of a platysma myocutaneous flap for the reimplantation of a severed ear: experience with five cases. Sao Paulo Med J 1999; 117(5): 218-23.
[http://dx.doi.org/10.1590/S1516-31801999000500007] [PMID: 10592135]

[23]   Turpin IM, Altman DI, Cruz HG, Achauer BM. Salvage of the severely injured ear. Ann Plast Surg 1988; 21(2): 170-9.
[http://dx.doi.org/10.1097/00000637-198808000-00016] [PMID: 3178126]

[24]   Anous MM, Hallock GG. Immediate reconstruction of the auricle using the amputated cartilage and the temporoparietal fascia. Ann Plast Surg 1988; 21(4): 378-81.
[http://dx.doi.org/10.1097/00000637-198810000-00015] [PMID: 3232926]

[25]   Brent B, Byrd HS. Secondary ear reconstruction with cartilage grafts covered by axial, random, and free flaps of temporoparietal fascia. Plast Reconstr Surg 1983; 72(2): 141-51.
[http://dx.doi.org/10.1097/00006534-198308000-00003] [PMID: 6878488]

[26]   Mladick RA, Horton C, Adamson J, Cohen B. The pocket principle: a new technique for the reattachment of a severed ear part. Plast Reconstr Surg 1971; 48(3): 219-23.
[http://dx.doi.org/10.1097/00006534-197109000-00004] [PMID: 5566470]

[27]   Bai H, Tollefson TT. Treatment strategies for auricular avulsions: best practice. JAMA Facial Plast Surg 2014; 16(1): 7-8.
[http://dx.doi.org/10.1001/jamafacial.2013.1622] [PMID: 24136398]

[28]   Steffen A, Katzbach R, Klaiber S. A comparison of ear reattachment methods: a review of 25 years since Pennington. Plast Reconstr Surg 2006; 118(6): 1358-64.
[http://dx.doi.org/10.1097/01.prs.0000239539.98956.b0] [PMID: 17051106]

[29]   Rubin JA, Kim SE, Bacon NJ. Traumatic tympanic bulla fracture. J Small Anim Pract. (20).

[30]   Bar-am Y, Pollard R, Kass PH, Verstraete FJM. The diagnostic yield of conventional radiographs and computed tomography in dogs and cats with maxillofacial trauma. Vet Surg 2008; 37(3): 294-9.
[http://dx.doi.org/10.1111/j.1532-950X.2008.00380.x] [PMID: 18394078]

[31]   Pratschke KM. Inflammatory polyps of the middle ear in 5 dogs. Vet Surg 2003; 32(3): 292-6.
[http://dx.doi.org/10.1053/jvet.2003.50036] [PMID: 12784207]

[32]   Devitt CM, Seim HB III, Willer R, McPHERRON MELISSA, Neely M. Passive drainage *versus* primary closure after total ear canal ablation-lateral bulla osteotomy in dogs: 59 dogs (1985-1995). Vet Surg 1997; 26(3): 210-6.
[http://dx.doi.org/10.1111/j.1532-950X.1997.tb01486.x] [PMID: 9150559]

[33]   Travetti O, Giudice C, Greci V, Lombardo R, Mortellaro CM, Di Giancamillo M. Computed tomography features of middle ear cholesteatoma in dogs. Vet Radiol Ultrasound 2010; 51(4): 374-9.
[http://dx.doi.org/10.1111/j.1740-8261.2010.01682.x] [PMID: 20806867]

[34]   Olivry T, Mueller RS. Critically appraised topic on adverse food reactions of companion animals (1): duration of elimination diets. BMC Vet Research, vol. 11, p225.

[35]   Mueller RS, Olivry T, Prelaud P. Critically appraised topic on adverse food reactions of companion animals (2): common food allergen sources in dogs and cats. BMC Vet Research, vol. 12, p9.

[36]   Olivry T, Mueller RS. Critically appraised topic on adverse food reactions of companion animals (3): prevalence of cutaneous adverse food reactions in dogs and cats. BMC Vet Research, vol. 13, p51.

[37]   Mueller RS, Olivry T. Critically appraised topic on adverse food reactions of companion animals (4):

can we diagnose adverse food reactions in dogs and cats with *in vivo* or *in vitro* tests? BMC Vet Research, vol. 13, p275.

[38] Mueller RS, Olivry T. Critically appraised topic on adverse food reactions of companion animals (6): prevalence of noncutaneous manifestations of adverse food reactions in dogs and cats. BMC Vet Research, vol. 14, p341.

CHAPTER 9

Diseases of Pinna and its Clinical Management

Jigar Raval[1], **Pranav Anjaria**[2], **Santanu Pal**[3,*] and **Tanmoy Rana**[4]

[1] *National Dairy Development Board, Anand-388001, Gujarat, India*

[2] *College of Veterinary Science & Animal Husbandry, Kamdhenu University, Anand-388001, Gujarat, India*

[3] *Indian Veterinary Research Institute, Izatnagar-243122, India*

[4] *Department of Veterinary Clinical Complex, West Bengal University of Veterinary & Animal Sciences, Kolkata-700094, India*

Abstract: Understanding pinna diseases is essential for veterinarians, pet owners, and anyone caring for dogs. The pinna, or external ear, plays a vital role in a dog's health and well-being, serving as a protective barrier for the sensitive inner ear, aiding in sound localization, and enhancing auditory perception. However, its anatomical features make it susceptible to various diseases, including infections, parasites, allergic reactions, traumatic injuries, and neoplastic conditions. Bacterial and fungal infections can cause inflammation, pain, and discharge in the pinna, necessitating proper diagnosis and treatment with antibiotics or antifungal medications. Parasitic infestations, such as ear mites and ticks, also target the pinna and require specific antiparasitic treatment. Allergic and immunologic disorders manifest as redness, swelling, and itching on the pinna, demanding accurate diagnosis and management strategies such as allergen avoidance, medications, or immunotherapy. Traumatic injuries, like hematomas, lacerations, and avulsion injuries, may affect the pinna, necessitating immediate attention to prevent infections and promote healing. Neoplastic diseases, both benign and malignant, require precise diagnosis and treatment planning. Understanding congenital and developmental disorders of the pinna is vital, as certain breeds may be predisposed to specific malformations leading to chronic ear problems. Genetic disorders affecting the pinna can contribute to hearing impairment or structural abnormalities, emphasizing the need for thorough assessment and management strategies. Recognizing the significance of pinna diseases enables early detection, intervention, and prevention strategies, emphasizing the importance of regular ear care and veterinary attention. By comprehending the anatomy and function of the pinna in dogs, optimal ear health and overall well-being for canine companions can be ensured.

* **Corresponding author Tanmoy Rana:** Department of Veterinary Clinical Complex, West Bengal University of Veterinary & Animal Sciences, Kolkata-700094, India; E-mail: tanmoyrana123@gmail.com

Keywords: Allergic reactions, Canine ear health, Diagnostics, Ear infections, Hearing impairment in dogs, Immunologic disorders, Infectious diseases, Medical treatment, Neoplastic conditions, Otitis externa, Parasitic infestations, Pinna diseases, Prevention, Surgical interventions, Symptomatic relief, Therapeutic management, Traumatic injuries, Veterinary care, Wound healing, X-ray imaging.

INTRODUCTION

Understanding pinna diseases is of paramount importance for veterinarians, pet owners, and anyone involved in the care of dogs. The pinna, also known as the external ear or ear flap, plays a vital role in a dog's overall health and well-being. As an external structure, the pinna is susceptible to a variety of diseases and disorders that can significantly impact a dog's quality of life. By comprehending the significance of pinna diseases and familiarizing ourselves with the intricate anatomy and function of the pinna in dogs, we can better diagnose, treat, and prevent these conditions, ensuring optimal ear health for our canine companions.

The pinna serves several essential functions in dogs. Firstly, it acts as a protective barrier, shielding the sensitive structures of the middle and inner ear from external elements. This includes preventing foreign objects, dust, and debris from entering the ear canal, which could potentially cause irritation or injury. Additionally, the pinna aids in sound localization, allowing dogs to determine the direction of sounds and facilitating their auditory perception. Through its intricate structure and position, the pinna captures and funnels sound waves, enhancing a dog's ability to detect and interpret auditory stimuli [1]. However, the unique anatomical features of the pinna also makes it susceptible to various diseases. Infections, both bacterial and fungal, can easily take hold in the warm, moist environment of the ear canal, spreading to the pinna and causing inflammation and discomfort. Parasitic infestations, such as ear mites, ticks, or fleas, can also target the pinna, leading to irritation, itchiness, and potential secondary infections. Moreover, allergic and immunologic disorders can manifest on the pinna, as it is a site prone to allergic reactions and hypersensitivity. Conditions like atopic dermatitis or contact dermatitis can result in redness, swelling, and the development of lesions on the pinna.

Traumatic injuries are another concern for the pinna. Hematomas, which are collections of blood under the skin, can occur from trauma or excessive shaking of the head, causing swelling and pain [2]. Lacerations, puncture wounds, and avulsion injuries may also affect the pinna, requiring immediate attention to prevent infection and promote proper healing. Neoplastic diseases, both benign and malignant, can develop on the pinna, necessitating accurate diagnosis, staging, and treatment planning. Early identification and intervention are crucial for achieving the best possible outcomes.

Understanding the congenital and developmental disorders of the pinna is equally important. Certain dog breeds may be predisposed to specific pinna malformations, such as folded or curled pinnae, which can lead to chronic ear problems. Genetic disorders affecting the pinna can also contribute to hearing impairment or structural abnormalities, emphasizing the need for thorough assessment and appropriate management strategies. By understanding the importance of pinna diseases and delving into the intricate anatomy and function of the pinna in dogs, we can enhance our ability to recognize, diagnose, and effectively treat these conditions. Additionally, prevention strategies can be implemented to mitigate the risk of pinna diseases, emphasizing the significance of regular ear care and prompt veterinary attention. Through a comprehensive understanding of pinna diseases, we can strive to ensure optimal ear health and overall well-being for our beloved canine companions [2].

IMPORTANCE OF UNDERSTANDING PINNA DISEASES

Understanding pinna diseases holds immense importance for veterinarians, pet owners, and anyone involved in the care of dogs. The pinna, or external ear, is a complex structure that can be affected by a wide range of diseases and disorders. By recognizing the significance of pinna diseases, we can better advocate for the health and well-being of dogs, improve diagnostic accuracy, provide effective treatment, and prevent complications associated with these conditions (Fig. **1**).

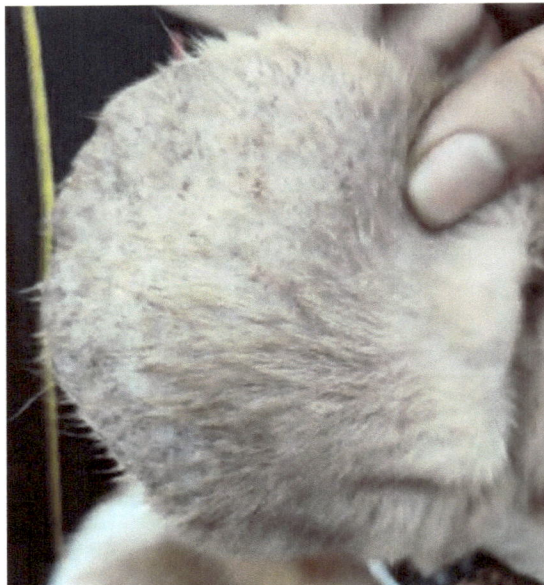

Fig. (1). Depicting ear infection in e.

The primary reasons to understand the pinna diseases is, it is crucial to ensure the overall health and comfort of dogs. The pinna is highly innervated and richly supplied with blood vessels, making it a sensitive and vital part of the auditory system. When the pinna is affected by diseases or disorders, it can cause significant discomfort, pain, and distress to the affected dog. By being knowledgeable about pinna diseases, we can promptly identify symptoms, seek appropriate veterinary care, and alleviate the dog's suffering. Pinna diseases can have various consequences and complications -if left untreated or misdiagnosed [3]. For instance, untreated infections can spread from the pinna to the middle or inner ear, leading to more severe complications such as otitis media or otitis interna. These conditions can result in hearing loss, balance issues, and potentially serious secondary infections. Understanding pinna diseases enables early detection and intervention, preventing the progression of diseases and minimizing potential complications. Another critical aspect of understanding pinna diseases is the impact they can have on a dog's quality of life. Dogs rely heavily on their sense of hearing to navigate their environment, communicate, and interact with both humans and other animals. Pinna diseases, such as chronic infections or structural abnormalities, can impair a dog's hearing ability, leading to reduced sensory perception and potential behavioural changes [4]. By recognizing and managing pinna diseases effectively, we can help dogs maintain their sensory functions and preserve their overall well-being (Fig. **2**).

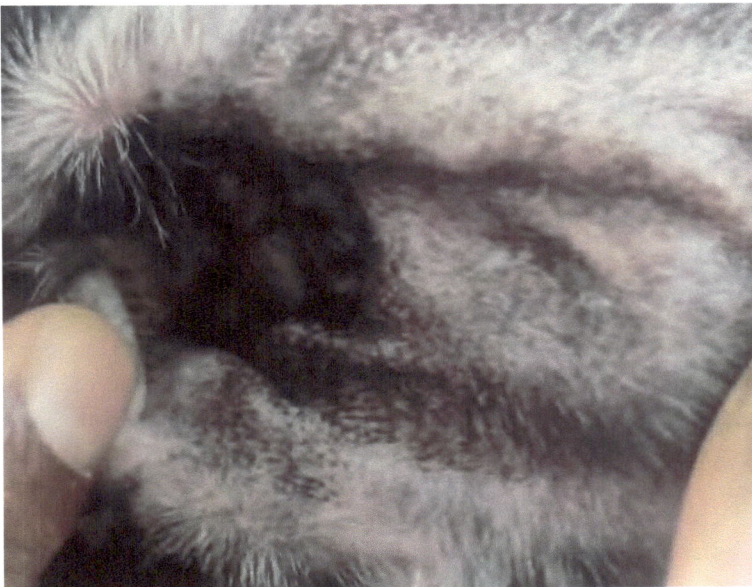

Fig. (2). Depicts ear rashes and black scales in the ear pinna

Furthermore, pinna diseases can serve as indicators or manifestations of underlying systemic conditions or health issues. For example, certain autoimmune disorders may present with pinna abnormalities or lesions. By recognizing these signs, veterinarians can investigate further and potentially diagnose and treat the underlying systemic condition. Thus, understanding pinna diseases can serve as a valuable diagnostic tool for identifying broader health concerns in dogs. Prevention is always better than cure, and this holds true for pinna diseases as well. By understanding the risk factors, predispositions, and causes of these conditions, we can implement preventive measures to minimize their occurrence. Regular ear cleaning, proper hygiene practices, routine veterinary check-ups, and appropriate parasite control can all contribute to reducing the likelihood of pinna diseases. Educating pet owners about these preventive measures is vital in ensuring the long-term health and well-being of their dogs [5].

Moreover, understanding pinna diseases contributes to the advancement of veterinary knowledge and research. By studying the etiology, pathogenesis, and treatment outcomes of various pinna conditions, researchers can enhance their understanding of these diseases and develop more effective treatment strategies. This knowledge can ultimately lead to improved veterinary care, better treatment outcomes, and advancements in veterinary medicine as a whole.

ANATOMY AND FUNCTION OF THE PINNA IN DOGS

The pinna, also known as the auricle or external ear, is a prominent feature of a dog's head and plays a crucial role in their auditory system. The pinna consists of cartilage covered by skin and is attached to the side of the dog's head. Its shape and size can vary greatly between different dog breeds and individuals, with some having erect ears while others have floppy or pendulous ears [6]. The pinna is composed of several distinctive anatomical components, each contributing to its form and function. Starting with the outermost layer, the skin covering the pinna is typically thin and hair-bearing. The skin's surface may have different pigmentation patterns, such as spots or patches, depending on the breed. Hair follicles present on the pinna can contribute in maintaining the temperature and protecting the underlying structures. Beneath the skin lies a layer of subcutaneous tissue, which provides cushioning and support to the pinna. This layer contains blood vessels and nerves that supply the pinna and play a vital role in its overall function. The rich blood supply helps maintain the health and vitality of the pinna's tissues, while the nerves allow for sensory perception and facilitate the dog's auditory capabilities. The core framework of the pinna is made up of elastic cartilage. This cartilage gives the pinna its characteristic shape and flexibility, allowing it to maintain its form while also being capable of slight movements [7]. The cartilage structure provides stability to the pinna and helps funnel sound waves towards the ear canal, optimizing the dog's ability to detect and localize sounds.

The pinna is anatomically divided into various regions and features. The most prominent and visible part is the auricular conch, which forms the cup-shaped portion of the pinna. The conch aids in collecting and directing sound waves into the ear canal, enhancing a dog's auditory perception. The pinna also includes additional structural components, such as ridges, folds, and notches. These features contribute to the pinna's unique shape and help in capturing and focusing sound waves towards the ear canal entrance. Moreover, these structural variations can impact the susceptibility of certain specific breeds to pinna diseases or conditions. The diverse array of pinna deformities, as presented in Table **1**, showcases the range of unique characteristics that can affect the external ear in dogs [8].

Table 1. Unique pinna deformities and their characteristics.

Pinna Deformity	Description	Characteristics
Macrotia	Abnormally large pinna	Oversized, disproportionate to the head size
Microtia	Abnormally small pinna	Underdeveloped, small in size
Cryptotia	Hidden or partially hidden pinna	Folded or partially covered by skin or hair
Stahl's Ear	Pointed or elf-like appearance	Excessive curvature or folding in the upper pinna
Cauliflower Ear	Deformity due to trauma or repeated injury	Swollen, irregular, and distorted shape
Cup Ear	Flat or cup-shaped pinna	Lack of normal pinna contour, concave appearance
Cocker Spaniel Ear	Pendulous, long and drooping pinna	Pinna extends below the jawline
Anotia	Absence of the pinna	Complete absence of the external ear
Lop Ear	Floppy or droopy pinna	Lack of normal rigidity or upright position

The main function of the pinna is to collect and funnel sound waves into the ear canal. Its shape and positioning allow for the localization of sound sources, helping dogs to determine the direction from which sounds are coming. By detecting and interpreting auditory stimuli, dogs can effectively communicate, navigate their environment, and respond to various sounds, including vocalizations, warnings, or potential threats. In addition to its role in hearing, the pinna also serves as a protective barrier for the dog's middle and inner ear structures. It helps to prevent foreign objects, debris, and insects from entering the ear canal, reducing the risk of irritation, infections, or injuries. The pinna's ability to direct sound waves and shield the ear canal contributes towards maintaining optimal ear health and function [9].

COMMON INFECTIOUS DISEASES OF THE PINNA

The pinna, or external ear, is susceptible to various infectious diseases that can cause discomfort, irritation, and potential complications in dogs (4). Understanding these common infectious diseases of the pinna is crucial for accurate diagnosis, appropriate treatment, and prevention strategies. Let's explore the four primary categories of infectious diseases that affect the pinna: bacterial infections, fungal infections, parasitic infections, and viral infections. To provide a comprehensive overview, Table **2** summarizes unique pinna diseases, their characteristics, and the available treatment options (Fig. **2**).

Table 2. Unique pinna diseases and their characteristics and treatment options.

Pinna Disease	Description	Symptoms	Treatment Options
Pemphigus foliaceus	Autoimmune disorder affecting the pinna	Crusty lesions, erosions, scaly skin	Immunosuppressive medications, topical treatments
Ceruminous gland tumors	Tumors originating from ceruminous glands	Masses or lumps on the pinna	Surgical excision, radiation therapy
Calcinosis cutis	Calcium deposits in the pinna skin	Hard nodules, ulceration, discomfort	Symptomatic treatment, surgical removal if needed
Otitis externa	Inflammation of the external ear canal	Redness, swelling, itching, discharge	Topical/Oral antibiotics, antifungal medications
Pinna abscess	Collection of pus within the pinna	Swelling, pain, warmth, discharge	Surgical drainage, antibiotics, wound management
Squamous cell carcinoma	Malignant skin tumor affecting the pinna	Ulcers, bleeding, slow-healing wounds	Surgical excision, radiation therapy
Chondritis	Inflammation of the pinna cartilage	Pain, swelling, tenderness	Anti-inflammatory medications, supportive care
Auricular hematoma	Collection of blood within the pinna	Swelling, "balloon-like" appearance, pain	Drainage, pressure bandaging, underlying cause treatment
Zoonotic dermatoses	Pinna diseases transmissible between animals and humans	Rash, lesions, itching, redness, discomfort	Appropriate treatment for the specific zoonotic disease

Bacterial Infections

Bacterial infections of the pinna can occur due to opportunistic pathogens or secondary infections resulting from underlying conditions. Common bacterial agents involved in pinna infections include *Staphylococcus* spp., *Streptococcus* spp., *Pseudomonas* spp., and *Escherichia coli* [10]. Factors such as trauma, allergies, or anatomical abnormalities can predispose the pinna to bacterial colonization and infection. Bacterial pinna infections typically manifest as redness, swelling, pain, discharge, and sometimes crusting or ulceration. Treatment involves identifying the causative bacteria through cytology or culture and administering appropriate antibiotics, often in the form of topical ointments or oral medications.

Fungal Infections

Fungal infections of the pinna, also known as otomycosis, are commonly caused by organisms such as *Malassezia* spp., *Candida* spp., and *Aspergillus* spp. These fungi thrive in warm and moist environments, making the pinna an ideal breeding ground. Factors such as excessive moisture, ear canal inflammation, or immune system imbalances can predispose dogs to fungal infections. Symptoms may include itchiness, redness, wax accumulation, and a characteristic musty odor. Diagnosis is achieved through microscopic examination and fungal culture. Antifungal medications, both topical and systemic, are employed to eliminate the fungal infection and restore the pinna's health [8].

Parasitic Infections

Parasitic infections affecting the pinna commonly include infestations of ear mites (*Otodectes cynotis*) and ticks. Ear mites are microscopic parasites that reside in the ear canal and pinna, causing intense itching, head shaking, and dark discharge. Tick infestations, although more commonly found on the body, can also attach to the pinna, leading to irritation, redness, and the risk of disease transmission. Treatment for ear mites involves specific parasiticides, such as acaricides, applied topically or administered systemically. Removal and prevention of ticks from the pinna require careful tick removal techniques and effective tick prevention measures [7].

Viral Infections

Viral infections affecting the pinna in dogs are relatively less common compared to other infectious agents. However, certain viruses can impact the pinna and cause discomfort or skin lesions. For example, canine papillomavirus (CPV) infections can lead to the formation of warts or papillomas on the pinna. Additionally, some viral diseases, such as canine distemper virus (CDV), can cause generalized skin inflammation and affect the pinna along with other areas of the body. Managing viral infections primarily involves supportive care, antiviral medications when available, and addressing any secondary bacterial or fungal complications (Fig. **3**).

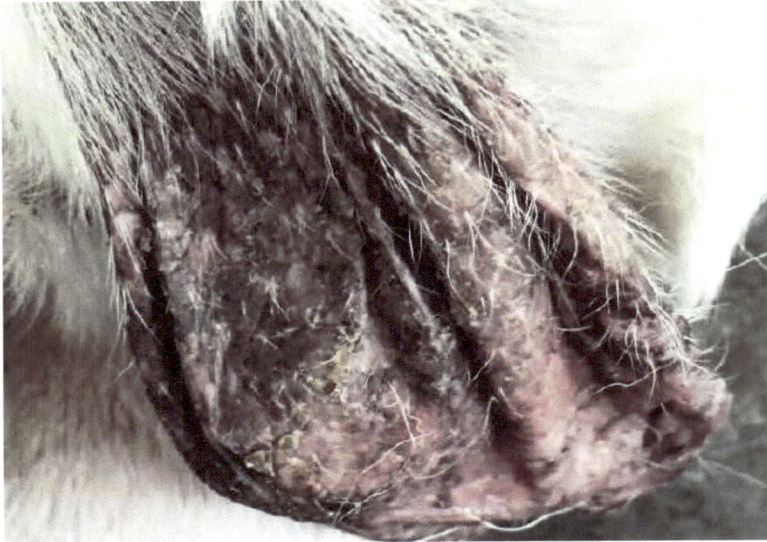

Fig. (3). Severe infection stages of pinna of a dog.

ALLERGIC AND IMMUNOLOGIC DISORDERS OF THE PINNA

Allergic and immunologic disorders encompass a group of conditions that can affect the pinna of dogs. These disorders arise due to abnormal immune responses to certain allergens or the body's own tissues. Understanding these disorders is crucial for diagnosing and managing pinna-related symptoms effectively. The three main categories of allergic and immunologic disorders that can impact the pinna are atopic dermatitis, contact dermatitis, and autoimmune disorders. Atopic dermatitis is a common allergic skin condition in dogs, and it can affect the pinna along with other areas of the body. It is typically triggered by environmental allergens such as pollen, dust mites, or certain foods. Dogs with atopic dermatitis may exhibit symptoms on the pinna, including redness, swelling, itchiness, and the development of papules or crusts. Identifying the underlying allergens through allergy testing can help manage the condition. Treatment options often involve allergen avoidance, medications to control itching and inflammation, and immunotherapy to desensitize the dog's immune system. Contact dermatitis occurs when the pinna comes into direct contact with an irritating or allergenic substance. Common culprits include certain plants, cleaning products, or topical medications. Dogs with contact dermatitis may display redness, swelling, itching, and possibly blisters or ulceration on the pinna. Diagnosis involves a thorough examination and identification of the offending substance. Treatment primarily focuses on removing the source of contact and providing symptomatic relief, which may include topical medications, anti-inflammatory drugs, and supportive care [6].

Autoimmune disorders affecting the pinna occur when the immune system mistakenly targets and attacks the body's own tissues in the pinna. Conditions such as pemphigus, lupus erythematosus, and vasculitis can lead to inflammation, ulceration, and damage to the pinna. Dogs with autoimmune disorders may experience pain, crusting, and scarring on the affected areas. Accurate diagnosis typically involves a combination of clinical examination, histopathology, and specific antibody testing. Treatment aims to control the immune response and reduce inflammation through immunosuppressive medications, corticosteroids, or other immunomodulatory drugs. Understanding these allergic and immunologic disorders of the pinna enables veterinarians to differentiate them from other conditions and provide targeted treatment [4, 5]. It is essential to establish an accurate diagnosis through comprehensive assessments, which may include clinical examinations, medical history, allergy testing, or specialized laboratory tests. Tailored treatment plans can then be implemented, considering the specific disorder and its severity. In some cases, ongoing management and long-term therapy may be necessary to control symptoms and prevent recurrences (Fig. **4**).

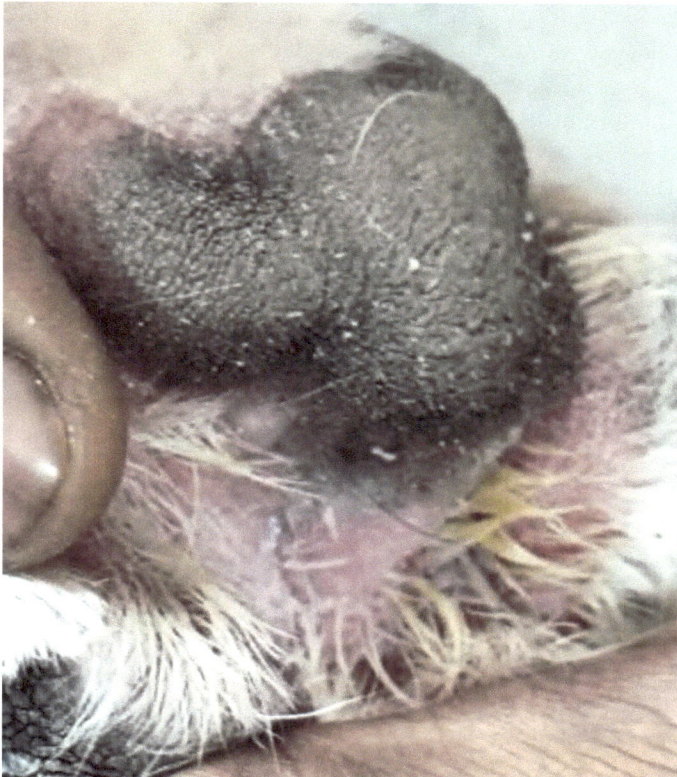

Fig. (4). Nodular lesion in the pinna.

TRAUMATIC INJURIES TO THE PINNA

Traumatic injuries to the pinna, or external ear, can occur in dogs due to various factors such as accidents, fights, or excessive scratching or head shaking. These injuries can range from mild to severe and may require immediate attention to prevent complications and promote proper healing. Understanding the types of traumatic injuries that can affect the pinna is crucial for prompt recognition, appropriate treatment, and optimal outcomes. One common traumatic injury to the pinna is a hematoma. A hematoma occurs when blood accumulates within the pinna, usually because of trauma or vigorous shaking of the head. The blood collects between the layers of the pinna, causing swelling, pain, and a characteristic "balloon-like" appearance. If left untreated, hematomas can lead to discomfort, infection, and potential permanent disfigurement. Treatment often involves draining the accumulated blood, providing appropriate pain relief, and applying pressure dressings or splints to prevent reaccumulation.

Lacerations and puncture wounds are another type of traumatic injury that can affect the pinna. Dogs may sustain lacerations or puncture wounds from fights with other animals, accidental injuries, or sharp objects. These injuries can vary in severity, from superficial cuts to deep, extensive wounds. Treatment typically involves thorough cleaning of the wound, removal of any foreign bodies, and closure of the laceration through sutures or other appropriate wound closure techniques. Antibiotics may also be prescribed to prevent infection. Avulsion injuries, although less common, can occur in situations where there is forceful tearing or shearing of the pinna. Avulsion injuries involve the partial or complete separation of a portion of the pinna from the rest of the ear. These injuries are often accompanied by significant tissue damage, bleeding, and potential nerve or blood vessel injury. Immediate veterinary attention is crucial for avulsion injuries. Treatment may involve surgical reattachment of the avulsed portion of the pinna, wound management, and appropriate pain management.

In all cases of traumatic injuries to the pinna, it is essential to thoroughly assess the extent of the injury and evaluate for any underlying damage to the cartilage, blood vessels, or nerves. Veterinary professionals may perform diagnostic tests, such as X-rays or ultrasound, to assess the full extent of the injury and guide treatment decisions.

NEUROLOGICAL DISORDERS AND SENSORY DYSFUNCTION OF THE PINNA

Neurological disorders and sensory dysfunction affecting the pinna can have significant implications for a dog's auditory perception and overall well-being. The pinna, or external ear, plays a crucial role in capturing and funneling sound waves, aiding in sound localization and contributing to a dog's ability to hear and interact with its environment. Understanding the neurological disorders and sensory dysfunction related to the pinna is vital for accurate diagnosis, appropriate management, and ensuring the best possible quality of life for affected dogs. One example of a neurological disorder that can impact the pinna is vestibular disease. Vestibular disorders involves dysfunction of the vestibular system, which is responsible for maintaining balance and spatial orientation. When the vestibular system is affected, dogs may experience symptoms such as head tilt, loss of balance, circling, and abnormal eye movements. These symptoms can indirectly impact the pinna, leading to changes in the dog's ability to accurately detect and localize sounds. Management of vestibular disease typically involves addressing the underlying cause, providing supportive care, and implementing strategies to help the dog adapt to changes in balance and coordination [8].

Nerve damage or neuropathies can also result in sensory dysfunction of the pinna. Trauma, infections, or certain medical conditions can lead to damage or impairment of the nerves that supply the pinna. Sensory dysfunction may manifest as reduced sensitivity to auditory stimuli or even complete hearing loss in the affected ear. Dogs may exhibit signs such as reduced responsiveness to sound, failure to react to auditory cues, or changes in behavior. Depending on the underlying cause and extent of nerve damage, management strategies may include treating the underlying condition, providing supportive care, and exploring options for hearing aids or assistive devices if appropriate. Sensorineural hearing loss refers to a type of hearing loss that originates in the inner ear or auditory nerve pathways. While the pinna itself is not directly involved in this type of hearing loss, it is an integral part of the auditory system that can be affected by the consequences of sensorineural hearing loss. Dogs with sensorineural hearing loss may have difficulty localizing sounds accurately or distinguishing certain frequencies. Management of sensorineural hearing loss often focuses on providing environmental accommodations, such as visual cues or training techniques, to help the dog navigate its surroundings and communicate effectively [1, 2].

Diagnosing neurological disorders and sensory dysfunction related to the pinna requires a comprehensive evaluation by a veterinary professional. This may involve a thorough physical examination, neurologic assessment, specialized tests such as auditory evoked response testing, and possibly imaging studies to assess the underlying cause. Treatment and management strategies for these conditions vary depending on the specific disorder, underlying cause, and individual dog. They may involve addressing any underlying medical conditions, providing supportive care, implementing environmental modifications to optimize the dog's quality of life, nd potentially exploring assistive devices or hearing aids in cases of hearing loss [7].

BREED-SPECIFIC AND AGE-RELATED PINNA DISEASES

Breed-specific and age-related pinna diseases encompass a range of conditions that can affect certain breeds or arise as a dog grows older. Understanding these specific diseases are crucial for early recognition, targeted management, and appropriate care for affected dogs [9]. Let's explore breed-specific and age-related pinna diseases in more detail.

Breed-Specific Pinna Diseases

Certain dog breeds are predisposed to specific pinna diseases due to inherited traits or genetic factors. For example, breeds with long, pendulous ears such as Basset Hounds or Cocker Spaniels are more prone to ear infections, as the shape of their pinnae can restrict airflow and create a favorable environment for bacterial or fungal growth [10]. Breeds with folded or curled pinnae, such as Scottish Folds or American Curl cats, may be susceptible to cartilage abnormalities or chronic ear problems. Understanding breed-specific risks enables veterinarians and owners to implement preventive measures, such as regular cleaning and ear care, to minimize the likelihood of pinna diseases in these susceptible breeds.

Age-Related Pinna Diseases

As dogs age, changes in the pinna can occur, leading to age-related pinna diseases. One common condition is senile or age-related pinna atrophy, where the pinna gradually loses its firmness and elasticity. This can result in pinna folding, curling, or drooping, making the dog more prone to infections and irritations. Additionally, elderly dogs may experience thinning or loss of hair on the pinna, making it more susceptible to sunburn and other environmental factors. Providing proper care, such as regular cleaning, sun protection, and monitoring for signs of infection, can help manage age-related pinna changes and promote the dog's comfort and well-being. Other age-related conditions that can affect the pinna include tumors or growths, such as benign polyps or malignant cancers. Elderly dogs may be more prone to developing various types of pinna tumors, which can present as lumps, ulcers, or changes in the pinna's appearance. Early detection and appropriate management, which may involve surgical removal, biopsy, or other treatments, are crucial for addressing these age-related growths effectively [6].

DIAGNOSTIC TECHNIQUES FOR PINNA DISEASES

Diagnostic techniques for pinna diseases involves a comprehensive approach to accurately identify the underlying cause of the condition. A combination of clinical examination, history taking, specialized tests, and imaging modalities may be employed to reach a definitive diagnosis. Let's delve into the various diagnostic techniques in detail:

Clinical Examination

A thorough clinical examination of the pinna is crucial to evaluate its overall appearance, symmetry, color, texture, and presence of any abnormalities. The veterinarian will visually inspect the pinna for signs of inflammation, swelling, lesions, discharge, or structural deformities. Palpation may also be performed to assess for tenderness, masses, or changes in tissue consistency.

History Taking

Gathering a detailed history from the pet owner is important in understanding the progression, duration, and potential triggers of the pinna disease. Information about the onset of symptoms, any previous treatments or medications, and exposure to allergens or irritants can provide valuable insights into the underlying cause.

Cytology and Culture

Cytology involves obtaining a sample of material from the pinna, such as discharge or crusts, and examining it microscopically. This technique helps identify the presence of bacteria, fungi, parasites, or abnormal cells. If an infection is suspected, culture and sensitivity testing may be performed to determine the specific causative organism and its sensitivity to different antibiotics or antifungal agents.

Biopsy and Histopathology

In cases where a neoplastic or suspicious lesion is present, a biopsy may be performed. This involves the surgical removal of a small portion of the affected tissue for microscopic examination. Histopathology then analyzes the tissue sample to determine the nature of the lesion, whether it is benign or malignant, and provides insights into the disease process and prognosis [4].

Imaging

Imaging modalities, such as X-rays or ultrasound, may be used to assess the underlying structures of the pinna, especially in cases of trauma, suspected foreign body, or tumors. X-rays can help evaluate bone integrity, while ultrasound can provide detailed images of soft tissues, blood vessels, and any abnormalities within the pinna.

Allergy Testing

In cases where allergic conditions are suspected, allergy testing may be performed to identify specific allergens triggering an allergic response. This can involve intradermal testing or blood tests to detect the presence of allergen-specific antibodies.

Endoscopy

In certain situations, endoscopy may be utilized to examine the ear canal and the deeper structures of the pinna. This technique allows for direct visualization of the area, detection of foreign bodies, evaluation of the middle ear, or collection of samples for further analysis.

Diagnostic Imaging (MRI/CT)

In more complex cases or when there is a need for detailed assessment, advanced imaging techniques such as magnetic resonance imaging (MRI) or computed tomography (CT) scans may be employed. These imaging modalities can provide high-resolution images of the pinna and surrounding structures, aiding in the diagnosis and treatment planning.

The selection of diagnostic techniques will depend on the individual case and the suspected underlying cause of the pinna disease. The veterinarian will determine the most appropriate diagnostic approach to obtain accurate information for an effective treatment plan.

TREATMENT APPROACHES FOR PINNA DISEASES

The treatment approaches for pinna diseases depend on the specific condition and underlying cause. The primary goals of treatment are to alleviate symptoms, eliminate the underlying cause, promote healing, and prevent recurrences. The treatment modalities can include medical management, surgical interventions, and supportive care. In cases of bacterial infections, appropriate antibiotics are administered to target the specific bacteria identified through culture and sensitivity testing. Topical antibiotics, such as ointments or ear drops, are commonly used to directly address the infection. In more severe or systemic cases, oral antibiotics may be prescribed to eliminate the bacteria and prevent further complications. For fungal infections, antifungal medications are employed to combat the overgrowth of fungi. Topical antifungal creams, ointments, or ear drops are frequently used to target the affected areas. In some cases, systemic antifungal drugs may be necessary to address deeper or more persistent infections [2, 3].

Parasitic infections, such as ear mites or ticks, require specific antiparasitic treatment. Acaricides or medications targeting the specific parasites are administered topically or orally to eliminate the infestation. Regular cleaning and maintenance of the pinna may also be recommended to prevent reinfestation. Inflammation associated with pinna diseases can be managed with anti-inflammatory medications. These medications help reduce redness, swelling, itching, and discomfort. Nonsteroidal anti-inflammatory drugs (NSAIDs), corticosteroids, or other immunomodulatory medications may be prescribed, depending on the severity and nature of the inflammation. Surgical interventions may be necessary in certain cases. For example, in traumatic injuries or lacerations, surgical repair may be performed to suture or reconstruct the damaged tissues. In cases of tumors or growths, surgical removal or excision may be recommended to eliminate the abnormal tissue [1, 2].

Supportive care plays an essential role in the overall management of pinna diseases. This can include regular cleaning and hygiene practices to maintain the cleanliness of the pinna, especially in cases of chronic infections or recurrent issues. Environmental modifications, such as avoiding allergens or irritants, can help minimize symptoms in allergic conditions. Providing pain management strategies, such as analgesics or local anesthetics, may be necessary to alleviate discomfort associated with certain pinna diseases. Additionally, ongoing monitoring, follow-up visits, and adherence to treatment protocols are crucial for successful outcomes. This allows for evaluation of treatment effectiveness, adjustment of medications if needed, and timely intervention in case of any complications or recurrence.

PREVENTION AND PROGNOSIS OF PINNA DISEASES

Prevention and prognosis are important considerations when it comes to pinna diseases. Taking proactive measures to prevent these conditions can significantly reduce the risk of their occurrence, while understanding the prognosis helps manage expectations and guide treatment decisions. Let's explore prevention and prognosis of pinna diseases in detail. Prevention of pinna diseases involves several key strategies. Regular ear care and hygiene practices are paramount, including routine cleaning to remove debris and excess moisture that can contribute to infections. Avoiding exposure to irritants or allergens, such as certain plants, chemicals, or environmental triggers, can help minimize the risk of contact dermatitis or allergic reactions affecting the pinna. Protecting the pinna from excessive sun exposure is crucial to prevent sunburn and potential long-term damage, especially in dogs with light-colored or thin-haired pinnae. Additionally, routine veterinary check-ups and monitoring of the pinna's health can help detect any early signs of disease or underlying conditions, enabling prompt intervention [6, 7].

Prognosis for pinna diseases varies depending on the specific condition, severity, and underlying cause. With early recognition and appropriate treatment, many pinna diseases have a good prognosis. Bacterial and fungal infections, when treated promptly and effectively, often resolve with minimal long-term consequences. However, chronic or recurring infections may require ongoing management to prevent relapses. Traumatic injuries to the pinna, such as lacerations or hematomas, can generally heal well with appropriate medical or surgical interventions [4]. Prognosis for pinna tumors or growths depends on factors such as the type of tumor, its location, and the extent of infiltration. Early detection and surgical removal, when feasible, can improve the prognosis in such cases. For age-related changes or certain breed-specific pinna conditions, management focuses on providing supportive care and minimizing discomfort.

CONCLUSION

It is important to note that the prognosis can vary from case to case, and some pinna diseases may have more complex or chronic courses. The involvement of underlying systemic conditions or complications can also impact the prognosis. Regular follow-up visits with the veterinarian, adherence to treatment plans, and ongoing monitoring of the pinna's health are crucial to evaluate progress, adjust treatment if needed, and manage any potential recurrences or complications effectively.

REFERENCES

[1]   Mak SL, Au SL, Tang WF, Li CH, Lee CC, Chiu WH. A Study on Hearing Hazards and sound measurement for Dogs. In: ISPCE-ASIA 2022 - IEEE International Symposium on Product Compliance Engineering - Asia 2022. Institute of Electrical and Electronics Engineers Inc.; 2022.
[http://dx.doi.org/10.1109/ISPCE-ASIA57917.2022.9970899]

[2]   Brown C. Surgical management of canine aural hematoma. Lab Anim (NY) [Internet]. 2010; 39(4): 104–5.
[http://dx.doi.org/10.1038/laban0410-104] [PMID: 20305632]

[3]   Cole LK. Anatomy and physiology of the canine ear. Vet Dermatol [Internet]. 2009; 20(5–6): 412–21.
[http://dx.doi.org/10.1111/j.1365-3164.2009.00849.x] [PMID: 20178478]

[4]   Matousek JL. Diseases of the ear pinna [Internet]. Vol. 34, Veterinary clinics of north america - small animal practice. 2004; p. 511–40. Available from: https://www.vetsmall.theclinics.com/article/S0195-5616(03)00165-7/abstract
[http://dx.doi.org/10.1016/j.cvsm.2003.10.014] [PMID: 15062622]

[5]   Rosser EJ. Causes of otitis externa [Internet]. Vol. 34, Veterinary Clinics of North America - Small Animal Practice. 2004; p. 459–68. Available from: https://www.vetsmall.theclinics.com/article/S0195-5616(03)00157-8/abstract
[http://dx.doi.org/10.1016/j.cvsm.2003.10.006] [PMID: 15062619]

[6]   Moller C, Neel JA, Marcia MK. Aural cytology. In: Small Animal Cytologic Diagnosis [Internet]. 2016; p. 407–31. Available from: https://books.google.com/books?hl=en&lr=&id= WcDBDAAAQBAJ&oi=fnd&pg=PA407&dq=in+dogs+Fungal+infections+of+the+pinna,+also+kno wn+as+otomycosis,+are+commonly+caused+by+organisms+such+as+Malassezia+spp.,+Candida+spp .,+and+Aspergillus+spp&ots=W-OCKs62FV&sig=9J
       [http://dx.doi.org/10.1201/9781315373560-16]

[7]   Newton H. Parasitic Skin Diseases. Clinical Atlas of Canine and Feline Dermatology. Wiley 2019; pp. 111-31.
       [http://dx.doi.org/10.1002/9781119226338.ch7]

[8]   Noxon JO. Otitis in the Allergic Dog. Veterinary Allergy. Wiley Blackwell 2013; pp. 175-82.
       [http://dx.doi.org/10.1002/9781118738818.ch27]

[9]   Harvey R. A Review of Recent Developments in Veterinary Otology [Internet]. Vol. 9, Veterinary Sciences. 2022. Available from: https://www.mdpi.com/2306-7381/9/4/161

[10]   Kumar S, Hussain K, Sharma R, Chhibber S, Sharma N. Prevalence of canine otitis externa in jammu. J Anim Res. 2014; 4(1): 121. Available from: https://www.indianjournals.com/ijor.aspx?target= ijor:jar&volume=4&issue=1&article=015
       [http://dx.doi.org/10.5958/2277-940X.2014.00083.7]

CHAPTER 10

Food Allergy and Otitic Pruritus

Abhishek Kalundia[1,*]

[1] *Cornerstone Pet Clinic, Hyderabad-500089, India*

Abstract: Otitis due to allergy induced by dietary protein is a common problem in dogs and cats. Topical treatment mostly seems to be successful as temporary relief, but chronic recurrence of inflammation and infection can lead to permanent inflammatory changes, discomfort and anatomical dis-arrangements, with anti-microbial resistance. This makes the otitis condition difficult to treat by a veterinarian. Eventually, the changes can become irreversible and require a total ear canal ablation/lateral bulla osteotomy or ablative laser surgery. Proper diagnosis of subtle changes in an animal's lifestyle, diet and skin pattern is very important to be noticed. Most importantly, clinicians must appreciate that all recurrent ear infections in dogs are secondary. Treatment are usually in 2-3 phases: treating the root cause of the allergy, treating the ongoing damage and inflammation and pruritus, and elimination of secondary infections/ organisms. This will typically involve ear cleaning, topical anti-microbial therapy, and topical or systemic glucocorticoids. Novel treatments including herbs and special animal extracts for infection and inflammation may offer additional options in the future. Understanding the underlying causes and pathogenesis of the disease condition, diagnosing it at the right time and addressing the treatment in collaboration and association with primary veterinarian, referral dermatologist and pet parents can make a huge difference in the treatment outcome of food allergy induced otitis.

Keywords: Atpy dermatitis, Allergens, Cats, Cyclosporin, Dogs, Food allergy, Hypothyroidism, Licorice root extracts, Otitis, Palmitoylethanolamide.

INTRODUCTION

An allergy is an immune response where a pet's body responds to a stimuli/trigger allergen. Often these are environmental or food related [1, 2]. Be it any allergen, any pet parent, guardian and the veterinary clinician would always prefer to get to the bottom of the route of causative allergen.

Allergy induced ear infections in dogs can be painful and recurrent in nature. Allergies cause the skin barriers within the ears to break down. This leads to increased wax production which allows yeast, bacteria and inflammation of the

---

[*] **Corresponding author Abhishek Kalundia:** Cornerstone Pet Clinic, Hyderabad-500089, India;
E-mail: dr.abhimed@rediffmail.com

ear, which is termed as otitis. Clinically allergy induced otitis are similar to otitis externa. When we tilt the ear flap and investigate the ear canal, they appear red, itchy and, pruritus, due to the allergy manifestation. Pain with discharge of various degrees and nature can be seen. In many of the cases this ear condition leads to stenosis of the ear canal. Most of the dogs with allergic otitis due to canine adverse food reaction will also have generalized skin infection. Groin and axilla regions may have erythematous spots with small pustules [3, 4].

CANINE ADVERSE FOOD REACTIONS - BRIEF

Canine food allergy is an undesired immunological reaction, when a certain protein ingredient of the pet's food is either changed or converted into molecules which are considered foreign molecules by the immune system. This triggers inflammatory and hypersensitivity reactions to various organs. In dogs and cats it's mostly in skin. Common food allergens (Jackson, 2023) known in canine pets are chicken, corn, eggs, potatoes and lentils. Dogs and cats with chronic otitis due to food allergy may also have dermatological manifestations of erythema, focal alopecia with discharges, rashes, and generalized alopecia. Many studies have reported a more close association of allergic diseases such ascontact allergy, food allergy, and atopic dermatitis, and also predisposition to be more prone to develop an otitis in many breeds, including the Dalmatian, Labrador retrievers, Pugs, American cocker spaniel, golden retriever, Chinese shar-pei, German shepherd dog, beagle, French bulldog, and Jack Russell terrier [5, 6].

In dogs, symptoms include facial itching, foot or limb chewing, itchy anal area, and recurrent ear infections.

1. No response to steroid therapy.

2. Five signs of canine food allergy.

3. Non seasonal generalized pruritus.

4. Accompanying signs of gastrointestinal disorders.

5. Recurrent ear and anal region infection and irritation.

6. Age of onset is either less than six months or more than five years.

One study of dogs with atopic dermatitis, food hypersensitivity, or both, showed that 58 of 120 dogs (48%) had inflamed ears without exudation and 62 dogs (52%) had otitis with an infectious component [7, 8].

CANINE FOOD ALLERGIC OTITIS - BRIEF

In recent years, canines and felines usually tend to have far more frequency of otitis than expected, sometimes as constant as throughout the year. It is often of multifactorial aetiology and may be part of a generalized skin disease or underlying systemic illness. Although initial symptomatic therapy is appropriate for early, acute cases of otitis externa, a systematic and thorough approach involving detailed history taking, complete physical and dermatological examinations, and appropriate diagnostic work-up is required when investigating and treating chronic otitis externa.

The internal ear canal structure pre-disposes the ears of cats and specially dogs. Unlike in humans, dogs ears are composed of two components - vertical component and horizontal component. This "J" shape of the dog's ear creates a predisposition to ear infections as debris must work its way upward rather than straight out [9, 10]. If ear wax cannot get out, it accumulates. Accumulation of earwax, skin oil, and other debris feed the bacteria and fungi that live in the normal ear canal leading them to proliferate. Other predisposing factors for chronic otitis are the presence of dense hair in the ear canal, a long and narrow ear canal, pendulous ears flaps, and climate or seasonal factors such as increased temperature and humidity are examples of predisposing factors [11, 12]. Both bilateral and unilateral otitis externa may be seen with food adverse reactions. Allergic skin disease affecting the ears is the most common cause for recurring increased ear wax production/ear infection. Allergens further facilitate the accumulation of the wax and infection [13]. A study reported that 52% of dogs with chronic otitis will end up with Otitis. With the deep internal structure of the ears are associated some important nerves. Damage of which can lead to signs and symptoms of a vestibular disease. Many studies have documented that *Malassezia* spp. yeast or cocci, and other infections like rods have been commonly found as secondary infectious organisms in dogs with food allergic otitis [14, 15].

The cause of otitis externa is often multifactorial. There have been several different classification schemes proposed to explain the pathogenesis of otitis [16]. Many studies have reported that of the allergy like atopy dermatitis with otitis in animals and have focused on the changes seen on the pinnae, specifically the erythema. Pinnal erythema is the predominant ear change seen in early and mild cases of allergic otitis [17, 18]. After chronicity of the allergic otitis, most dogs are found to have developed secondary bacterial with or without yeast infections, resulting to a more severe erythema, exudation, and proliferative changes characterized by hyperplasia of the epithelium and stenosis of the ear canal [19, 20].

Atopic dermatitis (also referred to as non-food- induced atopic dermatitis) has the strongest association of allergy with otitis, with several studies confirming a high incidence of otitis in dogs with atopic dermatitis [21, 22]. Most of the studies have documented that the age of onset of allergic otitis coincides with the age of onset of clinical signs of atopic dermatitis in dogs. It can go as high as 31% among the less than one year old dogs with their first onset of otitis along with atopic dermatitis lesions [23, 24].

DIAGNOSIS OF FOOD ALLERGIC OTITIS

Allergic otitis, especially otitis externa, is one of the most clinical presentations in a small animal clinic/hospital. Unlike other diseased conditions where there are some sort of tests which can indicate and confirm the diseases, there is no definite test for food allergy otitis. Hence canne food allergy induced otitis is totally based on clinical signs and symptoms and clinician's skill of collecting a comprehensive detailed anamnesis. It is very important for a veterinary dermatologist to rule out all the possibilities of other disorders and allergens like airborne inhalant allergens, atopy dermatitis, scabies and flea allergy dermatitis, before concluding that the pet has food allergy induced otitis [25, 26].

Food allergic induced otitis needs a thorough history about the pets lifestyle, diet, husbandry, travel history, boarding, tick and flea prevention, any current medications in use, any other clinical history of the animal, accompanying pets history and their well being and exposure to outdoor grass, play area is very necessary. Food hypersensitivity should be strongly considered when otitis or pinnal erythema/pruritus is the only clinical sign [27, 28].

Clinical signs upon preliminary physical examination [29]:

1. Pododermatitis

2. Perianal alopecia.

3. Constant head shaking.

4. Red, bronze or brown nail beds.

5. Yeast and musty foul odor from the ears.

6. Bronzing around the lips with yeast infection.

7. Pruritus and ventral abdomen erythema and dull hair coat.

8. Bilateral or occasional unilateral epiphora or conjunctivitis.

9. Chronic recurrent ear infection more than two to three times a year.

10. Pink skin with pustules or epidermal collarettes which do not go despite medicated shampoo baths.

An expert usage of portable otoscopy followed by a deep ear cleaning or flushing is mandated for a complete examination of the ear. To keep the pet comfortable, a veterinarian may decide to sedate or anesthetize for the procedure. Then the infection and its lesions can be more easily seen with an otoscope, up to the level of the eardrum.

Above mentioned signs have been found more in breeds (Bhagat, *et al.*, 2017) with drooping pendulous ears. The anatomy in these breeds is such that the ear canal doesn't get fresh air to breath. Which later gives a favorable environment for the germs to grow more and cause secondary inflammation and pus. Author agrees with many previous documents which support this fact. In case of chronic end stage ear infections, vestibular disease signs (head tilt, abnormal eye ball movement with or without ataxia) is seen [30, 31].

Certain labs may claim to do a complete allergy profile test but they aren't 100% useful. These blood tests can only detect antibodies against certain food proteins, but this does not necessarily mean the pet has an allergy. It may mean nothing more than the patient has eaten that type of protein before. Elimination dietary trial where in the pet is fed the hypoallergenic diet for a period of about two months is done. Once the pet has recovered from the ear and other skin lesions completely, or when the decided period of time is over, the pet is again made to undergo a challenge of exposure to the old die and seen for a maximum of about two weeks (Table **1**). If the itching recurs then the diagnosis is confirmed and the pet is advised to give the same hypoallergenic diet indefinitely [32, 33].

Table 1. Differential diagnosis of chronic otitis due to food allergy.

S. No.	Condition	Comments
1	Atopy Dermatißtis	Usually seasonal and good response to immunosuppressive therapies and steroids.
2	Scabies	Crusting seen along the Edges and lateral aspects of pinnae
3	Otodectic mites	Coffee grounds appearance of debris in the ear canals
4	Foreign body	Mostly unilateral ear lesion and acute onset.

(Table 1) cont.....

S. No.	Condition	Comments
5	Hyperadrenocorticism	Serum biochemistry revelas = Elevated SAP, Elevated cholesterol . Elevated ALT. Elevated glucose, Reduced urea, Hemograms reveals = leukocytosis, neutrophilia, lymphopenia and eosinopenia Urinalysis = Low specific gravity and Elevated, cortisol:creatinine ratio Radiographs = hepatomegaly, osteoporosis, mineralization of adrenal glands Low-dose dexamethasone suppression test, ACTH assays, Ultrasonography = Increased adrenal gland size ACTH stimulation test
6	Pemphigus foliaceus	Intraepidermal pustule forrnation due to pemphigus antibodies against antigens in the intercellular connections. Good response to steroid therapy.
7	Ceruminous gland adenomas (Cats and dogs) and adenocarcinomas (Dogs)	Unilateral, older animals, Otoscopy.
8	Hypothyroidism	Lymphocytic thyroiditis Serum biochemistry = Elevated SAP, elevated cholesterol, elevated ALT) Hemograms = anemia Thyroid tests = free T4, total T4 and TSH
9	Idiopathic seborrhea	Excessive wax formation even with topical medication. Ear cleaners, retinoids, corticosteroids.

TREATMENT

Main constraints in treating otitis due to adverse food reaction is that not only it takes time to diagnose and find which list of food ingredients are allergic to the pet, but also that it takes a lot of patience to see the repair to the damage which has already happened to the skin.

To date, numerous authors and literature have suggested excellent strategies to approach such conditions. And also, many literature have advised remarkable remedies for the elimination of clinical signs of allergy otitis. In general, a deep flushing technique using sterile saline is recommended to achieve a thorough cleaning of the external ear [34, 35].

Ear flushing with antiseptic mixed with local topical anesthetics would be required as the first line of treatment. Rarely sedation may be required too to ensure patients comfort. Presence of secondary bacterial infection has always been a concomitant finding in chronic recurrent otitis infection. In chronic recurrent otitis, it is always recommended to take the ear flush sample for culture fungal and/or bacterial and antibiotic sensitivity tests. Based on the culture and sensitivity report, a dermatologist can choose to flush the affected ears with a high concentration of selected and suitable antimicrobial medicine with or without corticosteroid,directly into the affected ear canal. In most of the chronic recurrent infectious otitis conditions, specific therapy should always be based on cytological findings [36, 37].

There are various home remedies one can choose to use for the emergency relief of allergic otitis. Twice a day 3-4 drops of a home remedy mixture consisting of two tablespoons of concentrated green tea water with one tablespoon of apple cider vinegar mixed with half teaspoon boric acid powder has been successfully used by the author for the past ten to fourteen years with satisfactory results. Green tea has anti-bacterial and anti-inflammatory properties [38, 39]. Boric acid is a well known anti-inflammatory component with immediate soothing effect. The apple cider vinegar has both antibacterial and antifungal properties. Most common causes of allergy induced otitis have been shown good relief by the above mentioned mixture [40, 41].

Licorice root extracts have been used (@ 0.5 ml per kg body weight twice a day for ten to maximum fourteen days) successfully by the author for severe inflammatory reactions induced by the various food ingredients allergic to a dog or cat. Licorice root is not meant to be used for long term in dogs and cats [42, 43].

Concentrated curcumin (@ 30-50 mg per kg) has also been known to be beneficial in many ailments in dogs and cats [44]

Cannabinoid oil (CBD) is also a well-known herbal medicine which has been extensively used as anti-inflammatory and anti-allergic medicines in dogs for various ailments. The author has been using it @ 3mg (2-3 drops) per 5 kg dog twice a day both orally or topically [44, 45].

Antihistamines like cetrizine (@ 0.5mg per 10 kg dog once a day) and Nettle leaf (half a cup concentrated solution twice a day orally) have also been used extensively in dogs with a satisfied access rate [46].

Along with above mentioned remedies, essential fatty acids have their own vital role to increase the defense mechanism of skin against the allergic reactions from food.

Bioactive Quercetin EMIQ has been also shown to have a good antioxidant and anti-inflammatory property for dogs with food induced allergic otitis . It also modulates the skin immune system to reduce allergies in dogs [47].

Beta Sitosterol is one of the few natural products which have shown a promising result in dogs with atopic dermatitis . generally used with a standard dose for 3-4 weeks [48].

Essential fatty acids such as olive oil, coconut oil, corn oil, cod liver oil and salmon oil are known to disrupt the production of inflammatory chemicals within the skin and reduce the need of antihistamines and steroids for the animal during its treatment. But a clinician should educate the pet parent that it will take about six weeks to build up enough omega 3 fatty acids in the body to see a difference [49].

Plants and animals make a natural substance called Palmitoylethanolamide (PEA). In animals, it helps restore balance to the skin's under sired biochemical reactions and immunological responses and prevents release of the biochemical causes of itching. Presently soybean extrats are available as concentrated form [50].

Systemic therapy with antibiotics, antifungals, and corticosteroids [51] may also be used, depending on the infection. A proper follow up and monitoring the ear infection is advisable for a successful outcome [52]. Some dogs and cats with allergic otitis may develop secondary infections and systemic complications even while receiving appropriate treatment for the allergic disease, sometimes due to secondary diseases or medicines used to treat the serious allergies. Hence, routine diagnostic tests should be performed to monitor such complications as a preventive measure [53].

Regular checkup for the pet's external ear canal and tympanic membrane every 10-14 days is a good practice. (Usually, a ruptured tympanic membrane will generally begin to heal within 21-35 days.) Topical medications should be continued for the affected ear canal until the appearance on physical examination is normal, until the pet has no more history of head shaking or other relevant clinical signs of the allergic otitis and until cytology of the ear canal reveals no infection. Systemic therapy may typically go for about 4-6 weeks, provided the patient is not diagnosed for any other ailment like hypothyroidism or the necessary novel protein diet, which may be included as the part of the therapy life long for an indefinite period of time [52].

PROGNOSIS

In general, the prognosis for dogs and some cats is good if appropriate therapy is started at the right time. The prognosis is not as good if the infection is resistant to the medications; if the pet develops the allergy to an unknown source of food; if the pet's body changes or modifies the protein in the regular food ingredient at some point of time; if the concurrent otitis externa is not managed adequately; if there is significant ulcerated fungal infection; or if there is no response to hyposensitization / hypersensitization therapy. In addition, some neurologic signs (*e.g.,* facial nerve problems, Horner syndrome) and malformed misshapen ear flap post healing due to negligence (aural hematomas) may be permanent [50,51].

PREVENTION

Ear infections will create clinical signs that can mask any clinical improvement from a dietary trial; therefore, some type of maintenance programme to prevent recurrence of infection is necessary. It is always necessary to keep the animals ears clean on a daily basis. Especially when they come in after the walks from outdoors or in the peak time of the year when there is abrupt change in the weather which becomes intolerable for the pets. However, it is not always possible to prevent every infection in some animal patients [51,52].

CONCLUSION

Allergy is one of the most preeminent important factors and etiology use of otitis and otic pruritus, commonly seen in case of canine atopic dermatitis (CAD), food hypersensitivity, and contact allergic reactions. The most common perpetuating and secondary factors also include bacterial and yeast infections, hyperplastic changes along the ear canals, and otitis media. Ear pinnal erythema and hyperkeratosis / hyperplasia is the predominant ear change seen in early and mild cases of allergic otitis in routine clinical practice in dogs. Food hypersensitivity is the second most common hypersensitivity to affect the ear after fore limb paws and skin. The goal of treatment should be to clear the infection from the dog as the first step. This may be done following standards of care for infectious otitis and should include cleaning of the ear canal to remove depositions accumulated within the ear canal and also the infectious agents; followed by specific treatment focused to identify and eradicate the infectious organism identified in the animal's ear. After the secondary infections are controlled in allergic animals with the allergic otitis, pruritus and pain directed at the ears may decrease to comfortable levels if not completely resolved.

REFERENCES

[1] Noxon J O. Otitis in the allergic dog. Veterinary allergy, 2013, 175-182.

[2] Scott DW. Observations on canine atopy. J Am Anim Hosp Assoc 1981; 17: 91-100.

[3] Hillier A. Definitively diagnosing atopic dermatitis in dogs. Vet Med 2002; 97: 198-208.

[4] Favrot C, Steffan J, Seewald W, Picco F. A prospective study on the clinical features of chronic canine atopic dermatitis and its diagnosis. Vet Dermatol 2010; 21(1): 23-31.
[http://dx.doi.org/10.1111/j.1365-3164.2009.00758.x] [PMID: 20187911]

[5] Griffin CE. Otitis externa and otitis media. In: Griffen CE, Kwochka KW, MacDonald JM, Eds. Current Veterinary Therapy: The Science and Art of Therapy. St. Louis: Mosby Year Book 1993; pp. 244-62.

[6] Rosser EJ Jr. Causes of otitis externa. Vet Clin North Am Small Anim Pract 2004; 34(2): 459-68.
[http://dx.doi.org/10.1016/j.cvsm.2003.10.006] [PMID: 15062619]

[7] Zur G, Lifshitz B, Bdolah-Abram T. The association between the signalment, common causes of canine otitis externa and pathogens. J Small Anim Pract 2011; 52(5): 254-8.
[http://dx.doi.org/10.1111/j.1748-5827.2011.01058.x] [PMID: 21539570]

[8] Zur G, Skorinsky I, Bdolah-Abram T. Canine atopic dermatitis in the Middle East: clinical signs, signalment and common allergens. Vet Med (Praha) 2012; 57(8): 410-9.
[http://dx.doi.org/10.17221/6309-VETMED]

[9] Logas DB. Diseases of the ear canal. Vet Clin North Am Small Anim Pract 1994; 24(5): 905-19.
[http://dx.doi.org/10.1016/S0195-5616(94)50108-6] [PMID: 7817493]

[10] Willemse T. Atopic skin disease: a review and a reconsideration of diagnostic criteria. J Small Anim Pract 1986; 27: 771-8.
[http://dx.doi.org/10.1111/j.1748-5827.1986.tb02119.x]

[11] Zur G, Ihrke PJ, White SD, Kass PH. Canine atopic dermatitis: a retrospective study of 266 cases examined at the University of California, Davis, 1992–1998. Part I. Clinical features and allergy testing results. Vet Dermatol 2002; 13(2): 89-102.
[http://dx.doi.org/10.1046/j.1365-3164.2002.00285.x] [PMID: 11972892]

[12] Saridomichelakis MN, Farmaki R, Leontides LS, Koutinas AF. Aetiology of canine otitis externa: a retrospective study of 100 cases. Vet Dermatol 2007; 18(5): 341-7.
[http://dx.doi.org/10.1111/j.1365-3164.2007.00619.x] [PMID: 17845622]

[13] Picco F, Zini E, Nett C, *et al.* A prospective study on canine atopic dermatitis and food-induced allergic dermatitis in Switzerland. Vet Dermatol 2008; 19(3): 150-5.
[http://dx.doi.org/10.1111/j.1365-3164.2008.00669.x] [PMID: 18477331]

[14] Muse R, Griffin C, Rosenkrantz WS. The prevalence of otic manifestations and otitis externa in allergic dogs. Proceedings of the AAVD/ACVD Annual Meeting. Las Vegas, NV, USA. 1996; pp. 33-6.

[15] Fraser MA, McNeil PE, Girling SJ. Prediction of future development of canine atopic dermatitis based on examination of clinical history. J Small Anim Pract 2008; 49(3): 128-32.
[http://dx.doi.org/10.1111/j.1748-5827.2007.00439.x] [PMID: 18005107]

[16] Griffin CE. Canine atopic disease. In: Griffin CE, Kwochka KW, MacDonald JM, Eds. Current Veterinary Therapy: The Science and Art of Therapy. St. Louis: Mosby Year Book 1993; pp. 99-120.

[17] White SD. Food hypersensitivity in 30 dogs. J Am Vet Med Assoc 1986; 188(7): 695-8.
[PMID: 3700223]

[18] Carlotti DN, Remy I, Prost C. Food allergy in dogs and cats. A review and report of 43 cases. Vet Dermatol 1990; 1(2): 55-62.
[http://dx.doi.org/10.1111/j.1365-3164.1990.tb00080.x] [PMID: 34233395]

[19]   Harvey RG. Food allergy and dietary intolerance in dogs: A report of 25 cases. J Small Anim Pract 1993; 34(4): 175-9.
[http://dx.doi.org/10.1111/j.1748-5827.1993.tb02647.x]

[20]   Chesney CJ. Food sensitivity in the dog: a quantitative study. J Small Anim Pract 2002; 43(5): 203-7.
[http://dx.doi.org/10.1111/j.1748-5827.2002.tb00058.x] [PMID: 12038852]

[21]   Chesney CJ. Food sensitivity in the dog: a quantitative study. J Small Anim Pract. 2002 May;43(5):203-7.

[22]   Jaeger K, Linek M, Power HT, *et al.* Breed and site predispositions of dogs with atopic dermatitis: a comparison of five locations in three continents. Vet Dermatol 2010; 21(1): 119-23.
[http://dx.doi.org/10.1111/j.1365-3164.2009.00845.x] [PMID: 20187918]

[23]   Loeffler A, Soares-Magalhaes R, Bond R, Lloyd DH. A retrospective analysis of case series using home-prepared and chicken hydrolysate diets in the diagnosis of adverse food reactions in 181 pruritic dogs. Vet Dermatol 2006; 17(4): 273-9.
[http://dx.doi.org/10.1111/j.1365-3164.2006.00522.x] [PMID: 16827671]

[24]   Nuttall T, Cole LK. Ear cleaning: the UK and US perspective. Vet Dermatol 2004; 15(2): 127-36.
[http://dx.doi.org/10.1111/j.1365-3164.2004.00375.x] [PMID: 15030561]

[25]   Colombo S, Hill PB, Shaw DJ, Thoday KL. Requirement for additional treatment for dogs with atopic dermatitis undergoing allergen-specific immunotherapy. Vet Rec 2007; 160(25): 861-4.
[http://dx.doi.org/10.1136/vr.160.25.861] [PMID: 17586789]

[26]   Abraham G, Gottschalk J, Ungemach FR. Evidence for ototopical glucocorticoid-induced decrease in hypothalamic-pituitary-adrenal axis response and liver function. Endocrinology 2005; 146(7): 3163-71.
[http://dx.doi.org/10.1210/en.2005-0080] [PMID: 15802495]

[27]   Aniya JS, Griffin CE. The effect of otic vehicle and concentration of dexamethasone on liver enzyme activities and adrenal function in small breed healthy dogs. Vet Dermatol 2008; 19(4): 226-31.
[http://dx.doi.org/10.1111/j.1365-3164.2008.00680.x] [PMID: 19086122]

[28]   Meyer DJ, Moriello KA, Feder BM, Fehrer-Sawyer SL, Maxwell AK. Effect of otic medications containing glucocorticoids on liver function test results in healthy dogs. J Am Vet Med Assoc 1990; 196(5): 743-4.
[http://dx.doi.org/10.2460/javma.1990.196.05.743] [PMID: 1968451]

[29]   Saridomichelakis MN, Farmaki R, Leontides LS, Koutinas AF. Aetiology of canine otitis externa: a retrospective study of 100 cases. Vet Dermatol 2007; 18(5): 341-7.
[http://dx.doi.org/10.1111/j.1365-3164.2007.00619.x] [PMID: 17845622]

[30]   Jackson HA. Food allergy in dogs and cats; current perspectives on etiology, diagnosis, and management. J Am Vet Med Assoc 2023; 261(S1): S23-9.
[http://dx.doi.org/10.2460/javma.22.12.0548] [PMID: 36917613]

[31]   Kennis R. Otitis Externa. Small Animal Soft Tissue Surgery, 2023, 846-850.

[32]   Bellah J R. Anatomy of the Ear. Small Animal Soft Tissue Surgery, 2023, 817-827.

[33]   Yang Y, Ding F, Xu T, *et al.* Double-stapled anastomosis without "dog-ears" reduces the anastomotic leakage in laparoscopic anterior resection of rectal cancer: A prospective, randomized, controlled study. Front Surg 2023; 9: 1003854.
[http://dx.doi.org/10.3389/fsurg.2022.1003854] [PMID: 36684218]

[34]   Mehmedov T N, Vacheva I B, Genova K I. Comparative analysis of different methods of treatment of atopic otitis in dogs. Bulgarian Journal of Animal Husbandry/Životnov Dni Nauki, 2023; 60(1).

[35]   Tinsley J, Griffin C, Sheinberg G, *et al.* An open-label clinical trial to evaluate the efficacy of an elemental diet for the diagnosis of adverse food reactions in dogs. Vet Dermatol 2023.
[PMID: 37621253]

[36] Wills J, Harvey R. Diagnosis and management of food allergy and intolerance in dogs and cats. Aust Vet J 1994; 71(10): 322-6.
[http://dx.doi.org/10.1111/j.1751-0813.1994.tb00907.x] [PMID: 7848179]

[37] Gotthelf LN. Diagnosis and treatment of otitis media in dogs and cats. Vet Clin North Am Small Anim Pract 2004; 34(2): 469-87.
[http://dx.doi.org/10.1016/j.cvsm.2003.10.007] [PMID: 15062620]

[38] Tiffany S, Parr JM, Templeman J, *et al.* Assessment of dog owners' knowledge relating to the diagnosis and treatment of canine food allergies. Can Vet J 2019; 60(3): 268-74.
[PMID: 30872849]

[39] Ghaly MF, Shaheen AA, Bouhy AM, Bendary MM. Alternative therapy to manage otitis media caused by multidrug-resistant fungi. Arch Microbiol 2020; 202(5): 1231-40.
[http://dx.doi.org/10.1007/s00203-020-01832-z] [PMID: 32108246]

[40] Levi JR, Brody RM, McKee-Cole K, Pribitkin E, O'Reilly R. Complementary and alternative medicine for pediatric otitis media. Int J Pediatr Otorhinolaryngol 2013; 77(6): 926-31.
[http://dx.doi.org/10.1016/j.ijporl.2013.03.009] [PMID: 23562352]

[41] Adriztina I, Adenin LI, Lubis YM. Efficacy of boric acid as a treatment of choice for chronic suppurative otitis media and its ototoxicity. Korean J Fam Med 2018; 39(1): 2-9.
[http://dx.doi.org/10.4082/kjfm.2018.39.1.2] [PMID: 29383205]

[42] Leung AKC, Wong AHC. Acute otitis media in children. Recent Pat Inflamm Allergy Drug Discov 2017; 11(1): 32-40.
[http://dx.doi.org/10.2174/1874609810666170712145332] [PMID: 28707578]

[43] Ural K, Gültekïn M, Erdoğan S, Erdoğan H. Antipruritic armamentarium with short term nutritional support solution involving slymarin and curcumin for atopic dermatitis in dogs. Vet J Meh Ak Ers Uni 2021; 6(1): 8-13.
[http://dx.doi.org/10.24880/maeuvfd.762776]

[44] Gaspar MIDC. 2021.A survey of the attidues, beliefs and knowledge about medical cannabis among vegetarians, veterinary students and atopic dog owners

[45] Tshiteya RM. Herbal medicines for common ailments: a quick reference guide. Natural Remedies, Inc. 2007.

[46] Salas, A. L., Ordóñez, R. M., Silva, C., Maldonado, L., Bedascarrasbure, E., Isla, M. I.

[47] Zampini, I. C. Antimicrobial activity of Argentinean propolis against Staphylococcus isolated of canine otitis. 2014.

[48] Varghese KJ, Anila J, Nagalekshmi R, Resiya S, Sonu J. Dasapushpam: The traditional uses and the therapeutic potential of ten sacred plants of Kerala state in India. Int J Pharm Sci Res 2010; 1(10): 50.

[49] Sævik BK, Bergvall K, Holm BR, *et al.* A randomized, controlled study to evaluate the steroid sparing effect of essential fatty acid supplementation in the treatment of canine atopic dermatitis. Vet Dermatol 2004; 15(3): 137-45.
[http://dx.doi.org/10.1111/j.1365-3164.2004.00378.x] [PMID: 15214949]

[50] Noli C, della Valle MF, Miolo A, Medori C, Schievano C. Efficacy of ultra-micronized palmitoylethanolamide in canine atopic dermatitis: an open-label multi-centre study. Vet Dermatol 2015; 26(6): 432-440, e101.
[http://dx.doi.org/10.1111/vde.12250] [PMID: 26283633]

[51] Nuttall T. Managing recurrent otitis externa in dogs: what have we learned and what can we do better? J Am Vet Med Assoc 2023; 261(S1): S10-22.
[http://dx.doi.org/10.2460/javma.23.01.0002] [PMID: 37019436]

[52] Zwueste DM, Grahn BH. A review of Horner's syndrome in small animals. Can Vet J 2019; 60(1): 81-8.

[PMID: 30651655]

[53]   Ahirwar V, Chandrapuria VP, Bhargava MK, Shrivastava OP, Shahi A, Jawre S. A study on etiology and occurrence of canine aural haematoma. Indian J Vet Surg 2007; 28(2): 137-8.

CHAPTER 11

Ceruminous Otitis and its Clinical Management

S.K. Maiti[1]**, Shraddha Sinha**[1,*] **and Varun Kumar Sarkar**[2]

[1] *Department of Teaching Veterinary Clinical Complex, Anjora, Durg, Chhattisgarh, India*

[2] *Division of Medicine, ICAR-IVRI Izatnagar, Bareilly (UP), India*

Abstract: Ceruminous otitis is the most common type of multifactorial disorder in dogs and is commonly associated with bacterial and/or yeast infections. The main diagnostic workup for Ceruminous otitis requires a detailed history, thorough physical as well as ear examinations, and cytologic evaluation. Diagnostic imaging may be essential tool for assessing the extent of mineralization of cartilage in the external ear and destruction of bone in the middle ear. If the ear canals are severely inflamed, pretreatment with systemic anti-inflammatory drugs is needed before flushing. Frequent ear cleaning with appropriate topical medication can control the odor associated with this condition. Steroids, cytotoxic drugs, and retinoic acid have variable effects to control ceruminous otitis.

Keywords: Ceruminous otitis, Chronic inflammation, Dog, Hyperplasia, Treatment.

INTRODUCTION

An inflammatory condition affecting the external ear canal, including the ear pinna, is known as otitis externa. Acute or chronic otitis externa can occur which is, Recurring or persistent otitis, and can last three months or more—. Chronic inflammation can cause changes in the external ear canal, such as glandular dilatation, glandular hyperplasia, hyperplasia of the epithelium, and hyperkeratosis. These alterations typically lead to an increase in the development of cerumen along the external ear canal, which raises the external ear canal's pH and local humidity and puts the ear at risk for secondary infection [1]. *Staphylococcus* species are the bacteria that are most frequently isolated from the ear canals of dogs that have otitis. Other bacteria that are frequently linked to otitis are *Corynebacterium*, *Pseudomonas*, *Proteus*, *Enterococcus* and *Streptococcus*. Certain bacteria, like *Staphylococcus* and *Pseudomonas*, have the ability to form biofilm, which can cause an infection to persist even in the face of

* **Corresponding author Shraddha Sinha:** Department of Teaching Veterinary Clinical Complex, Anjora, Durg, Chhattisgarh, India; E-mail: sinhashraddha220@gmail.com

Tanmoy Rana (Ed.)

appropriate treatment. This is because any antimicrobial therapy that aims to eradicate the infection must first break down the biofilm. Another prevalent cause of canine otitis externa is *Malassezia* yeast. It seems that certain dogs react allergically to *Malassezia* species, causing severe itching and pain. Treatment for acute and simple otitis externa is frequently successful; while more difficult for chronic or recurring otitis externa. Usually, there are underlying fundamental causes—including secondary otic infection—as well as predisposing and perpetuating variables at work. In addition to causing patient discomfort, severe glandular alterations, fibrosis, stenosis, and calcification along the external ear canal cause otitis media to evolve from acute to chronic and from simple to complex otic illness. These alterations are suggestive of end-stage ear disease, which is typically preventable with early intervention for both primary and secondary diseases [2].

ETIOLOGY

Chronic irritation of the ear canal's sebaceous and ceruminous glands can lead to hyperplasia, cystic dilatation of the ceruminous glands, and an increase in the activity of the sebaceous glands that cover them. The surplus cerumen secreted by ceruminous glands creates an ideal environment for the development of yeast and secondary bacteria. These organisms, which include *Pseudomonas* species, *Proteus* species, and *Malassezia pachydermatis*, are typical members of the ear flora. While some breeds with pendulous ears, can cause these organisms to develop excessively inside the ear canal as pendulous ears prevents air circulation and leads to incorrect drainage [3].

The external ear canal is obstructed by epidermal hyperplasia and inflammatory response in the majority of ceruminous otitis patients, making visual inspection challenging. Hyperplasia of the ear canal in dogs and cats can mimic neoplastic diseases, potentially resulting in incorrect diagnosis and therapy. Surgical surgery is frequently the preferred course of treatment when hyperplasia is unresponsive to medication and the ear canal becomes harder. Correct drainage is made possible by opening the ear canal surgically. For surgery to be successful, underlying infections must be found and treated.

Principal Elements

Primary factors include endocrine disorders like hypothyroidism, otic neoplasia, and foreign bodies. Otic parasites like *Otodectes cyanotis* and hypersensitivity diseases like food allergies, atopic dermatitis, and contact hypersensitivity are examples of diseases that directly affects the external ear canal and can cause otitis. The most frequent primary cause of canine otitis media is underlying hypersensitivity illness.

Contributing Variables

Predisposing circumstances are those that change the environment in the ear canal locally and raise the possibility of developing otitis externa. Excessive hair growth in the ears, stenotic ears, elevated cerumen production in the canals, otic masses, regular ear cleanings, variations in the outside temperature, and high levels of humidity may serve as risk factors [4].

Perpetuating Factors

Even after the underlying cause of the ear illness have been found and addressed, there are still elements that might exacerbate the inflammatory process without causing the disease itself. These factors are known as perpetuating factors. Common sustaining factors are bacteria like *Staphylococcus* and *Pseudomonas*, as well as yeast like *Malassezia*. The presence of the infection in the middle ear may also serve as a sustaining factor for repeated external ear infections if it spreads to the tympanic bulla. When treating dogs with recurrent otitis externa, perpetuating factors are frequently the primary cause of therapy failure (Fig. **1**).

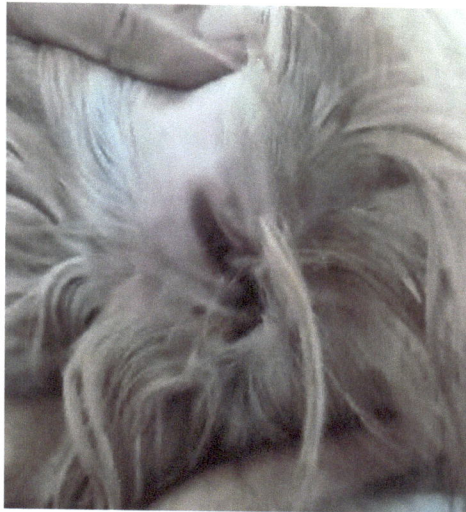

Fig. (1). Ceruminous otitis in dog.

DIAGNOSIS

The history, otoscopic examination, and cytology are used to make the diagnosis.

Otitis externa is not associated with any particular sex distribution. More often affected animals are younger ones. Otitis media reflects the same breed tendencies as skin diseases (allergies in retrievers and terriers, for example). Any combination of head shaking, ear manipulation pain, mal-odour, exudate, erythema, erosion, ulceration, oedema, or ceruminous gland hyperplasia can be considered as clinical symptom [5].

The ears should be inspected (the least affected/painful initially) followed by a thorough physical examination and dermatological evaluation. Sedation or systemic glucocorticoids may be necessary in exceptionally painful patients for a few days before to an otoscopic examination. The pinna and ear canals can be palpated to detect the presence of discomfort, mineralization (from chronicity), and oedema. Individuals who have significant, long-term alterations in their ear canals may require more sophisticated ear imaging. It is important to assess the pinnae for exudate presence, lichenification, ulceration, crusting, erosion, and erythema. Pinnae can be sampled *via* dermatophyte culture, skin scrapes/mineral oil preps (Demodex, Sarcoptes), or surface cytology (yeast, bacteria, inflammatory cells).

If possible, otoscopic assessment needs to be carried out on all patients with dermatology. Most of the time, a handheld otoscope will do, however video otoscopes can offer more magnification, which improves visibility of the tympanic membrane and canals.

Examining the canal should include looking for lumps, exudate (quantity and quality), glandular hyperplasia, erythema, erosion/ulceration, and stenosis. Whenever possible examining the tympanic membrane for bulging, rupture, or colour changes should be done . However, because of the exudate in the horizontal canal, the membrane is frequently invisible, necessitating cleaning or flushing. Prior to doing any cleaning, samples (cytology, mineral oil preps) should be taken.

Most dogs and cats have tiny amounts of commensal gram-positive cocci and yeast in their external ear canals. In the event that the microenvironment is altered and these organisms are encouraged to proliferate, they could turn pathogenic. A cotton-tipped applicator can be used to collect exudate, which can then be rolled onto a glass slide, stained with a modified Wright's stain or 3-step fast stain, and viewed under a microscope. (A study has demonstrated that ear swab cytology can be performed without heat fixing.) Microscopically examining smears at 4x, 10x, and oil immersion magnification will reveal the following: the quantity and shape of keratinocytes, bacteria, yeast, and WBCs; signs of microorganism phagocytosis; fungal hyphae; and acantholytic or neoplastic cells [6].

A Diff- Quick stained smear can be used to detect the presence of microbial overgrowth. Typically, *Streptococci* or *Staphylococci* are the coccal types, where as the typical rod-shaped organisms are *Proteus mirabilis*, *Escherichia coli*, or

Pseudomonas aeruginosa. Since many gram-negative rods (*Pseudomonas*) respond better to specific antibiotic classes (fluoroquinolones, aminoglycosides), a gram stain may be helpful if numerous rods are discovered. An infection with *Pseudomonas* is strongly suggested by ear canal ulcers, a slimy green discharge, and cytology that reveals only rods if a gram stain is not available. A very strong smell may also be connected to otitis externa that is primarily caused by infections with gram-negative rods. Although cultures from the horizontal canal can also be done in these situations, most of the time ear cultures are not needed because even resistant bacteria will usually respond to topical therapy as the antibiotics are being given at much higher levels than those assessed in susceptibility reports. The fact that numerous neutrophils are phagocytosing bacteria indicates that the organisms are harmful [7].

In an healty ears of dog's and cat's, yeast (*Malassezia pachydermatis*) may be present in small amounts, which usually multiplies during an ear infection occurs. In surface cytology samples taken from ears that are impacted, they are occasionally observed on the surface of exfoliated squamous epithelial cells. Topical treatment for yeast otitis usually involves an antifungal and a steroid to help in reducing the inflammation [8].

Otic exudate should be checked for eggs, larvae, while in adults for ear mites *Otodectes cynotis* and *Demodex* spp. in dogs and cats, and *Psoroptes cuniculi* in rabbits and goats, in addition to stained cytology. *Otodectes cynotis* in cats should raise serious suspicions when dark, 'coffee-ground' exudate is present [9]. On a glass slide, smears are made by mixing otic discharge and cerumen with a tiny amount of mineral oil. It is recommended to use a cover glass and observe the smear with low-power magnification. In rare cases, refractory ceruminous otitis externa in dogs and cats may be the only affected area of the body and be linked to a localised growth of *Demodex* spp. in the external ear canals [10].

The histopathologic alterations linked to persistent otitis externa are frequently non-specific.

Biopsies are often recommended in cases where an ear canal tumour is impeding it. There may be additional clinical indications in addition to those detected in the ear if the underlying issue is an allergy, endocrine, or autoimmune illness [11].

When proliferative tissues impede sufficient visualisation of the tympanic membrane, when otitis media is suspected of being the source of relapsing bacterial otitis externa, and when neurologic symptoms coexist with otitis externa, radiography of the osseous bullae is recommended. Proliferative or lytic osseous alterations, along with fluid densities, are frequently indicative of middle ear involvement. Regrettably, in many otitis media cases, radiographs are normal

[12]. When adequate treatment fails to alleviate severe, chronic otitis media, a CT or MRI scan, if one is available, should be conducted. On the other hand, some clinically normal dogs have middle ear fluid visible on CT or MRI scans [13].

TREATMENT

- Address the underlying causes of the external otitis.
- Choose antibiotics according to cytology and history.

Otitis externa can be successfully treated with owner compliance, inflammation control, targeted antibiotic therapy, and underlying cause. Owners must set realistic expectations and be aware that treating or improving otitis externa may take some time.

Many patients first need their discomfort and/or itching to be managed. Glucocorticoids lessen pain, oedema, and inflammation, which eventually improves the owner's capacity to properly care for and clean the ears at home. Most frequently utilised medications are prednisone and triamcinolone; dosage and length of usage vary according to disease severity and chronicity. Owners may occasionally need to wait a few days for the glucocorticoids to start working before they may clean their ears at home.

Cleaning infected ears with thick, dry, or waxy debris two - three times a week using a ceruminolytic solution such dioctyl sodium sulfosuccinate (DSS) or carbamide peroxide may be necessary. It may be necessary to clean infected ears with abundant purulent discharge once or twice a day. Squalene should be included in the ear cleaner if rods are observed, as *Pseudomonas* may be the reason. These bacteria can create a biofilm that shields microorganisms from antibiotics. Rinse the ears well with warm water to get rid of any remaining ear cleanser. Detergents and DSS should not be used if the tympanic membrane is torn; instead, the ear should be flushed with milder cleansers such as saline, saline plus povidone iodine, or Tris EDTA.

Effective treatment may involve topical and systemic antibacterial and anti-inflammatory therapy in addition to cleansing. Depending on the diagnosis, the course of treatment could last anywhere from seven to ten days to several months. Topical antibacterial drugs combined with corticosteroids minimise exudation, discomfort, oedema, and glandular secretions in the treatment of acute bacterial otitis externa. It is best to use the least potent corticosteroid that will lessen inflammation. Many over-the-counter topical medications combine glucocorticoids, antibiotics, and antifungals. Cytology should be taken into consideration while selecting specific products (for example, gram-negative rod infections may call for an aminoglycoside or fluoroquinolone).

Additionally, when purulent discharge is reduced by glucocorticoids, aminoglycosides—the most frequent antibiotics used in ear medications—work better. Dogs with chronic, highly stenotic ears may need to take prednisone at doses equal to 2 mg/kg/day for two weeks, then taper off. By using a large dose, the likelihood that the ear can be treated medically rather than requiring surgery, such as a complete ear canal ablation, is increased. However, this dose cannot be sustained over an extended period; instead, appropriate treatment of underlying illnesses and secondary infections is needed. When otitis externa is suspected, systemic antibiotics should be given; however, in situations of otitis media, they are not necessary. Nevertheless, as many gram-negative rods are resistant to common first-tier dermatologic antibiotics like cephalexin, the systemic antibiotic must be chosen based on cytology. Topical treatments are usually effective in treating yeast-related otitis externa; however, systemic antifungals like terbinafine (for dogs) or ketoconazole (for cats) may also be useful.

If both otitis externa and otitis media are suspected, a CT or MRI scan can help determine whether a middle ear flush and myringotomy are necessary. After the myringotomy creates an opening into the middle ear, topical ear medicine is applied in sufficient quantities to reach the middle ear.

Treatment duration varies depending on each instance, but it should go on until re-examination and repeat cytology shows that the infection has been cured. Animals suffering from infections caused by bacteria and yeast should undergo physical examinations, and their cytologies should be assessed every week or every other week until no infection is visible. This takes 2-4 weeks for most acute cases. In certain circumstances, a maintenance treatment must be administered indefinitely, and chronic cases may take months to resolve. Evaluation for otitis media should be taken into consideration if cases of otitis externa do not resolve after treating underlying problems, administering the proper therapy, and ensuring owner compliance.

Prevention strategies are the best way to manage chronic otitis. Topical and, in rare instances, systemic medications should be selected based on cytology and history in addition to determining the cause of acute otitis. These medications should have a narrow spectrum and be specific for the current condition, taking into consideration the medications that have been used to treat the current infection. An appropriate first line of treatment is neomycin. Although fluoroquinolone and aminoglycoside antibiotics are the most prevalent components in topical otic medicines, they should not be used unless absolutely necessary for successful therapy.

The owner must be instructed on the use (frequency and duration) of topical products, as many of them combine antibiotic, antifungal, and glucocorticoid drugs. When the ear "looks better," many owners stop taking their medication before the infection is completely cured. When resistance to a given antibiotic has been observed by a failure to respond clinically, the most effective treatments for *Pseudomonas* infections have been polymyxin B and fluoroquinolone drugs.

PREVENTION

Owners should be shown how to properly clean the ears. The frequency of cleaning usually decreases over time from daily to once or twice weekly as a preventive maintenance procedure. The ear canals should be kept dry and well ventilated. Using topical astringents in dogs that swim frequently and preventing water from entering the ear canals during bathing should minimize maceration of the ear canal.

Prolonged maceration damages the skin's protective layer, making the skin more vulnerable to opportunistic infections. In moist ear canals, preventive otic astringents may reduce the incidence of bacterial or fungal infections. Removing hair from the external auditory meatus, concave side of the pinna, and hair-rich ear canals promotes better ventilation and lowers relative humidity. However, if the hair is not bothering you, you shouldn't regularly remove it from the ear canal because doing so can create an acute inflammatory response.

CONCLUSION

Erythemato-ceruminous otitis externa (ECOE), the most common type of otitis in dogs is normally associated with bacterial and/or yeast infections. ECOE is closely associated with a mild or moderate secondary infection. Proper management of inflammation, directed antimicrobial therapy, proper ear cleaning, clipping of hairs around the ear and improvement of ventilation with decrease in humidity in the ears can prevent the occurrence of the ear infection.

REFERENCES

[1]   Gotthelf LN. Small Animal Ear Diseases-E-Book: An Illustrated Guide. Elsevier Health Sciences 2004.

[2]   Huang HP, Little CJL, McNeil PE. Histological changes in the external ear canal of dogs with otitis externa. Vet Dermatol 2009; 20(5-6): 422-8.
[http://dx.doi.org/10.1111/j.1365-3164.2009.00853.x] [PMID: 20178479]

[3]   Zamankhan Malayeri H, Jamshidi S, Zahraei Salehi T. Identification and antimicrobial susceptibility patterns of bacteria causing otitis externa in dogs. Vet Res Commun 2010; 34(5): 435-44.
[http://dx.doi.org/10.1007/s11259-010-9417-y] [PMID: 20526674]

[4]   Saridomichelakis MN, Farmaki R, Leontides LS, Koutinas AF. Aetiology of canine otitis externa: a retrospective study of 100 cases. Vet Dermatol 2007; 18(5): 341-7.

[http://dx.doi.org/10.1111/j.1365-3164.2007.00619.x] [PMID: 17845622]

[5]   Morgan JL, Coulter DB, Marshall AE, Goetsch DD. Effects of neomycin on the waveform of auditory-evoked brain stem potentials in dogs. Am J Vet Res 1980; 41(7): 1077-81.
[PMID: 7436102]

[6]   Mason CL, Paterson S, Cripps PJ. Use of a hearing loss grading system and an owner-based hearing questionnaire to assess hearing loss in pet dogs with chronic otitis externa or otitis media. Vet Dermatol 2013; 24(5): 512-e121.
[http://dx.doi.org/10.1111/vde.12057] [PMID: 23829225]

[7]   Tsuprun V, Cureoglu S, Schachern PA, *et al.* Role of pneumococcal proteins in sensorineural hearing loss due to otitis media. Otol Neurotol 2008; 29(8): 1056-60.
[http://dx.doi.org/10.1097/MAO.0b013e31818af3ad] [PMID: 18833010]

[8]   Cole LK, Rajala-Schultz PJ, Lorch G. Conductive hearing loss in four dogs associated with the use of ointment-based otic medications. Vet Dermatol 2018; 29(4): 341-e120.
[http://dx.doi.org/10.1111/vde.12542] [PMID: 29664150]

[9]   Eger CE, Lindsay P. Effects of otitis on hearing in dogs characterised by brainstem auditory evoked response testing. J Small Anim Pract 1997; 38(9): 380-6.
[http://dx.doi.org/10.1111/j.1748-5827.1997.tb03490.x] [PMID: 9322176]

[10] Shell LG. Otitis media and otitis interna. Etiology, diagnosis, and medical management. Vet Clin North Am Small Anim Pract 1988; 18(4): 885-99.
[http://dx.doi.org/10.1016/S0195-5616(88)50088-8] [PMID: 3264962]

[11] Belmudes A, Pressanti C, Barthez PY, Castilla-Castaño E, Fabries L, Cadiergues MC. Computed tomographic findings in 205 dogs with clinical signs compatible with middle ear disease: a retrospective study. Vet Dermatol 2018; 29(1): 45-e20.
[http://dx.doi.org/10.1111/vde.12503] [PMID: 28994490]

[12] Hnilica KA. Otitis Externa Small Animal Dermatology: A Color Atlas and Therapeutic Guide. 3rd ed. St. Louis, Missouri: Elsevier Saunders 2011; pp. 395-8.

[13] Cole LK, Kwochka KW, Kowalski JJ, Hillier A. Microbial flora and antimicrobial susceptibility patterns of isolated pathogens from the horizontal ear canal and middle ear in dogs with otitis media. J Am Vet Med Assoc 1998; 212(4): 534-8.
[http://dx.doi.org/10.2460/javma.1998.212.04.534] [PMID: 9491161]

[14] Rohleder JJ, Jones JC, Duncan RB, Larson MM, Waldron DL, Tromblee T. Comparative performance of radiography and computed tomography in the diagnosis of middle ear disease in 31 dogs. Vet Radiol Ultrasound 2006; 47(1): 45-52.
[http://dx.doi.org/10.1111/j.1740-8261.2005.00104.x] [PMID: 16429984]

[15] Gotthelf LN. Small Animal Ear Diseases-E-Book: An Illustrated Guide. Elsevier Health Sciences 2004.

CHAPTER 12

Ceruminoliths and its clinical Management

S.K. Maiti[1], Varun Kumar Sarkar[2] and Shraddha Sinha[1,*]

[1] *Department of Teaching Veterinary Clinical Complex, Anjora, Durg, Chhattisgarh, India*

[2] *Division of Medicine, ICAR-IVRI Izatnagar, Bareilly (UP), India*

Abstract: Epithelial migration plays a crucial role in maintaining the health of the ear canal and tympanic membrane. This process involves the movement of keratinocytes, and it serves to eliminate debris, prevent cerumen (earwax) buildup, and facilitates the healing of tympanic membrane damage. Keratinocytes not only acts as a physical barrier but also have immunological capabilities to protect the ear canal from contaminants. Failure of epithelial migration can lead to ceruminoliths, which are hard earwax concretions that can cause discomfort and even hearing loss. Ceruminoliths are commonly associated with factors like over production of cerumen, obstruction in the ear canal, and damage to the germinal epithelium. Diagnosis of ceruminoliths typically involves otoscopic examination and otic cytology. Management options include cerumenolytic agents, irrigation, and manual removal under vision, each with its own considerations and precautions. Treatment of the underlying cause, such as ear mite infestations, may also be necessary to prevent ceruminolith formation. This comprehensive review sheds light on the mechanisms, causes, diagnosis, and management of ceruminoliths, emphasizing the importance of ear health and the various strategies for effective removal.

Keywords: Abnormalities, Anatomy, Auditory, Balance organ, Canine, Causes, Cerumen, Ceruminoliths, Diagnosis, Ear, Ear canal, Earwax, Epithelial migration, Ear irrigation, Feline, Otic exam, Otoscopy, Pinnae, Treatment, Tympanic membrane.

INTRODUCTION

Normal Anatomy of Ear Canal in Dog and Cat

The ear serves as both an auditory and a balance organ [1]. The structure of the canine and feline ear can be subdivided into several components, which include the pinnae, external ear canals (external acoustic meatuses), middle ear, and internal ear. Understanding the typical anatomy and function of the ear is essential

---

* **Corresponding author Shraddha Sinha:** Department of Teaching Veterinary Clinical Complex, Anjora, Durg, Chhattisgarh, India; E-mail: sinhashraddha220@gmail.com

Tanmoy Rana (Ed.)

for identifying any abnormalities that may affect or originate within these ear compartments [2, 3]. The shape of the pinna is designed to capture sound waves and direct them into the ear canal towards the eardrum. In dogs and cats, the pinnae are flexible and can move independently of each other. The size and configuration of the pinnae differ among breeds. In dogs, the ear canal is notably deeper than in humans, which enhances its capability to effectively channel sound towards the eardrum. However, this deeper canal is more prone to accumulating dirt and wax, potentially resulting in inflammation and secondary infections [4, 5]. The pinnae are constructed from auricular cartilage, which is enveloped on both sides by skin containing apocrine sweat glands, sebaceous glands, and hair follicles. In comparison to the inner, concave surface, which is thinner, the pinna's rounder exterior has more hair follicles per square inch [6]. There are numerous muscles in the pinna, each with specific functions to move the ear in particular directions. The external ear canal's opening is oriented dorso-laterally. The upper part of the auricular cartilage takes on a funnel shape, giving rise to the vertical ear canal. This vertical canal then curves inward just above the level of the eardrum to become the horizontal ear canal [7, 8]. There is a notable cartilaginous ridge that acts as a separation between the vertical and horizontal ear canals. In its normal position, this ridge can obstruct the examination of the horizontal ear canal, requiring the ear pinna to be grasped and lifted to access it. The epidermis lining of the external ear canal shares a similar histological structure to that of the pinna; however, in most breeds, there are fewer hairs, and these hairs do not extend the entire length of the ear canal [9]. A sparse number of fine hairs can be observed beyond the tympanic membrane. These hairs serve as a valuable reference point when performing ear flushing, aiding in the identification of the tympanic membrane in cases of abnormal ears. Additionally, the external ear canal houses sebaceous glands and ceruminous glands, which are specialized apocrine glands. Cerumen is a protective emulsion that lines the ear canal. It consists of shed keratinized squamous epithelial cells, in combination with the secretions from both the sebaceous and ceruminous glands within the ears. A remarkable characteristic of the tympanic membrane is its capacity to maintain an exceedingly thin and robust structure, even in the presence of ongoing secretions from the dermal adnexal glands. "Epithelial migration" is the principal mechanism responsible for maintaining the external ear's typanic membrane thinness and self-cleaning ability [10].

Epithelial Migration

Epithelial migration serves as a mechanism for both eliminating debris and facilitating the healing of any damage to the tympanic membrane [11]. The lateral (external auditory canal) surface keratinocytes of the tympanic membrane and the auditory canal epithelium migrate in a process known as epithelial migration [12,

13]. Within the ear canal, cerumen is created when these desquamated epithelial cells interact with the secretions of the apocrine and sebaceous glands [14]. This process functions as a self-cleaning mechanism, effectively removing debris from both the external auditory canal and the tympanic membrane. During this process, cerumen is carried away from the tympanic membrane and towards the opening of the distal auditory canal, thus preventing the buildup of cerumen that might otherwise cause conductive hearing loss [15, 16]. Additionally, the migratory process plays a significant role in the healing of post-operative tympanic membrane incisions and spontaneous tympanic membrane perforations [17]. The keratinocytes have been proven to have immunological capabilities in addition to serving as a mechanical barrier to protect the ear canal from outside contaminants. Keratinocytes store interleukin-1 (IL-1). When these cells are harmed, IL-1 is produced, which prompts further cells to generate IL-1. This leads to a series of immunologic events that cause granulocytes, monocytes, and macrophages to migrate to the site of injury. Loss of this protective immune system permits unregulated bacterial colonisation when a section of the ear canal has been damaged by trauma or ulcer formation, encouraging the development of otitis externa (Gotthelf, 2005). In many species, including humans [18, 19], gerbils [20], rats [21], and guinea pigs [22], the epithelial migration rate and pattern have now been described. For typical feline tympanic membranes, there is, little information on epithelial migration. However, canine tympanic membrane epithelial migration has, been studied [23].

CERUMINOLITHS

Skin flakes may build up in the ear canal as a result of failure in epithelial migration. But more frequently, wax and keratin buildup at the eardrum's base results in either soft wax plugs or large, hard concretions known as ceruminoliths. On the horizontal ear canal's floor, ceruminoliths appear lying adherent to the eardrum [24]. They are most frequently observed because of allergic otitis or ear mite infestations. This debris may cause the tympanum to become perforated, act as a nidus for infection, cause discomfort, block the passage of medicine to the deeper parts of the ear canal, and serve as a source of infection [25]. Hearing is hampered by ceruminoliths that block the horizontal ear canal. The weight of the ceruminolith pushes against the eardrum in certain head postures, which may raise air pressure in the middle ear cavity and result in vestibular disorder symptoms [26]. Due to its closeness to the tympanic membrane and movement into the middle ear when the dog shakes its head, the ceruminolith can not only cause discomfort but also tear the membrane and result in otitis media [27].

Causes of Ceruminolith

The main factor for development of ceruminoliths are following:

Overproduction

When the rate of cerumen production surpasses the rate of cerumen migration out of the ear, it can lead to cerumen impaction or ceruminoliths.

Obstruction

Differences in the structure of the ear canal can result in the buildup of cerumen. For example, benign bony growths in the ear canal, such as exostoses or osteomas, can hinder the migration of cerumen. Soft tissue abnormalities can also lead to obstructions, as seen in patients with a history of otitis externa or ear canal trauma [28]. Certain dog breeds are prone to excessive hair growth within their ear canals, while others have congenital anatomical characteristics like small, narrow ear canals or a propensity for overproducing cerumen. These factors can contribute to cerumen impaction in these breeds [29, 30].

Failure of Epithelial Migration

In cases where the germinal epithelium of the eardrum is harmed due to infection or ear mite infestation, it can lead to a damage to the keratinocytes, which are on the surface of the tympanic membrane. When healing occurs, fibrosis may cause lasting alterations to the tympanic membrane. This can disrupt the normal process of epithelial migration. When epithelial migration fails, it may result in the accumulation of skin flakes in the ear canal [31].

Diagnosis

Otic Exam

A high-quality otoscope enables the assessment of various aspects of the ear, including the quantity and nature of exudate, the presence of ear mites, estimation of inflammation, hyperplasia, and stenosis in the ear canal, the condition of the tympanic membrane, and the presence of any masses or growths [32].

Sample for Mites

To identify ear mites (*Otodectes cynotis*), a sample of the exudate can be collected and smeared onto a slide with mineral oil, allowing for microscopic examination. This method is often used to diagnose ear mite infestations in the ear canal [33].

Otic Cytology

Performing this test is a crucial first step in assessing the presence of secondary infections and providing appropriate treatment. It's essential to identify any inflammatory or neoplastic cells, as well as determine the specific types of bacteria and yeast present. When collecting samples from the ear, care should be taken to minimize the risk of causing damage or trauma to the ear canal and tympanic membrane [32].

Video Otoscopy

Video otoscopes, while somewhat less convenient than traditional otoscopes, offers numerous advantages. Their magnification, illumination, and image quality make it possible to assess fine details within the ear. The working channels in video otoscopes significantly ease tasks like ear flushing, removing foreign objects, manipulating polyps, conducting minor surgical procedures, using lasers, and performing myringotomy. Additionally, the capability to capture images and videos not only enhances communication with clients but also aids in monitoring the progress of the cases [34].

Diagnostic Imaging

Computed tomography (CT) is highly sensitive and specific for detecting issues such as stenosis and occlusion of the ear canals, as well as bulging or rupture of the tympanic membrane. While CT scans may be more expensive, they offer the advantage of being quicker and easier to perform and interpret compared to other imaging methods. Ideally, the ear canals should exhibit thin walls, which remain open, and have a uniform diameter or a gentle taper toward the tympanic membrane when examined through CT scans. The density of material within the ear canals can be evaluated to distinguish between debris and stenosis, and contrast enhancement can be employed to identify inflamed soft tissues. Even small amounts of mineralization in the ear canals are readily visible. While magnetic resonance imaging may not be as effective for visualizing the ear canals, it can be beneficial for certain types of imaging beyond the ear canal [35].

Management

The primary methods for earwax removal includes the use of wax softeners like olive oil drops, sodium bicarbonate drops, or water to aid removal of the wax. This can be followed by mechanical removal through methods such as electronically controlled irrigation of the ear canal (flushing the wax out using water) or micro suction (using a vacuum to extract the wax). The effectiveness of these earwax removal techniques and the most suitable setting for each method are not definitively established, and it may vary depending on individual circumstances. It's advisable to consult with a healthcare professional or an ear specialist to determine the most appropriate approach for your specific situation [36]. When earwax treatment is warranted, there are three commonly recommended removal methods: cerumenolytic agents (which help soften the wax), irrigation (using water to flush out the softened wax), and manual removal (physical extraction of the softened wax). The choice of method depends on individual factors and the severity of the earwax impaction, and it's typically best determined by a healthcare professional [37].

Cerumenolytic agents - are liquid solutions designed to thin, soften, break up, and dissolve earwax. These solutions are typically either water-based or oil-based, with water-based solutions being more commonly used. Water-based cerumenolytics may contain ingredients such as hydrogen peroxide, acetic acid, docusate sodium, and sodium bicarbonate. Among these, docusate sodium appears to be particularly effective, especially when used as a pre-treatment before ear irrigation [38]. Oil-based cerumenolytics often contain ingredients like peanut, olive, or almond oils. Many of these drops can be obtained over the counter without a prescription. The typical dosing regimen involves using up to five drops per dose, administered one to two times daily for a duration of three to seven days. Carbamide peroxide is a commonly prescribed cerumenolytic, with dosages typically consisting of five to 10 drops applied twice daily for a period of up to four days. These drops function by releasing oxygen, which helps to soften the earwax and encourages its natural extrusion, and they also have a mild antibacterial effect [12].

Irrigation - is an alternative method for safely and effectively removing excess cerumen, but it should only be used when the tympanic membrane (eardrum) can be visualized to ensure safety. Ear irrigation entails the gentle flushing of earwax from the ear canal using either a syringe or an electronic irrigator. This process is typically performed by a healthcare professional to minimize the risk of injury to the ear [13, 15]. In a clinical setting, various irrigation methods can be employed to remove earwax. One common approach involves using warm water alone or a 50/50 mixture of water and hydrogen peroxide. These solutions are placed into a syringe and gently discharged into the ear canal, with a basin positioned underneath to catch the flushed-out earwax and liquid. This method can be effective in dislodging and removing earwax, but it should be done carefully to avoid injury or discomfort. It's important to have it performed by a healthcare professional or under their guidance [12, 14]. Heating the flushing solution can be beneficial as it helps to further soften the waxy debris for easier removal. In some cases, the use of a large bore suction catheter can be employed with care to assist in removing the softened earwax [18]. Using a cerumenolytic for the five days leading up to the irrigation procedure, or if that's not possible, applying the cerumenolytic agent for 15-30 minutes just before the procedure, can enhance the success of earwax removal through irrigation. The cerumenolytic softens the earwax, making it easier to flush out during the irrigation process. This pre-treatment step is a common practice to optimize the effectiveness of the earwax removal procedure [34, 35]. To prevent potential chronic effects and stimulation of the vestibular system, it's important to ensure that the water used for ear irrigation is close to body temperature. Water that is too cold or too warm can affect the inner ear and balance, so maintaining a comfortable and neutral temperature is essential for safe and effective ear irrigation [22, 23]. An alternative to using a syringe for ear irrigation is a standard oral jet irrigator, which may be used with or without a modified tip for this purpose. While these methods are generally affordable and considered safe, it's important to note that they can potentially cause trauma, including the perforation of the tympanic membrane (eardrum), if not used with care. There are also electronic irrigators available for earwax removal, but there are no controlled trials comparing the efficacy and safety of different ear irrigation methods. It's important to follow proper guidelines and have these procedures performed by trained healthcare professionals to minimize the risk and complications [12].

Manual removal under vision- Manual removal techniques provide an alternative approach for earwax removal, especially in cases where cerumenolytic agents have proven ineffective or when irrigation is not a suitable option. When dealing with a hardened concretion-type ceruminolith, the use of grasping forceps is necessary for extraction. The utilization of a video otoscope is particularly helpful in this process, as it allows the healthcare professional to clearly visualize the ceruminolith on a video monitor, aiding in its precise and safe removal. This method can be especially useful when dealing with more challenging or stubborn earwax obstructions [16, 17]. Common tools for manual earwax removal include wax hooks for hard wax, Jobson-Horne probes for softer foreign objects, crocodile forceps for various items, and suction (micro-suction). These tools are selected based on the type of obstruction and are typically used by healthcare professionals for safe and effective earwax removal [2, 18]. In cases where an endoscopic grasping tool is employed, it can be inserted through the biopsy channel of the video otoscope to carefully grasp and remove earwax concretions or other obstructions. After the removal of such concretions, it's not uncommon for the tympanic membrane (eardrum) to appear abnormal. This may be due to small holes or erosions in the tympanic membrane that occur during the removal process. However, these small holes in the tympanum tend to heal rapidly on their own. Healing of the tympanic membrane is generally a natural and efficient process, but it's still advisable to follow up with appropriate medical care to ensure proper healing and to monitor for any potential complications [37, 38].

Manual earwax removal offers several advantages. It takes place under direct observation, allowing instruments to gently extract earwax without pushing it against structures. As a result, the risk of causing physical harm to the external ear canal or the eardrum is diminished, and the procedure ensures more dependable and immediate confirmation of complete clearance [18, 19]. The enhanced visual clarity provided by magnified visualization simplifies the diagnosis of anatomical or other abnormalities. Manual earwax removal is favored in patients with conditions such as convoluted ear canals, or when irrigation is not advisable or contraindicated, as is the case with conditions like tympanic membrane perforation, the presence of ear tubes (grommets), a mastoid cavity, or individuals who have recently undergone ear surgery [12, 15].

Treatment of underlying cause - When there is a known risk factor for earwax impaction, additional treatment may be necessary. Ear mite infestation is a significant risk factor for increased earwax production and the formation of ceruminoliths, often associated with ceruminous otitis externa. Numerous products are effective for treating *Otodectes* mite infestation in cats. Historically, ear preparations have been used for treatment, but they often require repeated application in the ear, which can reduce patient compliance. Milbemycin oxime (0.1%, MilbeMite; Elanco) continues to be a valuable ear treatment option because it is approved for use in kittens as young as 4 weeks old. More recently, researchers have explored the use of isoxazolines in cats with *Otodectes cynotis* infestations. Afoxolaner, selamectin plus sarolaner (Revolution Plus; Zoetis), fluralaner (Bravecto; Merck), and fluralaner plus moxidectin (Bravecto Plus; Merck) have successfully resolved *Otodectes cynotis* infestations in cats with just a single application [30, 31]. Isoxazolines have shown high effectiveness in treating demodicosis in dogs, and there have been reports of both fluralaner and sarolaner (when used in combination with selamectin) being effective for the treatment of feline demodicosis [14, 15].

CONCLUDING REMARKS

In conclusion, the intricate processes of epithelial migration play a vital role in both maintaining ear health and facilitating healing. Epithelial migration eliminates debris and aids in the recovery of damaged tympanic membranes. This process, in conjunction with apocrine and sebaceous gland secretions, forms cerumen, which acts as a self-cleaning mechanism for the ear canal, preventing cerumen buildup and conductive hearing loss. Ceruminoliths, or earwax concretions, can develop due to overproduction, obstructions in the ear canal, and disruptions in epithelial migration. These concretions pose various risks, including tympanic membrane perforation, infection, discomfort, and even vestibular symptoms in certain head postures. Diagnosis of ear issues involves otic exams, microscopic examination of earwax for mites, otic cytology, and advanced techniques like video otoscopy and diagnostic imaging. Proper management includes methods such as cerumenolytic agents, ear irrigation, and manual removal, tailored to the specific case. Additionally, addressing underlying causes, such as ear mite infestations, is crucial in managing ceruminoliths and preventing their recurrence. The use of isoxazolines and other effective treatments can resolve otic issues, including demodicosis. In summary, understanding the mechanisms of epithelial migration, the causes of ceruminoliths, and the available diagnostic and treatment methods is essential for maintaining ear health in both humans and animals, ultimately ensuring optimal hearing and overall well-being.

REFERENCES

[1]   Aaron K, Cooper TE, Warner L, Burton MJ. Ear drops for the removal of ear wax. Cochrane Libr 2018; 2018(10): CD012171.
[http://dx.doi.org/10.1002/14651858.CD012171.pub2] [PMID: 30043448]

[2]   Beccati MB, Pandolfi PP, DiPalma AD. Efficacy of fluralaner spot-on in cats affected by generalized demodicosis: seven cases. Vet Dermatol 2019; 30: 454.

[3]   Becskei C, Reinemeyer C, King VL, Lin D, Myers MR, Vatta AF. Efficacy of a new spot-on formulation of selamectin plus sarolaner in the treatment of *Otodectes cynotis* in cats. Vet Parasitol 2017; 238 (Suppl. 1): S27-30.
[http://dx.doi.org/10.1016/j.vetpar.2017.02.029] [PMID: 28395753]

[4]   Brame B, Cain C. Chronic Otitis in Cats: Clinical management of primary, predisposing and perpetuating factors. J Feline Med Surg 2021; 23(5): 433-46.
[http://dx.doi.org/10.1177/1098612X211007072] [PMID: 33896249]

[5]   Calhoun ML, Stinson AW. Integument. In: Dellmann HD, Brown EM, Eds. Textbook of Veterinary Histology. 3rd ed. Philadelphia: Lea & Febiger 1987; pp. 382-415.

[6]   Deong KK, Prepageran N, Raman R. Epithelial migration of the postmyringoplasty tympanic membrane. Otol Neurotol 2006; 27(6): 855-8.
[http://dx.doi.org/10.1097/01.mao.0000231503.92275.12] [PMID: 16936572]

[7]   Gotthelf LN. Diagnosis and treatment of otitis media in dogs and cats. Vet Clin North Am Small Anim Pract. 2004 Mar;34(2):469-87.

[8]   Duangkaew L, Hoffman H. Efficacy of oral fluralaner for the treatment of *Demodex gatoi* in two shelter cats. Vet Dermatol 2018; 29(3): 262.
[http://dx.doi.org/10.1111/vde.12520] [PMID: 29388292]

[9]   Fraser G. The histopathology of the external auditory meatus of the dog. J Comp Pathol Ther 1961; 71: 253-IN21.
[http://dx.doi.org/10.1016/S0368-1742(61)80031-3] [PMID: 13701505]

[10]   Gotthelf L N. Failure of Epithelial Migration: Ceruminoliths. 2005; 221-234.

[11]   Gupta T, Bhutta MF. Ear Wax and Its Removal: Current Practices and Recommendations. Hear J 2023; 76(9): 22-5.
[http://dx.doi.org/10.1097/01.HJ.0000978464.61642.e6]

[12]   Hand C, Harvey I. The effectiveness of topical preparations for the treatment of earwax: a systematic review. Br J Gen Pract 2004; 54(508): 862-7.
[PMID: 15527615]

[13]   Hanger HC, Mulley GP. Cerumen: its fascination and clinical importance: a review. J R Soc Med

1992; 85(6): 346-9.
[PMID: 1625268]

[14]   Harvey RG, Harari J, Delauche AJ. The normal ear Ear Diseases of the Dog and Cat. Ames, IA: Iowa State University Press 2001; pp. 9-41.

[15]   Horton GA, Simpson MTW, Beyea MM, Beyea JA. Cerumen management: an updated clinical review and evidence-based approach for primary care physicians. J Prim Care Community Health 2020; 11
[http://dx.doi.org/10.1177/2150132720904181] [PMID: 31994443]

[16]   Kakoi H, Anniko M, Pettersson CÅV. Auditory epithelial migration: I. Macroscopic evidence of migration and pathways in rat. Acta Otolaryngol 1996; 116(3): 435-8.
[http://dx.doi.org/10.3109/00016489609137869] [PMID: 8790744]

[17]   Koch, S. N. Feline otitis: diagnosis and treatment. In Sponsors of the 8th world congress of veterinary dermatology, 2016, p. 230.

[18]   Lam A. Ear Infections in Dogs: Work Up and Treatment. 2018.

[19]   Machado MA, Campos DR, Lopes NL, *et al.* Efficacy of afoxolaner in the treatment of otodectic mange in naturally infested cats. Vet Parasitol 2018; 256: 29-31.
[http://dx.doi.org/10.1016/j.vetpar.2018.04.013] [PMID: 29887026]

[20]   Matricoti I, Maina E. The use of oral fluralaner for the treatment of feline generalised demodicosis: a case report. J Small Anim Pract 2017; 58(8): 476-9.
[http://dx.doi.org/10.1111/jsap.12682] [PMID: 28466558]

[21]   Meyer F, Preuß R, Angelow A, Chenot JF, Meyer E, Kiel S. Cerumen impaction removal in general practices: a comparison of approved standard products. J Prim Care Community Health 2020; 11
[http://dx.doi.org/10.1177/2150132720973829] [PMID: 33334227]

[22]   Miller SM. Epidermal migration in the external ear canal of the guinea pig. J Otolaryngol Soc Aust 1983; 5(2): 71-5.

[23]   Moriello KA. Ear Structure and Function in Dogs. MSD Veterinary Manual 2018.

[24]   Njaa BL, Cole LK, Tabacca N. Practical otic anatomy and physiology of the dog and cat. Vet Clin North Am Small Anim Pract 2012; 42(6): 1109-26.
[http://dx.doi.org/10.1016/j.cvsm.2012.08.011] [PMID: 23122171]

[25]   Nuttall, T. Diagnostic approach to otitis externa. In Sponsors of the 8 th world congress of veterinary dermatology, 2016, p. 88.

[26]   Nuttall T. Successful management of otitis externa. In Practice, 38, 17-21. O'Donoghue, G. M. (1983). Epithelial migration on the guinea-pig tympanic membrane: the influence of perforation and ventilating tube insertion. Clin Otolaryngol Allied Sci 2016; 8(5): 297-303.

[27]   Radford JC. Treatment of impacted ear wax: a case for increased community-based microsuction. BJGP Open 2020; 4(2): bjgpopen20X101064.
[http://dx.doi.org/10.3399/bjgpopen20X101064] [PMID: 32238391]

[28]   Rosychuck R. Feline ear disease: so much more than ear mites. Proceedings of the Southern European Veterinary Conference. 17-9.

[29]   Schwartz SR, Magit AE, Rosenfeld RM, *et al.* Clinical practice guideline (update): earwax (cerumen impaction). Otolaryngol Head Neck Surg 2017; 156(S1): S1-S29.
[http://dx.doi.org/10.1177/0194599816671491] [PMID: 28045591]

[30]   Sevy JO, Hohman MH, Singh A. Cerumen Impaction Removal. Simpson, A. C. (2021). Successful treatment of otodemodicosis due to *Demodex cati* with sarolaner/selamectin topical solution in a cat. J Feline Med Surg Open Rep 2017; 7(1): 2055116920984386.

[31]   Tabacca NE, Cole LK, Hillier A, Rajala-Schultz PJ. Epithelial migration on the canine tympanic membrane. Vet Dermatol 2011; 22(6): 502-10.

[http://dx.doi.org/10.1111/j.1365-3164.2011.00982.x] [PMID: 21535257]

[32]   Taenzler J, de Vos C, Roepke RKA, Heckeroth AR. Efficacy of fluralaner plus moxidectin (Bravecto® Plus spot-on solution for cats) against *Otodectes cynotis* infestations in cats. Parasit Vectors 2018; 11(1): 595.
[http://dx.doi.org/10.1186/s13071-018-3167-z] [PMID: 30449272]

[33]   Taenzler J, de Vos C, Roepke RKA, Frénais R, Heckeroth AR. Efficacy of fluralaner against *Otodectes cynotis* infestations in dogs and cats. Parasit Vectors 2017; 10(1): 30.
[http://dx.doi.org/10.1186/s13071-016-1954-y] [PMID: 28093080]

[34]   Tang IP, Prepageran N, Raman R, Sharizhal T. Epithelial migration in the atelectatic tympanic membrane. J Laryngol Otol 2009; 123(12): 1321-4.
[http://dx.doi.org/10.1017/S0022215109990806] [PMID: 19835642]

[35]   Tinling SP, Chole RA. Gerbilline cholesteatoma development Part I: Epithelial migration pattern and rate on the gerbil tympanic membrane: comparisons with human and guinea pig. Otolaryngol Head Neck Surg 2006; 134(5): 788-93.
[http://dx.doi.org/10.1016/j.otohns.2005.12.022] [PMID: 16647536]

[36]   UK, N. G. C. Management of earwax. In Hearing loss in adults: assessment and management. National Institute for Health and Care Excellence (NICE). 2018.

[37]   Wang W, Wang Z, Chi F. Spontaneous healing of various tympanic membrane perforations in the rat. Acta Otolaryngol 2004; 124(10): 1141-4.
[http://dx.doi.org/10.1080/00016480410022921] [PMID: 15768806]

[38]   Yi ZX, Shi GS, Huang CC. Age-related epithelial migration on the tympanic membrane of the Mongolian gerbil. Otolaryngol Head Neck Surg 1988; 98(6): 564-7.
[http://dx.doi.org/10.1177/019459988809800605] [PMID: 3138613]

CHAPTER 13

Ruptured Ear Drums and its Clinical Management

Amitava Roy[1] and **Tanmoy Rana**[2,*]

[1] *Department of Livestock Farm Complex, West Bengal University of Animal & Fishery Sciences, Kolkata, India*

[2] *Department of Veterinary Clinical Complex, West Bengal University of Animal & Fishery Sciences, Kolkata-700094, India*

Abstract: The nervous system's vestibular system is primarily in charge of preserving the animal's balance and orientation in reaction to gravity. It recognises the head's rotational movements, static position, acceleration, and deceleration. After then, it synchronises the head's movement and position with the position of the eyes, trunk, and limbs. The vestibular system's structure and the symptoms of malfunction is covered in part one of this article. Part two explores the various illnesses that may be at the root of this and gives in detail the proper diagnostic procedures, available treatments, and associated prognoses.

Keywords: Dog, Rupture eardrums, Vestibular diseases.

INTRODUCTION

The outer ear, middle ear, and inner ear are the three portions of a dog's ear. The smallest bones in the body, the malleus, incus, and stapes, are found in the middle ear. Due to its extraordinary fragility, the eardrum is readily harmed by ear infections or ear cleaning. The three middle ear bones and the labyrinth are reached by sounds that are transmitted from the environment by the eardrum. Any condition that affects the eardrum's integrity and structure, including an infection or perforation, can drastically reduce a dog's hearing. The changes in the external ear canal caused by persistent inflammation can include glandular hyperplasia, glandular dilation, epithelial hyperplasia, and hyperkeratosis [1]. These alterations typically lead to increased cerumen production throughout the external ear canal, which raises the external ear canal's pH and local humidity levels and puts the ear at risk for secondary infection. *Staphylococcus* species are the bacteria that are most frequently isolated from the ear canals of dogs with otitis [2]. Other bacteria that are frequently linked to otitis are *Corynebacterium, Pseudomonas, Proteus,*

---

*Corresponding author **Tanmoy Rana**: Department of Veterinary Clinical Complex, West Bengal University of Animal & Fishery Sciences, Kolkata-700094, India; E-mail: tanmoyrana123@gmail.com

Enterococcus, and *Streptococcus*. Certain bacteria, like *Staphylococcus* and *Pseudomonas*, have the ability to form biofilms, which can cause an infection to persist even in the face of appropriate treatment. This is because any antimicrobial medication used to treat the illness must first break down the biofilm. Another frequent cause of canine otitis externa is *Malassezia* yeast. Any problems with the ear drum should be handled seriously and with quick veterinarian care.

HOW TO SPOT A RUPTURED EARDRUM IN THE DOG?

Dog's ear has three sections— The tympanic membrane, often known as the eardrum, divides the middle ear from the outer ear. It is a crucial component for sound transmission into r dog's ear.

The eardrum is a sensitive, fragile flap of tissue— Most frequently, chronic inflammation or infection that started in the outer ear canal and moved down to the eardrum will cause the eardrum to rupture.

Middle and inner ear infections can cause serious issues— The dog may lose their balance or go deaf if the eardrum ruptures and inflammation and infection spread further inside the ear.

WHAT IS EARDRUM RUPTURE?

Should seek veterinarian care if the dog's eardrum has ruptured. If an eardrum perforation is not treated, dog may experience long-term complications, including deafness in the afflicted ear. Dog's eardrum may rupture or perforate for a number of reasons, such as abrupt and significant changes in air pressure, middle ear infections, extremely loud noises, trauma, and foreign objects.

The tympanic membrane, a thin membrane that serves as a barrier between the middle and inner ear and the external ear, is r dog's eardrum. The tympanic membrane and eardrum are hidden deep inside the dog's ear canal, so anyone cannot see them. The primary function of the eardrum is to transmit sounds that are captured to the middle ear's ossicles. The ossicles are three small bones that then transmit the sounds that have been captured to the labyrinth [3].

Symptoms of Eardrum Rupture in Dogs

Pain

Pain is one of the most blatant indications of a perforated eardrum. There are various ways that ear pain might present. When the damaged ear is handled, many dogs may whine, some may continue to scratch or rub the ear, while others may tilt their heads or continually shake them. Because opening and closing the jaw tends to make the ear ache worse, affected dogs may also refuse to eat or open their jaws.

Discharge

The middle ear and the dog's ear canal are separated by the eardrum, also referred to as the tympanic membrane. The thin, drum-like tympanic membrane may become compressed by fluid accumulation in the middle ear, which can lead to rupture. This membrane may tear or develop a hole, allowing fluid from the middle ear to leak into the ear canal. This fluid may have the appearance of thick pus that is frequently tinted with blood. Note that the dog may experience improved comfort and reduced pain when pressure builds up and the eardrum bursts [4].

Neurological Signs

According to the Merck Veterinary Manual, paralysis of the facial nerves may be seen on the same side of the damaged ear because the dog's middle ear area is where the sympathetic and facial nerves travel through. As a result, a dog might not be able to blink, their eyes might totally close, and their lips and facial features might look drooping. A ruptured eardrum and an inner ear infection may also result in staggering, walking in circles, uncontrollable eye movements, and incoordination because the middle ear and inner ear both play a significant role in balance.

Hearing Loss

A damaged eardrum will impair the dog's hearing because it is the eardrum's job to transfer noises to the inner ear. However, if only one eardrum is harmed, the hearing loss might not even be visible. According to George M. Strain in his book Deafness in canines and Cats, even canines with unilateral hearing loss may still be able to respond to sound stimuli.

Visible Symptoms

Consult a veterinarian if you believe that a dog's eardrum is punctured. Aveterinarian may be able to detect a perforation or tear in the ear canal using an otoscope. Few dogs would consent to a complete eardrum examination, thus sedation or general anesthesia may be required. The tympanic membrane is visible once the otoscope has been placed into the ear canal. The jagged borders of the eardrum can be seen when this membrane is perforated. The eardrum may have a hole if it was torn [5].

Common Signs of a Ruptured Eardrum in Dogs

Pain

The majority of dogs enjoy having their ears scratched, but if a dog whimpers, yells, or even snaps when you reach for their ear, they can be suffering from a painful ruptured eardrum.

Otosclerosis of the ear canal

Ear infections frequently result in redness and irritation on the interior of the ear flap and ear canal.

Odour

Stinky ears on a four-legged pet may indicate an ear infection.

Hearing loss

It might be challenging to determine whether a dog is actually deaf or just experiencing age-related hearing loss. However, if a dog isn't responding to your calls, listening to usual orders, or running away when the treat container rattles, they probably have lost their hearing.

Ear discharge

Ear discharge that is caused by an infection is frequently thick, pus-like, and occasionally bloody. Check a dog's ears frequently for symptoms of discharge and infection [6].

Nystagmus

When a dog's eyes rapidly flicker back and forth, it is known as nystagmus. It can indicate an inner ear infection brought on by an eardrum rupture.

Stumbling

When the dog has an ear infection, it may lose coordination and stumble when walking.

Head tilt

The dog's head may incline towards the side of the affected ear if they have an inner ear infection.

Drooping face

Sometimes facial paralysis can happen, resulting in a drooping of the face and mouth on one side. Additionally, the eyelids may completely close or become incapable of blinking.

Causes of Eardrum Rupture in Dogs

There are several potential causes for the dog's eardrum to burst, but many of them can be avoided with caution. The following are typical reasons for eardrum ruptures:

• Extremely loud noises

• Severe and/or sudden changes in atmospheric pressure

• Middle ear infection

• Exposure to toxins

• Trauma

• Foreign objects that have invaded the ear canal

What to Know About the Eardrum

A dog's ear has three sections: The middle ear, the inner ear, and the exterior or outer ear. The pinna, or ear flap, and the ear canal make up the outer ear. Sound waves are captured and directed by the pinna through the ear canal to the eardrum. The outer ear canal of a dog is divided from the middle and inner ear by a thin membrane called the eardrum. The eardrum, which is stretched taut like a drum, vibrates in response to sound. These tremors cause the middle ear's small bones to move, which causes vibrations to go to the inner ear. The noises are transmitted to the brain for recognition from the inner ear [7].

Dog's middle and inner ears are prone to inflammation and infection if their eardrums are not entirely intact and functional. Additionally, if a dog's eardrum ruptures, they may lose their hearing.

Ear Infections

The most frequent cause of an eardrum rupture is ear infections. Long-lasting inflammation brought on by chronic ear infections may tear the eardrum. If the membrane tears, bacteria and yeast from the outer ear can enter the middle and inner ear, leading to a more serious infection.

Loud Noises

For instance, being too close to a gunshot or a fireworks show might cause an eardrum to rupture. Being too close to an excessively loud noise will injure, even though a loud noise from a distance won't.

Trauma

A violent injury, such as being hit by a car or falling from a tremendous height, can destroy a dog's eardrum.

Polyps or Masses

A polyp or lump in r dog's ear canal that gets too big can press up against the eardrum and cause it to burst.

Drastic Changes in Atmospheric Pressure

A sudden and dramatic change in air pressure, such as when flying, can burst an eardrum.

Foreign Object in the Ear

Dogs' eardrums are challenging to pierce because their ear canals are L-shaped rather than straight like ours. Rarely, migrating foxtail may burst the eardrum, although using a Q-tip or pharmaceutical applicator to do so would be difficult [2].

Diagnosis of Eardrum Rupture in Dogs

Before doing a physical examination, the veterinarian will first obtain r dog's medical history. To accurately identify a ruptured eardrum, an ear examination is required. Many dogs will require sedation in order to examine their ears. Some vets will do an antiquated test that checks for air bubbles that occur in r dog's ear canal while it breathes. Fluorescein can also be inserted into the ear canal and used as a test. The eardrum has burst if the fluorescein escapes *via* r dog's nose.

Additionally, a veterinarian should run standard diagnostic procedures such a complete blood count, biochemistry panel, and urinalysis. These will aid in eliminating further causes and assist in identifying whether an infection is present. If a middle ear infection is present, radiographs, CT scans, and MRI scans can reveal the extent of the infection [4].

Techniques to Assess the Eardrum

Veterinarians use a variety of ways to evaluate the eardrum's structural integrity. The integrity of the eardrum will determine which drugs and flushing treatments to employ, thus it should always be assessed.

Use of a Catheter

Until it stops, a catheter with a tiny diameter is placed into the ear canal. To feel the "stop", the catheter is extended and retracted. A soft feel to the "stop" denotes an intact eardrum, whereas a harsh feel is associated with a ruptured eardrum. The catheter's impact on the tympanic bulla's wall is what causes the sharp sensation.

Tympanometry

A sensor is used in tympanometry (also known as impedance audiometry) to gauge how the eardrum reacts to sound waves. However, using this in veterinary clinics is not practicable. It serves as an instrument for animal studies.

Fluorescein Solution or Diluted Povidone-iodine Solution

While the dog or cat is sedated, the warmed solution is injected into the ear canal. The eardrum is burst if the fluid comes out of the animal's nose or if it is snorted out *via* the oropharynx [2].

Video Otoscope

The video otoscope's tip is put into the ear canal of the suspected burst eardrum and the ear is filled with warmed saline. When a dog or cat is inhaling, air bubbles rising from the ear canal suggest a ruptured eardrum.

Positive Contrast Canalography

In dogs with otitis media, this technique is used to find a ruptured eardrum.

Treatment of Eardrum Rupture in Dogs

After determining that a dog has an ruptured eardrum, a veterinarian will go with the available treatment choices. Always heed to veterinarian's advice and administer any recommended medication as instructed.

Following a thorough evaluation of pet, veterinarian may carry out the following actions to solve the issue.

• Utilize the necessary drugs to clean out the afflicted ear.

• Based on the findings, administer supportive and symptomatic care. Steroids, a course of antibiotics, an immune system suppressant, and/or an antifungal drug may be recommended by r veterinarian.

• A veterinarian may undertake surgery to fix the dog's injured eardrum and restore its hearing [3].

The severity of the issue and the dog's response to the treatment determines the prognosis of a ruptured eardrum in dogs to a considerable extent. While minor occurrences may resolve in 3–4 weeks, some dogs may experience chronic hearing loss. Neurological symptoms like eye jerking, head tilting, and circling may continue. To be certain that any foreign objects or pus have been eliminated, veterinarian will need to do a complete ear flushing, usually while pet is sedated. Additionally, oral antibiotics and antifungal drugs may be prescribed for the dog. It may also be necessary to provide corticosteroids if dog is in pain or is inflamed. Unless vet has given the all-clear, never give the dog over-the-counter drugs. If a dog's eardrum has ruptured, many over-the-counter treatments can be hazardous. Otitis externa can cause dogs to lose their hearing. There are three types of hearing loss: mixed (a mix of sensorineural and conductive), conductive, and sensorineural. Sensorineural hearing loss can happen when otitis interna, ototoxic drugs (Morgan *et al.,* 1980), presbycusis, noise, physical trauma, general anaesthesia, or infection harm the brain's neurological (cochlea nerve) circuits (Mason *et al.,* 2013; Belmudes *et al.,* 2018). Stenosis, glandular hyperplasia, and otitis associated exudates can all cause conductive hearing loss (Cole *et al.,* 2018). Cleaning the exudates and debris out of the external ear canals helps dogs with otitis externa restore their hearing, which is measured (Shell, 1988). The patients' brain stem auditory evoked response (BAER) test values improved after using otic medicine [1].

In some cases, surgery may be necessary to restore serious harm that the ruptured eardrum may have caused. Dog's best surgical option will be discussed with veterinarian. Any over-the-counter medication should not be given without first visiting veterinarian. Be aware that the ear channel tissues are exceedingly delicate, and that some products will simply exacerbate the situation. Any drug can easily enter the inner ear when there is a rip or hole in the eardrum, which might potentially result in permanent hearing loss.

Recovering from a Ruptured Ear Drum

A ruptured eardrum will often recover without surgery in three to six weeks. Dogs that need surgery heal more slowly and require more frequent veterinary appointments. The extent of the rupture will determine whether the dog experiences neurological issues or irreversible hearing loss. Always pay attention to a vet and adhere to their recommended course of action [3].

How to Stop the Eardrum in R Dog from Rupturing

Use the following preventative advice to make sure dog doesn't experience the pain of a ruptured eardrum:

• **Don't shove objects in a dog's ear** — Only cleaning and medication solutions should ever be used in a dog's ears. When removing debris or administering medication, have to gentle. Do not bury a finger, cotton swab, or application tool so deeply that it is concealed.

• **Keep a dog's ears clean** — it's essential to keep a dog's ears clean if want to avoid an eardrum rupture. Moisture, debris, matted hair, and ear infections can all lead to inflammation that harms the tympanic membrane. a dog's ears can require weekly cleanings, depending on how they are. It's also beneficial to use a regular ear cleaner to clean a dog's ears after a swim or bath.

• To keep a dog's ears clean, read our guide to the best ear cleaners.

• **Find the cause of chronic ear infections** — Dogs who have chronic ear inflammation are more likely to have burst eardrums. A healthy ear depends on identifying and treating the underlying cause of chronic otitis. If a dog has food allergies, a diet change may be necessary, as may medicine to treat environmental allergies.

• **Avoid long-term exposure to very loud noises** — If frequently hunt with a gun or if you use loud power tools at home, restrict your dog to a calm area while you are doing so. To protect their ears, keep a four-legged friend's exposure to loud noises to a minimum [4].

CONCLUSION

Every doctor has had the unpleasant experience of being unable to prevent or treat an eardrum rupture, and they all consider surgery as a viable choice for treatment in these circumstances. It must be emphasized, though, that surgery might also be doomed to failure if the root problems are not identified and treated. Total canal ablation with bulla contents draining may be the only option in more severe cases where the morphological abnormalities show irreversible and the settlement of rupture of eardrums becomes impossible.

REFERENCES

[1] Belmudes A, Pressanti C, Barthez PY, Castilla-Castaño E, Fabries L, Cadiergues MC. Computed tomographic findings in 205 dogs with clinical signs compatible with middle ear disease: a retrospective study. Vet Dermatol 2018; 29(1): 45-e20.
[http://dx.doi.org/10.1111/vde.12503] [PMID: 28994490]

[2] Cole LK, Rajala-Schultz PJ, Lorch G. Conductive hearing loss in four dogs associated with the use of ointment-based otic medications. Vet Dermatol 2018; 29(4): 341-e120.
[http://dx.doi.org/10.1111/vde.12542] [PMID: 29664150]

[3] Huang HP, Little CJL, McNeil PE. Histological changes in the external ear canal of dogs with otitis externa. Vet Dermatol 2009; 20(5-6): 422-8.
[http://dx.doi.org/10.1111/j.1365-3164.2009.00853.x] [PMID: 20178479]

[4] Malayeri HZ, Jamshidi S, Zahraei Salehi T. Identification and antimicrobial susceptibility patterns of bacteria causing otitis externa in dogs. Vet Res Commun 2010; 34(5): 435-44.
[http://dx.doi.org/10.1007/s11259-010-9417-y] [PMID: 20526674]

[5] Mason CL, Paterson S, Cripps PJ. Use of a hearing loss grading system and an owner-based hearing questionnaire to assess hearing loss in pet dogs with chronic otitis externa or otitis media. Vet Dermatol 2013; 24(5): 512-e121.
[http://dx.doi.org/10.1111/vde.12057] [PMID: 23829225]

[6] Morgan JL, Coulter DB, Marshall AE, Goetsch DD. Effects of neomycin on the waveform of auditory-evoked brain stem potentials in dogs. Am J Vet Res 1980; 41(7): 1077-81.
[PMID: 7436102]

[7] Shell LG. Otitis media and otitis interna. Etiology, diagnosis, and medical management. Vet Clin North Am Small Anim Pract 1988; 18(4): 885-99.
[http://dx.doi.org/10.1016/S0195-5616(88)50088-8] [PMID: 3264962]

CHAPTER 14

Otitis Externa and its Clinical Management

G. Saritha[1,*]

[1] *Department of Veterinary Medicine, CVSc, Proddatur, SVVU, India*

Abstract: An ear is called a vestibule-cochlear organ since it enables to hear as well as sense of balance to animals. The external portion of the ear consist of a flap known as pinna and an opening at the base of the ear. Otitis externa is defined as an acute or chronic inflammation of the epithelium of the external ear canal which may also involve the pinna and it results from a combination of dynamic changes affecting the anatomical, psychological and microbiological status of the external ear canal. The etiological factors of the otitis externa can be categorised as predisposing factors, primary causes, perpetuating factors and secondary causes. Predisposing factors are those which increase the risk of developing otitis externa, whereas primary causes directly induces otitis externa. These long-term alterations causes the skin to be thicken, the canal to become stenosed, and a great deal of folds to form, all of which prevent the area from being cleaned effectively and serve as a breeding ground for secondary infections. Diagnosis of otitis externa is done by proper history and symptomatology, roll smear examination for mites and other cytological evidence, otoscopy, isolation and cultureantibiotic sensitivity test for selecting suitable antibiotic for treatment.

Generally otitis externa can be treated by application of suitable cleansers, topical antibiotic and anti fungal therapy along with corticosteroids. Sometimes it is difficult to treat chronic and recurrent otitis externa.

Keywords: Cerumen secretions, Cytology, Dog, Otits externa, Topical antibiotic, Wax.

INTRODUCTION

Vestibular-cochlear organ in the ear is the most important organ which enables to hear and also in balancing the body in animals. There are two parts in ear, a flap like organ called pinna and an external orifice into the ear canal.

At the external orifice of the ear, auricular cartilage begins to roll into a funnel shape that extends downwards forming a vertical ear canal which terminates with

---

* **Corresponding author G. Saritha:** Department of Veterinary Medicine, CVSc, Proddatur, SVVU, India;
E-mail: drsaritha.vet@gmail.com

Tanmoy Rana (Ed.)

the tympanic membrane or eardrum. This anatomical structure is predisposing factor for most of the ear infections. Ear infection in dogs results from irritation caused by excessive accumulation of ear wax, tissue debris and oil from skin. Generally, sebaceous and ceruminous glands in stratified squamous epithelium of the ear canal can secrets an odourless white fluid which later combines with desquamated epithelial cells and forms cerumen or ear wax which helps in protection of skin from various injuries or microorganisms. But sometimes the excessive secretion of cerumen helps in growth of *Malassezia pachydermatitis* [1].

Otitis externa is one of the most important and multifactorial disease accounting for 10-20% of all other clinical conditions of canines. Otitis externa brings dynamic changes in anatomical, microbiological as well as psychological status of the ear canal with involvement of ear pinna resulting in acute or chronic inflammatory changes of epithelium [2].

OTITIS EXTERNA

Otitis externa is an inflammatory condition that affects the pinna and external ear canal. Acute or chronic (permanent or recurrent otitis lasting three months or longer) otitis externa are both possible. It can be quite difficult to treat canine chronic as well as recurrent otitis externa, which calls for multifactorial as well as step-by-step strategic planning. Recognizing the causes, and the factors that contributes to otitis is a crucial first step towards effective diagnosis and treatment.

Changes that occur in external ear canal in response to chronic inflammation may include glandular hyperplacia, glandular dilation, epithelial hyperplacia and hyperkeratosis. These changes are responsible for increased cerumen production which in turn causes increase in pH and local humidity, thus predisposing to secondary infection.

Epidemiology

Various authors reported that otitis externa accounts for up to 15-20% of different ailments presenting to the clinics [3, 4]. It is very important to know the age, breed and sex predisposition of dogs to the otitis externa. The dogs aged between 1 and 3 years are more susceptible for otitis externa by Malasezia [5, 6].

Otitis externa occurs more commonly in males than in females. However according to some authors there is no sex predisposition for canine otitis externa [7].

Etiology and Pathogenesis

The multifactorial etiology of otitis externa can be categorized into predisposing factors, primary causes, secondary causes and perpetuating factors. Among these primary factors are the direct inducers of otitis externa, whereas predisposing factors are those to elevate the risk of otitis.

Perpetuating factors are those which prevent resolution of otitis whereas secondary causes are those which contribute to pathology only in the abnormal ear or in combination with predisposing factors.

Because the infection occurs typically only in a portion of the tissue, it is crucial to comprehend the multifaceted nature of otitis and pay attention to the various causes as well as contributing variables (Fig. **1**). After initiating the inflammatory process inside the ear canal, change the aural environment, and promote the growth of infections as secondary complicating factors. When a secondary complicating problem first appears, the owner or even the veterinarian may not be aware of the underlying reason, which may be extremely mild (Fig. **2**).

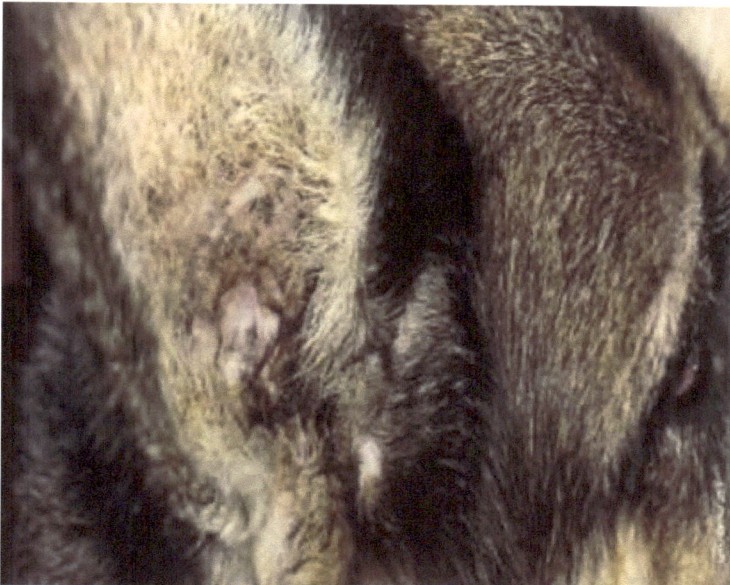

Fig. (1). Otitis externa in german shepherd dog.

Primary Causes

Hypersensitivities (atopic dermatitis, food hypersensitivity) [8], parasites (*Otodectes cynotis, Demodicosis, Sarcoptes*), foreign bodies (like plant awns), epithelialization disorders or autoimmune diseases (sebaceous adenitis, Vitamin A responsive dermatosis, pemphigus foliaceus, *etc.*), metabolic disorders (hypothyroidism and hyperadrenocorticism), foreign bodies (fox tail plant awns) [8, 9] (Fig. **3**).

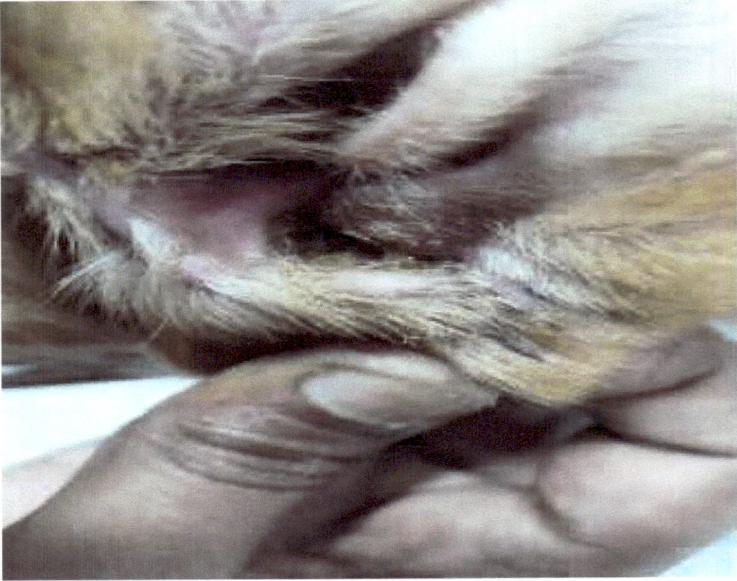

Fig. (2). Honey brown color discharge in stenosed ear.

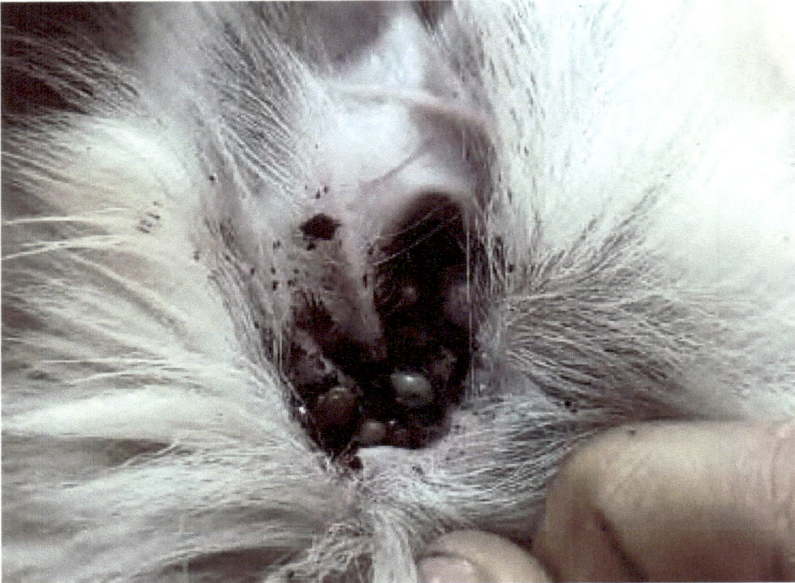

Fig. (3). Severe tick infestation in ear canal.

Sometimes acute allergic reactions like flea bite hypersensitivity, contact allergic dermatitis auto immune disorders also contributes to the condition of otitis externa. Conditions like vasculopathy, vasculitis, juvenile cellulitis, easonophillic dermatitis are also considered for the clinical outcome of otitis externa (Fig. **4**).

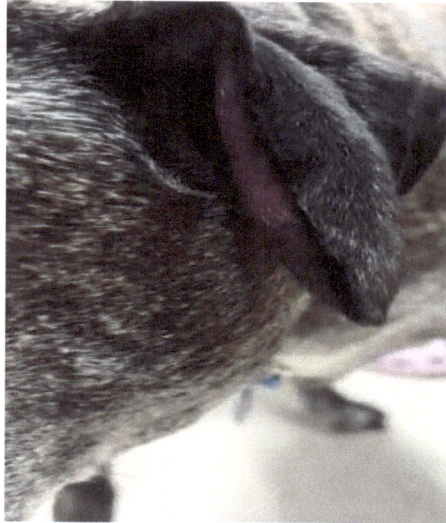

Fig. (4). Haematoma of ear pinna.

With chronic-recurrent (63%) otitis externa, allergic dermatitis (43/100 dogs) was the most frequent primary cause of otitis, followed by foreign bodies like awns of grass with the presence of acariasis. In 32 out of 100 cases, there were no identifiable primary factors. Unilateral or bilateral otitis can be accompanied by allergic and hormonal illnesses, but bilateral otitis is more typical. Although unilateral otitis is typically accompanied by foreign bodies, neoplasia, and polyps, bilateral issues have also been noted (Fig. **5**).

Secondary Causes

The bacteria most commonly isolated from canine otitic ear canals are *Staphylococcus* spp [2].

In addition to primary causes or predisposing conditions, secondary causes can also develop. Infections are the most prevalent secondary causes. Bacteria and yeast, such as *Malassezia pachydermatis*, *Staphylococcus*, *Streptococcus*, *Enterococcus*, *Pseudomonas*, *Proetus*, *Klebsiella*, and *Escherichia coli*, are secondary causes. Topical treatment is among the additional secondary reasons.

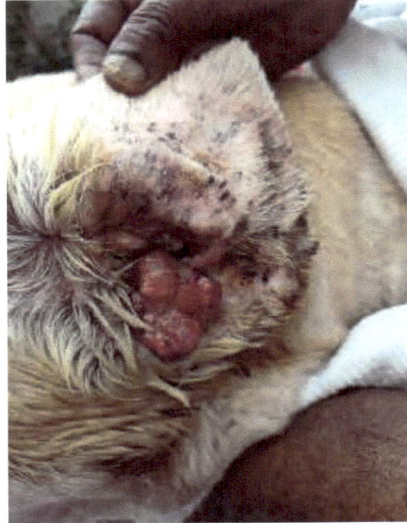

Fig. (5). Neoplacia in otits externa.

Reactions to topical medications and excessive cleaning, which can result in too much moisture and tissue maceration, are some additional secondary reasons. In general, once discovered, secondary matter of causes of otitis externa are simple to get rid of. It is typically the case that primary causes or perpetuating factors have not been fully addressed when they are chronic and challenging to treat (Figs. **6** & **7**).

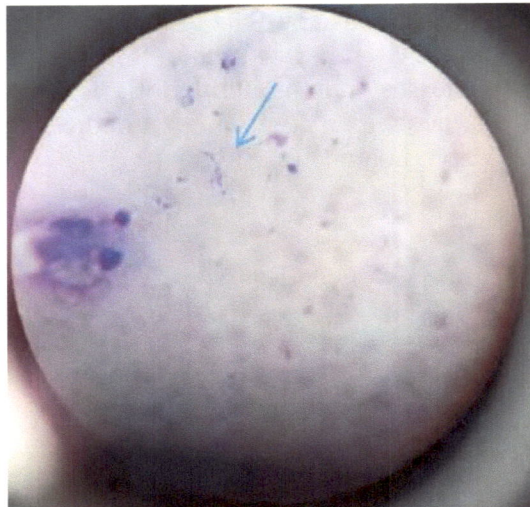

Fig. (6). Fungal buds presence in otitic roll smears.

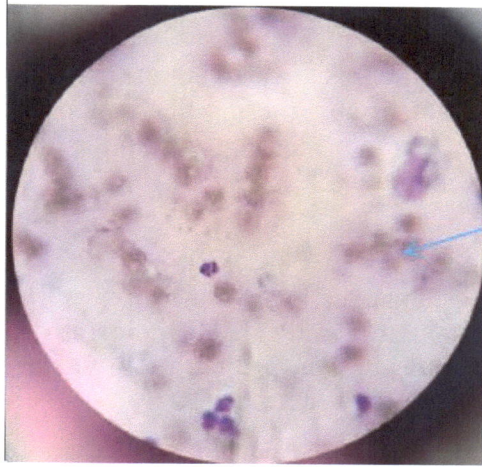

Fig. (7). Malasezia pachydermatitis.

Potential Risk Factors

The external ear canal's microenvironment is altered by predisposing conditions, which causes faster multiplication of most of the pathogenic and opportunistic bacteria or yeast.However they do not alone cause otitis externa. When combined with primary as well as secondary causes, these elements pose a serious issue. Predisposing variables in dogs include conformation (hairy ear canals, pendulous pinnae and ear canal stenosis), as well as excessive wetness from swimming or bathing. It is crucial, to observe the Hyper activity of the cerumen glands in German shepherds.

Hyperactivity of the cerumen glands, lower aural temperature, higher humidity and moisture levels were the most common reasons for higher incidence of otitis externa in german shepherd dogs [10].

If dog is spending more time in water like swimming, bathing for long duration may also causes the hyper activity of ceruminous glands, which in turn results in obstruction of the ear canal and increases the chance for otitis externa [11].

Perpetuating Factors

Otitis Media

Tympanic rupture arising from trauma or from tumours, or foreign bodies in the external ear can cause the development of otitis media. Otitis media develop with the extension of otitis externa or from any infection ascending through the Eustachian tube or from any haematogenous route.

Pyrexia and Systemic Diseases

Pyrexia as well as systemic diseases are also predisposing factors for bacterial and fungal otitis externa, presumably by altering the homeostasis within the resident microflora of the aural integument and by disrupting the epidermal barrier or suppressing cell mediated immunity [12].

Obstructive Ear Diseases

Proliferative inflammatory changes, extra luminal swellings and neoplacia may produce compression of external ear canal that in turn releases the secretions through external auditory meatus and suppuration which may extend in to the surrounding tissues owing to otitis externa.

The inflammatory process is sustained and aggravated by perpetuating variables, which also delay or exacerbate otitis externa. Once present, they serve as ideal settings and tiny niches that enhance or allows the development of secondary causes viz. infection. Chronic inflammation triggers alterations such as cerumen gland hyperplasia and dilatation, cutaneous edema and fibrosis, and epidermal hyperkeratosis and hyperplasia. Breed differences do exist; for example, compared to other breeds, the Cocker Spaniel develops higher cerumen gland hyperplasia and ectasia but less fibrosis (Table **1**).

Table 1. Categorisation of etilogy of otitis externa in canines.

1.	Predisposing factors (increase the risk)	Breed, conformation, excessive moisture, climatic changes, excessive cerumen production, neoplasms, systemic diseases (pyrexia, debilitation, immune suppression)
2.	Primary causes (directly induces)	Auto immune diseases, glandular diseases, hyperkeratinisation, foreign bodies, parasites and viral diseases.
3.	Secondary causes (causes pathology in the presence of abnormal ear)	Bacteria (*Staphylococci, Pseudomonas, Corynebacteria*), *Malassezia pachydermatitis, Candida albicans*
4.	Perpetuating factors (prevent resolution of otits)	Otits media, tympanic membrane changes

PROGRESSIVE PATHOLOGICAL CHANGES IN EAR CANAL

These long-term alterations cause the skin to thicken, the canal to become stenosed, and a great deal of folds to form, all of which prevent the area from being cleaned effectively and serve as a breeding ground for secondary infections. When just primary and secondary causes are treated for otitis externa, perpetuating factors frequently hinder remission of the condition. Although initially mild, these characteristics have the potential to become the most serious aspect of chronic ear disease. They are generally observed in chronic conditions and are not disease-specific [13]. The most frequent justifications for surgical intervention are perpetuating causes.

Essential Diagnostic Procedures

• Proper history taking to determine primary triggering factors.

• Complete clinical examination the ear.

• Appropriate tests by scrapings and tape impression smears.

History

Investigating the root cause and related causes requires a thorough and comprehensive history.

Symptomatology

Sweet smelling exudates, dark brown waxy appearance indicates *Malassezia* pachydermatitis infection. Dark brown to black, crumbly exudate resembling coffee grounds indicates *Otodectes cyanotis* infection.

Erythemato ceruminous otitis externa contains cerumen with intense pruritus.

Suppurative otitis externa contains greenish colour with *Pseudomonas aeruginosa* infection.

Malodorous, profuse purulent bilateral otic discharge with moderate to severe inflammation, ulceration and hypertrophy of the ear canal was indicative of *Pseudomonas* species [14] where intensive ear scratching, greasy otic discharge erythema, malodour, excoriations, swelling of pinnae and external ear canals were the clinical signs observed most frequently [15].

Examination for Mites

A drop of liquid paraffin is taken on to a glass slide and mixed with the exudate sample taken from affected ear and observed under low power microscope to examine the mites [16].

Cytological Examination

Cytological assay is most efficient method for identifying Malasssezia pachydermatits. Cytology is having presence of bacterial cocci, rods and neutrophils [17].

The most frequently associated micro organism from otitis ears was *Staphylococcus intermedius, Streptococus canis, Proteus* spp *and Escherichia coli.*

Canine chronic otits externa is commonly associated with the presence of *Pseudomonas* infections [19].

Otic Inspection

This can be used for examination as well as palpation of horizontal and vertical canals, there by the clinician can assess the quantity and type of exudate in the ear canals, gauge the degree of otic inflammation, look for masses, hyperplasia, and foreign bodies, and assess the condition of tympanic membrane (such as structural changes or rupture). Every time, it's best to undertake an otoscopic examination on both ears. To prevent the patient from becoming overly sensitive to the operation, it is best to check the unaffected ear first. In order to prevent cross contamination, it is crucial to switch cones between ears.

These results aid in deciding whether whole ear canal ablation with or without bulla osteotomy is the best course of action. Before doing an otoscopic examination, the patient may require sedation or general anesthesia if their ears hurt [20].

Otoscopy

Otoscopes that are often used (*i.e.*, handheld) should have a powerful light and power supply. If available, fiberoptic video-enhanced otoscopy (such as the video-otoscope) is incredibly beneficial for improving diagnosis and therapy because it not only makes it possible to see minute details that might not be visible with standard otoscopes but also makes it easier to flush the ears properly, assess the severity of the disease, and identify indications for further testing and treatment. Tympanic membraneent (such as myringotomy, otitis media). However, a dermatologist referral is advised due to the cost of purchasing and maintaining this equipment [18].

Visual Inspection

An extensive physical examination that includes a thorough dermatologic examination might aid in determining the underlying or root cause. A thorough neurologic examination is recommended because individuals with otitis media as well as otitis interna may also have concurrent neurologic abnormalities (such as facial paralysis, nystagmus, ataxia, and head tilt).

Orthotic Cytology

The choice of topical medication is aided by otic cytology, which determines whether an infection is persistent in the ears. Samples of cytology should be softly taken from the horizontal canal. To check for mites, exudate samples can be spread with mineral oil on a slide. *Staphylococcus pseudintermedius* is the most frequent form of rod bacteria and *Pseudomonas aeruginosa* is the most frequent type of coccoid bacteria discovered in the ears of dogs with otitis externa. *Malassezia* species are also common organisms1–5 (Fig. **8**).

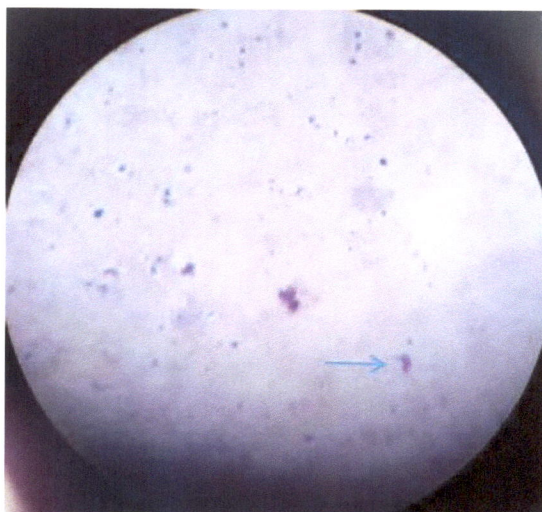

Fig. (8). Cytologic paradigm of *Malassezia* species (high-power oil immersion field 100× objective).

To determine the severity and enable monitoring at subsequent visits, it is crucial to describe the existence of any inflammatory or cancerous cells and quantify each type of bacteria or yeast under oil immersion field (100x). In one investigation, canine external ear canals with mean bacterial count of 25 per high-power dry field as well as mean *Malassezia* counts per high-power dry field of 5 were deemed abnormal. 5 Leukocytes are usually aberrant, and indicate bacterial infection.

Culture and Sensitivity of Bacteria

Statistics of antibiotic sensitivity test, represents the serum level needed globally and may not accurately predict the genuine susceptibility of otic bacteria, which makes culture and sensitivity (C/S) potentially beneficial in detecting specific otic pathogens and assisting with treatment decision on Topical antibiotics.

Cocci (Fig. **8**) and/or rods (Fig. **9**) observed on cytology, are indicators of chronic otitis due to bacteria. The rods involved in canine otitis externa are frequently *P. aeruginosa* and other gram negative bacteria such as *E. coli*, *Klebsiella* and *Enterobacter* spp. *P.aeruginosa* and *P. mirabilis* display high rate of resistance to most of the antimicrobials tested with very high resistance to Aminoglycosides, other than Penicillins and tetracyclines. A recent study has reported that administration of a topical bacteriophage mixture leads to lysis of *P. aeruginosa* in the ear canal and that might potentially became a convenient and effective treatment for *P.aerugenosa* associated otitis in dogs.

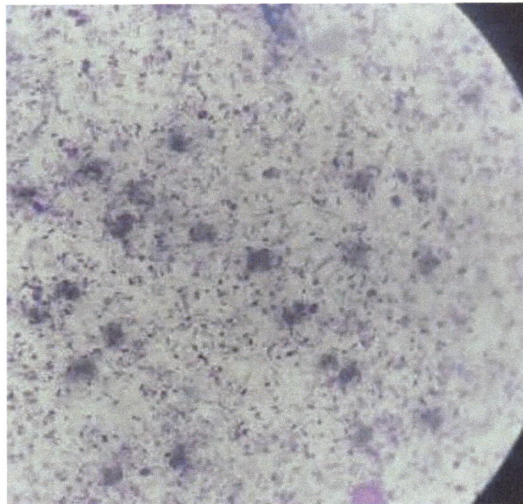

Fig. (9). Degenerate neutrophils, rods and cocci as seen *via* a high-power oil immersion field 100 objective.

Multidrug-resistant Bacterial History

Bacterial abundance on cytology despite apparently proper therapy with a history of prolong-term oral as well as topical antibiotic therapy (Fig. **9**).

Prior to aerobic cytological smear examination, cytology should always be carried out to help interpret the findings and identify any coexisting issues. Only 68% of the time, in one study, did cytologic and culture results accord.

Prior to aerobic C/S, cytology should always be carried out to help interpret the findings and identify any coexisting issues. Only 68% of the time, in one study, did cytologic and culture results accord. This may help to explain why, occasionally, there is a discrepancy between *in vitro* sensitivity results and *in vivo* responses to topical medication. Clinicians should be cautious since this data raises doubts about the effectiveness of C/S in choosing antimicrobials to treat otic infections.

Clinicians should be cautious and skeptical when interpreting the results of otic cytologic and culture tests since this study raises doubts about the efficacy of C/S for choosing antimicrobials for otic infections.

Because of the presence of mixed and commensal bacteria in external ear canal, *in vivo* antibiotic sensitivity test results are taken cautiously.

Imaging Techniques for Diagnostics

Diagnostic imaging is frequently necessary to identify contributing issues, such as middle ear disease (*e.g.*, neoplasia, otitis media), otitis interna, and pain upon opening the mouth in dogs with chronic, recurrent, and severe otitis as well as those with neurologic signs (*e.g.*, vestibular signs or facial nerve paralysis), para-aural swelling, or pain. Patients with otitis media may also have a tympanic membrane that seems to be normal. Otitis media is typical, with a reported prevalence of 50% to 88.9% [16]. Up to 89% of canines with recurrent otitis media for six months or more may have an intact but defective tympanic membrane. About 70% of these dogs also have recurring ear infections.

Deep Ear Irrigation

This process is very beneficial as a diagnostic tool and as a component of the therapy strategy. Before performing a deep ear flush, it may be necessary to administer an anti-inflammatory dose of oral as well as topical glucocorticoids for a brief period (two to three weeks) in order to reduce the ear canal inflammation and stenosis [14]. In order to thoroughly clean the ear and inspect the ear canal and tympanic membrane, this treatment should be carried out under general anesthesia. In addition, anesthesia enables the insertion of an endotracheal tube, which prevents fluids from entering the posterior pharynx *via* the auditory tube after passing through the middle ear.

There are several methods for flushing and cleaning the ears. After flushing, it's crucial to schedule follow-up treatments to assess the condition of the tympanic membrane and track treatment response [12, 15]. The tympanic membrane normally recovers from myringotomy within 30 days of the surgery. Referral to a dermatologist may be the best course of action because deep ear flush as well as myringotomy are procedures that are best carried out by skilled professionals with a video-otoscope.

Treatment

Acute and uncomplicated otitis externa can be treated successfully, but chronic or recurrent otitis externa is more challenging. Typically, because, underlying primary factors as well as predisposing and perpetuating factors all play a part, including secondary infection. Repeated bouts of inflammation and infection can cause lack of success in treating otitis. Infact otitis externa is a dermatological disease condition [10]. Treatment of the underlying skin disease is always essential for successful management of otitis externa.

Treatment for Otitis Externa has Five Main Objectives

• Put an end to agony and anguish.

• Take out the trash and discharge.

• Purge the exterior and middle ears of infection.

• Whenever feasible, reverse chronic pathologic alterations.

• Determine the root of the otitis and address it.

Topical Treatment

Topical treatment alone is usually sufficient for treating otitis externa and is chosen whenever possible. On the other hand, persistent, serious instances of otitis externa and otitis media frequently call for extra systemic treatment. The dosage of the drug is crucial. In general, depending on the size of the dog, it is advised to use between 10 and 20 drops (or 0.5 to 1 mL) per ear. The efficacy of topical dosage forms can be dependent on various factors such as pharmacology of active component, physic chemical properties of the formulation, including pH, viscosity, spreadability and bio-adhesion [5].

Ear Cleansers

Once the otitis and infection are under control, ear cleaners should be used as maintenance therapy (typically once to twice weekly) to help prevent further infections. The effectiveness of topical antimicrobials, particularly aminoglycosides and polymyxin B, is considerably enhanced by the removal of detritus and purulent material. Over cleaning should be avoided, as it can lead to ear infections and maceration. Owners should be instructed on the right way to clean their dog's ears and should avoid using cotton swabs or balls inside their ears. Drying agents, antiseptics, ceruminolytics, and combination treatment are among the ear cleaners that are readily available (Table **2**).

Table 2. Listing these ear cleaners.

-	Product	Type	Dilution	Usage
1.	Acetic acid	Flushing and drying	1:1 or 1:3 dilution	Maintenance
2.	Chlorehexidine (5%)	flushing	1:100 of water	Bacterial otitis
3.	Glacial acetic acid	drying	-	Maintenance for yeast otits
4.	Lactic acid/ salicylic acid	-	-	Ceruminolytic
4.	Povidone iodine	flushing	-	Flushing
5.	Saline	Flushing	-	Flushing
6.	Dioctyle sodium sulphosuccinate	Ceruminolytic	-	Flushing

Acaricidals

Treatment options for infections brought on by *Otodectes cynotis* (ear mites) and, less frequently, *Demodex* species include a wide variety of acaricidal products [10 - 13]. Ivermectin, selamectin, monosulfiram, milbemycin, fipronil, permethrin, piperonyl butoxide, pyrethrins, thiabendazole, and rotenone are examples of veterinary acaricidal medications for label and extra label usage antibiotics

Drug concentrations used topically could be 100–1000 times higher than the minimal inhibitory concentration [13]. For the majority of bacterial and/or yeast otic infections, antibiotics should be taken up to one week after negative cytologic results [10 - 13]. It's often advised to apply twice daily. I advise caring for the patient up till the infection is cleared up if it's a multidrug-resistant infection.

When an infection is present and cleaning methods are insufficient, antibacterial agents are recommended. Glucocorticoids and antifungals are also present in the majority of topical antibacterial treatments.

The first-line antibiotics that are most frequently used are gentamicin, neomycin alone or in combination with other drugs. All topical gentamicin products have been linked to ototoxicity. Similar to chlorhexidine, In one study, otic gentamicin given every 12 hours for 21 days to ears with ruptured tympanic membranes had neither vestibule toxic or ototoxic consequences [9, 11]. The topical antibiotic polymyxin B is also quite effective against many *Pseudomonas* infections.

Second-line antibiotics include ticarcillin-clavulanate potassium, which can be purchased from compounding pharmacies, injectable amikacin combined with saline at a final concentration of 25 mg/mL, and tobramycin (Tobrex ocular solution, alcon.com). Due to the recent discovery that dogs treated with topicals containing amikacin and tobramycin were more likely to experience ototoxicity, caution should be used when using specific topical aminoglycosides. This finding was based on brainstem auditory evoked response testing.

Mupirocin and fluoroquinolones are third-line antibiotics. When treating *Staphylococcus* infections that are methicillin- and multi-drug resistant, mupirozin should be used; one tube of the medication (30 g) should be mixed with 30 mL of sterile saline. In chronic, severe instances, enrofloxacin plus silver sulfadiazine is frequently unsuccessful [14].

Many other off-label recipes call for injectable enrofloxacin formulations, such as a 25% mixture of the drug (22.7 mg/mL diluted with water, saline, or other active ingredients with varying amounts of dexamethasone, not to exceed 0.1% to 1%). Posatex can be used to treat multidrug-resistant infections such those caused by *Staphylococcus* and *Pseudomonas*. It comprises orbifloxacin, posaconazole, and prednisone.

Antifungal medications can be utilized in any incidence of otitis linked to yeasts like *Malassezia* or *Candida* species [10 - 13]. Only antifungal medicines can be discovered, although many products on the market also contain glucocorticoids and antibiotics. Antifungal medications that are typically effective include clotrimazole, miconazole, thiabendazole, acetic acid, and TrizEDTA and ketoconazole flush.

Glucocorticoids

There are numerous topical products with varying potencies that can be used in the external ear canal [10 - 13] Topical glucocorticoids are helpful in cases of chronic otitis externa. Glucocorticoids contain anti-inflammatory and anti-pruritic properties, as well as a reduction in exudation and swelling, all of which contribute to a decrease in pain and discomfort. They also reduce glandular secretions and promote sebaceous atrophy. Scar tissue and proliferative alterations may be lessened by glucocorticoids, aiding in the promotion of drainage and ventilation. The majority of ear products are made up of different glucocorticoid, antibiotic, antifungal, and parasiticide mixtures [10].

Long-term topical glucocorticoids may be needed in allergic otitis externa cases, along with careful management for adrenal suppression or any local adverse effects, like hair loss on the pinnae. In these circumstances, products with lesser glucocorticoids should be used, such as those with 1.0% or 0.5% hydrocortisone. For many chronic, stenotic otitis, and hyperplastic cases, it is advisable to suggest fluocinolone and dimethyl sulfoxide, with excellent outcomes.

The suggestion is only to be used with undamaged tympanic membranes following ear cleaning. These are fantastic solutions for patients who refuse topical medication at home, helping to increase compliance and maybe benefiting cases of acute or mild otitis. Because significant hyperplasia and stenosis prevent ear washing and examination of the tympanic membrane, their use in chronic severe otitis patients is constrained.

Systemic Treatment

A severe case of otitis externa that is refractory to topical treatment alone, simultaneous otitis media along with otits externa, owner unable to use topical medication, topical treatment ruled out by unfavourable changes, marked chronic proliferative changes are certain conditions that needs implementation of systemic therapy [11].

Antibiotics

Animals with otitis in accordance of moderate to severe proliferative changes with probable otitis, or no response to suitable topical therapy and washing may be treated with these medications. Prior to choosing a systemic antibiotic, The length of treatment may vary, but typically continue to administer medication for 1 month after clinical symptoms have subsided. When *Pseudomonas species* with other pertinent gram-negative organisms, or extremely resistant gram-positive bacteria are recovered and susceptibility is proven following culture, fluoroquinolones may be administered. Sometimes, higher doses are required than are typically advised.

Enrofloxacin is one oral fluoroquinolone that may be used. When *Pseudomonas* species, other pertinent gram-negative organisms, or extremely resistant gram-positive bacteria are recovered and susceptibility is proven following culture, fluoroquinolones may be administered. Sometimes, higher doses are required than are typically advised.

Enrofloxacin at 10 to 20 mg/kg q24h, marbofloxacin at 5 to 10 mg/kg q24h, or orbifloxacin at 10 mg/kg q24h are oral fluoroquinolones that may be employed. Ciprofloxacin should not be used in dogs due to uneven and low oral absorption (58.4%) using oral tablets, which could result in inefficiency and bacterial resistance. Rarely, multidrug-resistant otitis patients may require the use of injectable antimicrobials like aminoglycosides, carbapenems, and ceftazidime sodium. These medicines' potential negative effects must be taken into account. referring a dermatologist to handle these cases [8, 10].

LED-illuminated gel contains chromophores illuminated by a LED lamp, reemit fluorescent light which can stimulate physiological responses, promoting healing and controlling bacteria in in canine otitis externa,.

Antifungals

Malassezia otitis cases with severe symptoms or those who don't respond well to topical treatment alone may occasionally benefit from antifungal medications. Fluconazole, itraconazole, and ketoconazole are some of the most popular oral antifungals. They are all dosed at 5 to 10 mg/kg q24 or q12 (split) hours. Additionally, 30 mg/kg q24h of terbinafine may be administered.

Glucocorticoids

Glucocorticoids are typically prescribed in cases of persistent pathologic alterations, such as significant hyperplasia and canal stenosis, and a highly irritated and painful otitis. Prednisone or prednisolone oral anti-inflammatory dosages (0.5 to 1 mg/kg q24h) can be administered initially before being decreased to the lowest alternate-day dosage that manages the clinical symptoms. In most cases of *Pseudomonas* otitis, it is advisable for oral glucocorticoids [5, 6].

A few days prior to the owners cleaning and medicating the ears, oral glucocorticoids may also assist to lessen pain and discomfort. In cases of extreme pain, combination of oral glucocorticoids with oral opioids, such as oral tramadol at 2 to 4 mg/kg every 4 to 12 hourly gives good results. Alternate-day glucocorticoid medication may be recommended with careful monitoring for side effects when longer-term treatment is anticipated.

Cyclosporine

When surgery is not an option, oral cyclosporine at a concentration of 5mg/kg body weight may be considered a medicinal alternative for otitis externa, resulting in improved temperament, hearing, and quality of life. In cases when surgery is not an option, oral cyclosporine may be tried.

Education of the Clients and Follow-Up Visits

The prolonged process of managing otitis, including the requirement for appropriate home therapy and numerous follow-up visits, long-term prognosis, quality of life, pain management, and medical costs, must be discussed with clients. Additionally, clients must be shown how to properly clean their ears and administer eardrops [8]. Every 2 to 4 weeks, depending on the severity, dogs with otitis should undergo a re-evaluation with an otic examination and cytology to determine how well the treatment is working. The majority of bacterial and yeast infections should be treated for at least a week after clinical improvement and negative ear cytologic results.

Home Care for Ear Maintenance and Prevention

A cleaning and drying agent (to prevent wax buildup in the ear canal), antimicrobial ear cleaners (for example, for recurrent ear infections), and occasionally topical glucocorticoids are all necessary forms of maintenance otic therapy.

Surgical Management

Surgical care may be suggested, especially in cases of otic tumors and chronic end-stage otitis, after thorough discussion and consideration of all available medical therapeutic options.

CONCLUDING REMARKS

Otitis externa, an inflammatory disease of the external ear canal with ear pinna. It is acute or chronic with glandular hyperplasia, glandular dilation, epithelial hyperplasia, and hyperkeratosis. Physical examination can help with early detection of mild and early cases of otitis externa. Proper effective treatment by controlling infection with inflammatory changes and identification of the underlying factors (that led to development of otitis externa) are important preventive strategies by counteracting the disease. Topical application as well as systemic use of anti-inflammatory therapy and/or anti-microbial therapy may be indicated for individual patients. Glucocorticoids can be applied for a short duration to help with reduction of pain and swelling.

REFERENCES

[1]   Agnihotri D, Sharma A and Khurana R 2014 XXXII Annual Convention of ISVM and International Symposium on the 21st Centuary Road map for Veterinary Practice, Education and research in India and Developing Countries, 6.P.21; PP 91.

[2]   Hawkins C, Harper D, Burch D, Änggård E, Soothill J. Topical treatment of *Pseudomonas aeruginosa* otitis of dogs with a bacteriophage mixture: A before/after clinical trial. Vet Microbiol 2010; 146(3-4): 309-13.
       [http://dx.doi.org/10.1016/j.vetmic.2010.05.014] [PMID: 20627620]

[3]   Cole LK, Kwochka KW, Kowalski JJ, Hillier A. Microbial flora and antimicrobial susceptibility patterns of isolated pathogens from the horizontal ear canal and middle ear in dogs with otitis media. J Am Vet Med Assoc 1998; 212(4): 534-8.
       [http://dx.doi.org/10.2460/javma.1998.212.04.534] [PMID: 9491161]

[4]   Diagnosis and treatment of otitis media in dogs and cats, Gotthelf, L. N. 2004.Small Animal Practice, 34(2), 469-487 in Veterinary Clinics.

[5]   Fernandez G, Barboza G, Villalobos A, Parra O, Finol G, Ramirez RA. Isolation and identification of micro organisms present in 53 dogs suffering otitis externa. Rev Cient (Maracaibo) 2006; 16: 23-30.

[6]   Gabal M A 1988 Preliminary studies on the mechanism of infection and characterization of *Malassezia* pachydermatis in association with canine otitis externa. Mycopathologia, Vol. 104, PP: 93-98.

[7]   Girão MD, Prado MR, Brilhante RSN, *et al. Malassezia pachydermatis* isolated from normal and diseased external ear canals in dogs: A comparative analysis. Vet J 2006; 172(3): 544-8.
[http://dx.doi.org/10.1016/j.tvjl.2005.07.004] [PMID: 16154787]

[8]   J. Bajwa. TreaTympanic membraneent options and side effects for canine otitis externa. The Canadian Veterinary Journal, 2019; 60(1), 97.

[9]   Lund EM, Armstrong PJ, Kirk CA, Kolar LM, Klausner JS. Health status and population characteristics of dogs and cats examined at private veterinary practices in the United States. J Am Vet Med Assoc 1999; 214(9): 1336-41.
[http://dx.doi.org/10.2460/javma.1999.214.09.1336] [PMID: 10319174]

[10]   Lyskova P, Vydrzalova M, Mazurova J. Identification and antimicrobial susceptibility of bacteria and yeasts isolated from healthy dogs and dogs with otitis externa. J Vet Med A Physiol Pathol Clin Med 2007; 54(10): 559-63.
[http://dx.doi.org/10.1111/j.1439-0442.2007.00996.x] [PMID: 18045339]

[11]   Mactaggart D. Assessment and management of chronic ear disease. In Pract 2008; 30(8): 450-8.
[http://dx.doi.org/10.1136/inpract.30.8.450]

[12]   Nuttall T, Cole LK. Evidence-based veterinary dermatology: a systematic review of interventions for treatment of *Pseudomonas* otitis in dogs. Vet Dermatol 2007; 18(2): 69-77.
[http://dx.doi.org/10.1111/j.1365-3164.2007.00575.x] [PMID: 17355420]

[13]   Nuttall TJ. Use of ticarcillin in the management of canine otitis externa complicated by *Pseudomonas aeruginosa*. J Small Anim Pract 1998; 39(4): 165-8.
[http://dx.doi.org/10.1111/j.1748-5827.1998.tb03624.x] [PMID: 9577757]

[14]   Patterson S. Ototoxicity. Proc WCVD 6 2008; 227-30.

[15]   Rosser EJ Jr. Evaluation of the patient with otitis externa. Vet Clin North Am Small Anim Pract 1988; 18(4): 765-72.
[http://dx.doi.org/10.1016/S0195-5616(88)50079-7] [PMID: 3264953]

[16]   Saridomichelakis MN, Farmaki R, Leontides LS, Koutinas AF. Aetiology of canine otitis externa: a retrospective study of 100 cases. Vet Dermatol 2007; 18(5): 341-7.
[http://dx.doi.org/10.1111/j.1365-3164.2007.00619.x] [PMID: 17845622]

[17]   Scott D W, Miller W H and Griffin C E 2001 Diseases of the eyelids, claws, anal sacs and ears. In Small Animal Dermatology, 6th Ed., Philadelphia, W B Saunders, PP: 71 - 1235.
[http://dx.doi.org/10.1016/B978-0-7216-7618-0.50023-7]

[18]   Tambella AM, Attili AR, Beribè F, *et al.* Management of otitis externa with an led-illuminated gel: a randomized controlled clinical trial in dogs. BMC Vet Res 2020; 16(1): 91.
[http://dx.doi.org/10.1186/s12917-020-02311-9] [PMID: 32192496]

[19]   Usui R, Usui R, Fukuda M, Fukui E, Hasegawa A. Treatment of canine otitis externa using video otoscopy. J Vet Med Sci 2011; 73(9): 1249-52.
[http://dx.doi.org/10.1292/jvms.10-0488] [PMID: 21597241]

[20]   Zur G, Lifshitz B, Bdolah-Abram T. The association between the signalment, common causes of canine otitis externa and pathogens. J Small Anim Pract 2011; 52(5): 254-8.
[http://dx.doi.org/10.1111/j.1748-5827.2011.01058.x] [PMID: 21539570]

CHAPTER 15

Otitis Media and its Clinical Management

Nidhi S. Choudhary²·*, H. K. Mehta¹, V. Agrawal², Sumit Gautam¹ and **Rakesh Dangi¹**

¹ *Department of Veterinary Medicine, College of Veterinary Science and A.H. Mhow, NDVSU Jabalpur (MP), India*

² *Department of Veterinary Parasitology, College of Veterinary Science and A.H. Mhow, NDVSU Jabalpur (MP), India*

Abstract: Otitis externa and otitis media are prevalent conditions in veterinary medicine, frequently encountered in dogs suffering from chronic ear ailments and in cats affected by upper respiratory diseases and polyps. Detecting otitis media necessitates a comprehensive evaluation of the patient's medical history and clinical manifestations, coupled with additional diagnostic techniques to ascertain the presence of disease within the bulla. In cases where the integrity of the eardrum cannot be definitively assessed, it is judicious to assume the presence of middle ear pathology and initiate appropriate management. An essential precaution is to abstain from employing potentially ototoxic ear cleansers and topical medications in suspected otitis media cases. The successful treatment of this condition often involves a combination of systemic and topical therapies within the thoroughly cleaned bulla.

Within the realm of veterinary practice, otitis media is an affliction that is all too common and frequently proves to be a vexing challenge. Its diagnosis can be a laborious and, at times, invasive process, incurring substantial costs. Otitis media typically emanates as an extension of external ear afflictions, often arising as a consequence of chronic otitis externa. Furthermore, the presence of otitis media can be a causative factor in cases where treatment for otitis externa has proven ineffective, underscoring the imperative of reaching a definitive diagnosis to guide appropriate therapeutic interventions. Otitis media, or middle ear pathology more broadly, poses a diagnostic conundrum, as the presenting clinical signs often mirror those of otitis externa, rendering differentiation difficult in the absence of evident facial and/or sympathetic nerve dysfunction. It is worth noting that otitis media can progress, in some instances, to otitis interna, giving rise to peripheral vestibular syndrome symptoms. This underscores the critical importance of recommending tomographic imaging in situations where chronic otitis externa manifests as a suppurative or proliferative condition.

---

* **Corresponding author Nidhi S. Choudhary:** Department of Veterinary Medicine, College of Veterinary Science and A.H. Mhow, NDVSU Jabalpur (MP), India; E-mail: drnidhichoudhary2002@gmail.com

Tanmoy Rana (Ed.)

Keywords: Eardrum, Otitis, Otitis media, Otitis externa, Tympanic membrane.

INTRODUCTION

Secondary ear infections result from the presence of commensal microorganisms like *Staphylococci* and *Malassezia* or environmental opportunistic pathogens, such as *Pseudomonas*. The primary etiological factor represents the true instigator of the inflammatory response within the ear, necessitating precise identification and effective management. While predisposing factors alone seldom incite otitis, they do heighten the susceptibility of a dog to ear inflammation or the progression to severe disease. Ongoing issues manifest as a consequence of recurring bouts of inflammation and infection, ultimately culminating in an advanced stage of otitis, compelling the need for surgical intervention.

The term otitis refers to an ear infection, however it does not specify which region of the ear is affected. Otitis media is an inflammation and/or infection of the middle ear, whereas otitis externa is an infection that develops in the external ear canal. Because some nerves are directly related with the middle ear, infection there can damage them, resulting in the neurologic symptoms seen with this illness: head tilt, loss of balance, and nystagmus (back-and-forth eye movements). These are known as vestibular indications. Middle ear infections can also induce facial nerve paralysis, resulting in a slack-jawed look on that side of the face.

Otitis media is most commonly caused by an existing otitis externa and moves from the external ear canal *via* the tympanic membrane and into the middle ear. The external ear canal infection causes inflammation and damage to the ear canal and tympanic membrane, allowing the infection to invade the middle ear.

Otitis media has been discovered in 16% of dogs with acute (short-term) otitis externa and 52% of dogs with chronic (long-term) otitis externa. In comparison, 63% of cats with otitis media/interna had no prior history of ear infection [1].

ETIOLOGY

Otitis media is a middle ear infection. The following are the most common causes of otitis media in dogs:

1) Otitis externa spreading through the eardrum into the bulla.

2) Bacterial migration from the pharynx to the middle ear through the Eustachian tube.

3) Aural tumour.

4) Foreign body (plant awn).

The migration of germs from the outer ear to the inner ear is the most prevalent cause of otitis media in dogs. This happens in chronic otitis externa situations. Maceration and eventual destruction of the tympanic membrane are caused by continuous moisture in the outer ear. The infection subsequently spreads into the bulla from the ear canal. If the outer ear infection is mostly gone, the eardrum will mend. Unfortunately, the mended eardrum traps infection and exudate in the middle ear (Fig. **1**).

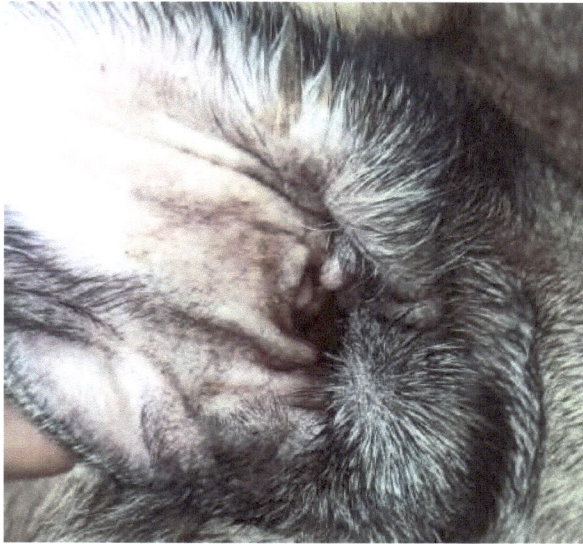

Fig. (1). Ear infection of a dog.

Other causes of otitis media can include infections in the nose and throat, trauma, foreign bodies, fungal infections, inflammatory polyps, cancer, *etc.* In addition, developmental abnormalities of the external ear canal and pharynx can lead to otitis media. It is generally agreed that most cases of otitis media are caused by bacteria. Although *Staphylococcus* and *Streptococcus spp.* are among the most commonly isolated organisms, they have also been isolated from the middle ears of healthy dogs thus; their role as primary inducers of inflammation is questionable.

Pseudomonas and *Proteus spp.* are also usually cited as etiologic agents of otitis media, however they have not been isolated from healthy dogs' middle ears. *Clostridium spp.* and *Escherichia coli* have also been linked to otitis media. Otitis medium is commonly caused by yeast infections such as *Malassezia canis* or *Candida spp.*

PATHOPHYSIOLOGY

In canine patients, secondary otitis media occurs when exudates and infectious agents flow from the external ear canal into the middle ear through an eroded or ruptured eardrum, becoming entrapped in the ventral portion of the bulla. The introduction of medications, substances found in ear flushing products, or debris from the external ear canal into the middle ear, resulting from a compromised eardrum, initiates a tissue response within the respiratory epithelial lining of the middle ear, known as secondary otitis media. The pathogenesis of this condition is intricate and frequently multifaceted in dogs. Due to the distinctive L-shaped structure of the canine external ear canal, proteolytic enzymes within the exudates produced as a consequence of otitis externa accumulate against the thinnest section of the eardrum. The ensuing inflammation and enzymatic degradation lead to necrosis of the epithelial layer and the underlying collagen, causing a thinning of the tympanic membrane (TM) and its subsequent weakening.

The ulceration along the ear canal can extend to the eardrum, resulting in the discharge of serum, which can induce maceration and excoriation of the epithelium. The release of bacterial proteases, collagenases, elastases, and lysozymes from phagocytic cells, combined with epidermal maceration caused by the excessive serum in the ear canal, disrupts the epithelial layers of the ear canal, potentially leading to eardrum erosion or rupture. Regardless of whether the condition is primary or secondary in nature, the ensuing inflammation causes the mucoperiosteum, the lining epithelium in the bulla, to transition from a cuboidal to a pseudostratified columnar ciliated configuration, accompanied by an increase in secretory cell and gland quantity, contributing to exudate accumulation. Prolonged inflammation results in mucosal ulceration and erosion of the epithelial lining. The lamina propria thickens in response to the inflammatory process, while enhanced vascularity leads to edema and granulation tissue formation. As otitis media becomes chronic, the lamina propria transforms into dense connective tissue, and bone spicules may develop within it. The cycle of inflammation, ulceration, infection, and granulation tissue formation may persist, causing destruction of the adjacent bone. The exudates and secretions thus generated in the bulla escape into the external ear through the ruptured eardrum, contributing to the existing exudates in the external ear canal. This substantial liquid volume fills the ear canal, occasionally overflowing onto the pinna during head shaking. When there is an obstruction like a polyp or tumor impeding the drainage of secretions and exudates from the middle ear, significant amounts of inspissated material can accumulate upon removal of the obstruction.

The fluid pressure gradient created by suppurative otitis media and heightened mucus production prevents the complete closure of the eardrum. As the fluid pressure elevates within the bulla, it exerts force against the healing eardrum, which possesses a thin and delicate covering. This pressure enables fluid to escape through the path of least resistance, leaving a small perforation in the tympanic membrane. As long as this eardrum aperture persists, the condition remains in a state of flux, with fluid capable of moving into or out of the bulla, carrying infectious agents and exudates in both directions.

Resolution of otitis media in dogs occurs when the quantity of middle ear secretions and exudate diminishes, the infection is effectively managed through therapy, and the fluid pressure decreases, enabling the eardrum to heal [2].

Secondary otitis media in dogs is caused by otitis externa that extends through the eardrum. Bacteria, yeast, hairs, cells, enzymes, and drugs all travel past the eardrum and into the middle ear bulla. The foreign substance causes irritation and promotes mucus output from the mucous membrane [3].

Otitis media, characterized by an inflammatory process affecting the middle ear, is a prevalent condition observed in small animal veterinary clinics, affecting both canine and feline patients. It leads to damage to the tympanic membrane and bulla and manifests through a spectrum of clinical indications, encompassing pain and vestibular symptoms. The development of otitis media can be attributed to either primary or secondary causative factors. In dogs, secondary otitis media often arises as a consequence of the extension of chronic otitis externa through the tympanic membrane. Nevertheless, primary factors, including the presence of foreign bodies, primary secretory otitis media (PSOM) in Cavalier King Charles Spaniels, or inadvertent rupture during ear cleaning, can also precipitate this condition. Neglected or inadequately treated otitis media can progress to otitis interna, an inflammatory disorder affecting the inner ear structures, resulting in damage to the auditory system, frequently leading to deafness and neurologic manifestations. In severe instances of otitis interna, there exists a risk of life-threatening otogenic intracranial infections and meningitis, facilitated by the passage of infectious agents from the inner ear to the brainstem *via* the nerves and vessels situated in the internal acoustic meatus [4].

CLINICAL SIGNS

In the context of otitis media in dogs, a frequent scenario involves a prior history of recurrent or chronic bacterial infections in the external ear. The mucous membrane lining the tympanic bulla responds to various foreign substances, such as infectious agents, hair, cells, cerumen from the external ear canal, and chemicals or pharmaceuticals applied externally, by generating a purulent exudate and elevating the secretion of protective mucus through activated goblet cells. Notably, mucus is not generated throughout the external ear but rather seeps from the tympanic bulla into the horizontal canal through any rupture in the tympanic membrane [2].

Sensitivity to palpation at the base of the ear canal or discomfort when manipulating the pinna should raise suspicions of otitis media in clinical practice. Patients afflicted by otitis media may also display a reluctance to have their mouths opened, potentially accompanied by a history of avoiding hard food due to inflammation, swelling, and pain within the adjacent bulla, near the temporomandibular joint. When otitis media influences the nerves surrounding the ear base or the tympanic bulla, subtle manifestations may include keratoconjunctivitis sicca on the same side, resulting from impairment of the palpebral branch of the facial nerve. Patients may be presented by their owners with concerns about hearing impairment. Such cases merit evaluation for otitis media, as the presence of fluid in the middle ear can diminish auditory acuity. In instances where this fluid results from prior flushing, it is typically reabsorbed within 7 to 10 days, and the patient's hearing capacity is restored. However, when the eardrum is perforated or when the ossicles in the middle ear have undergone sclerotic changes, air conduction hearing is compromised, particularly affecting the effective transmission of high-pitched sound waves from the ear canal to the cochlea [2].

Typical indications of otitis media encompass manifestations such as discharge emerging from the external ear canal, dogs frequently pawing or rubbing the affected ear, engaging in head-shaking behavior, experiencing auditory deficits, or encountering pain upon head contact. Some dogs may exhibit signs of depression, reduced appetite, and possibly fever [5].

As the condition progresses into chronicity, it gives rise to proliferative alterations resulting in the stenosis and occlusion of the ear canal, and in certain cases, even a rupture of the tympanic membrane. Consequently, fibrosis and mineralization of the ear canal occur, and, albeit infrequently, are accompanied by ulcerations of the canal, often accompanied by ongoing pain and impairment, particularly in instances involving *Psuedomonas aeruginosa* infections [6]. Particular clinical symptoms that signifies otitis media encompass the occurrence of facial nerve paralysis and Horner's syndrome. Damage to the facial nerve, which courses near the middle ear, elicits clinical signs like a drooping ear or lip, salivary drooling, and a reduced or absent palpebral reflex. Horner's syndrome is a consequence of harm to the sympathetic nerve fibers that travel in proximity to the middle ear, characterized by ptosis, miosis, enophthalmos, and protrusion of the nictitating membrane [7]. Additional signs encompass nerve-related keratoconjunctivitis sicca, a dry nose, hearing deficits, and sensitivity upon palpation of the tympanic bulla (TB), or discomfort upon opening the mouth [8].

DIAGNOSIS

Diagnosing otitis media in dogs poses a considerable challenge due to the unique, elongated, and conical shape of the canine ear canal, which impedes the clear observation of the tympanic membrane (TM). Furthermore, many dogs with otitis media maintain an intact TM, creating an illusion of normalcy within the middle ear. A substantial number of canine patients afflicted by otitis media also contend with chronic otitis externa, marked by pathological alterations to the ear canal, causing stenosis that renders a visual assessment of the TM unfeasible. A prevailing theory suggests that otitis media often extends from untreated, improperly managed, or treatment-resistant otitis externa, resulting in cumulative damage and gradual weakening of the eardrum over time.

Otitis Media, like other skin illnesses, is diagnosed based on symptoms, history, physical findings, and laboratory tests.

History

To identify the fundamental underlying dermatologic condition, get a complete history to determine the age of start, duration of clinical manifestations, and level of skin involvement (such as pruritus). Identify previous treatment procedures and responses to therapy to assist guide future treatment selections.

Physical Examination

A physical examination should be undertaken to detect systemic symptoms of sickness or localized infections that may indicate hematogenous infection disseminated to the middle ear. Swelling, lumps, or soreness should be palpated carefully around the temporomandibular joints and the base of the ears. The pharyngeal region should be examined for evidence of inflammation or tumors that may have traveled to the middle ear through the auditory tube. Schirmer tear strips should be used to measure tear production. The external auditory canal should then be inspected. In most situations, heavy sedation or general anesthesia is required to adequately inspect the external ear canal and tympanic membrane.

Otoscopic Examination

Conducting an otoscopic assessment is essential to examine the condition of the external ear canal and the tympanic membrane. This examination is carried out employing either a handheld otoscope or a video otoscope (Fig. **2**).

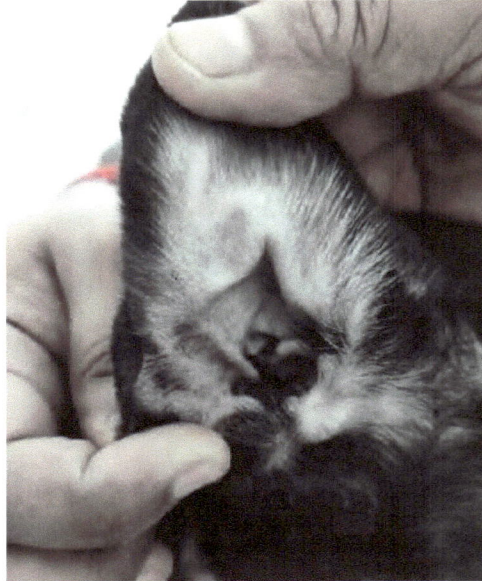

Fig. (2). Depicts Otitis Media of a dog.

Video-otoscopy

Conducting video otoscopy involves the utilization of specialized equipment such as an otoendoscope, camera, light source, and monitor. This approach results in the enhanced illumination and magnification of the vertical and horizontal ear canal and tympanic membrane, facilitating a more comprehensive assessment of these anatomical features in comparison to the conventional hand-held otoscope (Fig. **3**). The procedure is typically carried out under sedation or anesthesia, and it offers the advantage of allowing ear flushing through the otoendoscope's opening, retrieval of foreign objects, debris, or parasites using grasping forceps, obtaining biopsies with specialized biopsy forceps, and performing myringotomy *via* a catheter [7].

The most direct approach to diagnosing otitis media involves confirming the absence of the tympanic membrane (TM), which is most effectively accomplished using video otoscopy . In addition to visualizing the TM for assessing its condition and appearance, the video otoscope serves the purpose of detecting the emergence of air bubbles from the tympanic cavity (TC). To achieve this, the procedure entails placing the dog in lateral recumbency and filling the ear canal with saline, with a focus on observing the region of the TM. If, during the dog's breathing, air bubbles become evident in this area, it serves as confirmation of a ruptured TM.

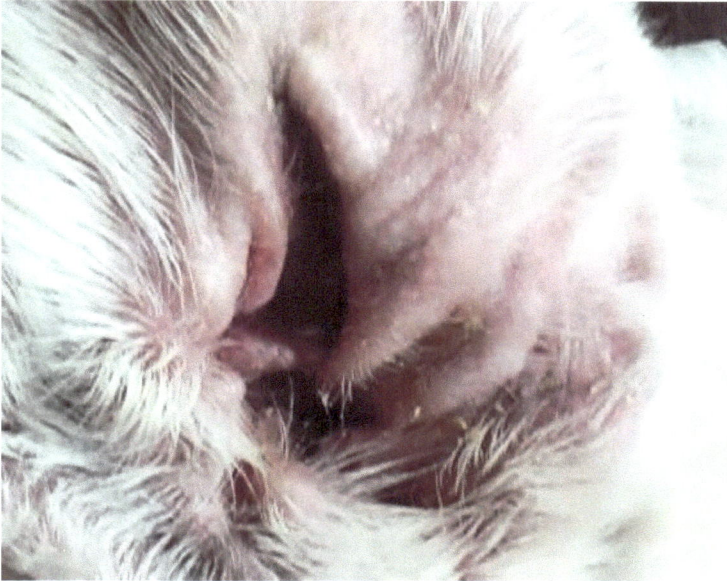

Fig. (3). History of chronic otitis externa that can lead to otitis media in dog if untreated.

Cytology and Bacterial Culture and Susceptibility Testing (C/S)

Cytology and culture/sensitivity (C/S) testing are crucial diagnostic procedures employed to guide the selection of appropriate systemic and topical antimicrobial treatments. Cytology is a cost-effective and swift examination recommended for all cases of otitis. The process involves swabbing and transferring the sample onto a glass slide, followed by heat fixation and staining with a modified Wright's stain (Diff-Quik) or a gram stain. At low magnification (100x), the search begins for keratinocytes and inflammatory cells. Upon their identification, immersion oil is applied to the slide, enabling examination at high magnification (1000x). The count and classification of bacteria, yeast, and inflammatory cells are meticulously recorded. When obtaining samples for cytology and C/S, it is advisable to do so from the horizontal ear canal prior to performing a deep otic flush. In cases of tympanic membrane abnormalities (such as bulging, discoloration, or opacity), samples can be directly collected from the middle ear cavity if the tympanic membrane is ruptured, or *via* a myringtomy if the membrane displays irregularities (Fig. **4**) [7].

Radiograph

Radiography serves as a widely accessible imaging technique and is typically the initial choice for assessing the status of the middle ear. To ensure optimal patient positioning for visualizing the tympanic bulla, the use of general anesthesia is often necessary [9]. Five standard projections are typically employed, including dorsoventral, latero-lateral, rostro 30° ventral caudo-dorsal open-mouth (rostro-caudal open-mouth), and left and right lateral 20° ventral-latero-dorsal aspects (lateral oblique) [10]. In cases involving a substantial presence of viscous exudate or the occurrence of tissue growths such as neoplasms, polyps, or cholesteatomas within the air-filled bulla tympanica, the entire bulla may exhibit a radiopaque appearance.

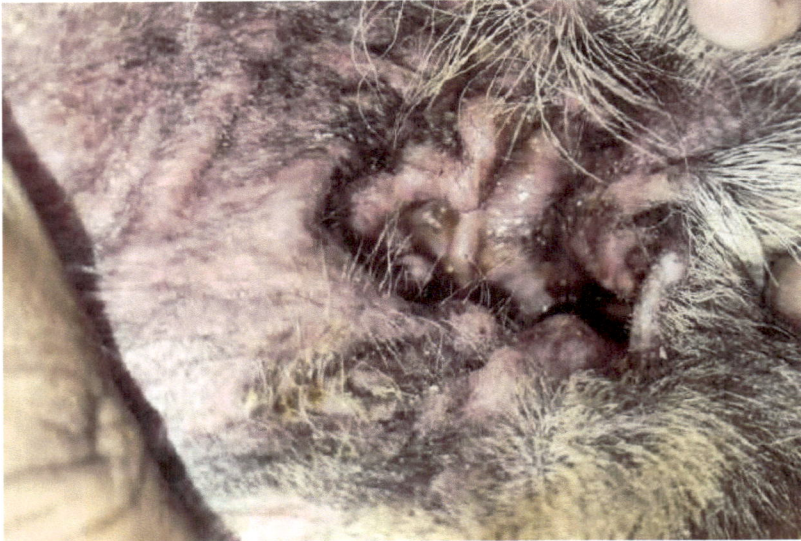

Fig. (4). Mucoid exudate in the ear canal.

Computed Tomography Scan

Imaging methods such as computed tomography (CT) and magnetic resonance imaging (MRI) offer complementary diagnostic approaches, exhibiting superior diagnostic capabilities when compared to alternative imaging techniques. CT primarily excels in providing precise delineation of bony structures, whereas MRI is particularly adept at defining soft tissue structures, including the inner ear labyrinth fluid and intracranial structures. Factors such as accessibility, cost-effectiveness, shorter scan duration, and the enhanced visualization of bony structures establish high-resolution CT as the preferred choice for middle ear imaging in human patients. Additionally, CT has been explored as a valuable option for evaluating middle ear structures in animals. This noninvasive diagnostic method allows the cross-sectional visualization of anatomical structures, eliminating the issue of superimposition experienced with radiographs. Consequently, CT appears to offer superior sensitivity and specificity when compared to radiography for the diagnosis of middle ear conditions [11].

Biopsy

Any mass discovered in the vertical, horizontal, or middle ear canals should be biopsied. Submit the formalin-fixed biopsy specimens for histopathologic examination.

TREATMENT

Planning treatment of otitis media requires a stepwise protocol for maximal effect. An organized approach allows the clinician to formulate treatment or to change existing treatment based on observations. The steps outlined provide a framework for treating otitis media:

1. Access middle ear.

2. Perform cytology and bacterial culture.

3. Flush bulla.

4. Infuse topical medications into the bulla.

5. Reduce inflammation with corticosteroids.

6. Administer systemic and topical antimicrobials.

7. Recheck weekly, and retreat for two to three times.

8. Consider surgery.

The objectives of treatment entail the cleansing of the external and middle ear, the elimination of infected, inflammatory, or foreign substances, and the facilitation of middle ear drainage. Otitis therapy consists of identifying and controlling all the factors involved and considering medical options, including topical and systemic therapy; these should be co-adjuvated by ear cleaning and, when needed, by ear flushing. Length of treatment and prognosis varies based on causes and factors.

In certain situations, empiric therapy becomes a necessity, particularly in healthcare facilities where access to microbiology laboratories is limited, and when invasive diagnostics are unfeasible, which is often the case with otitis media. While there are identifiable trends, noteworthy disparities in resistance rates have been documented across various medical institutions and geographical regions [12].

The active involvement of pet owners plays a pivotal role, as the majority of topical treatments are typically administered by clients at home, significantly influencing the overall treatment outcome. Furthermore, the importance of adhering to follow-up appointments for examinations and repeat cytology should be emphasized, as maintaining clients' commitment to consistent treatment can be a recurring challenge [13].

Accessing the Middle Ear

This entails otoscopic examination.

Flushing and Suctioning the Bulla

A vital technique in otitis media treatment involves flushing the bulla. Thick exudate that accumulates within the middle ear during otitis media can impede the penetration of topical otic medications. Hence, the exudate and secretory material need to be removed. Hydrating the mucus with a flushing solution renders it less dense and more amenable to suction. This technique effectively separates mucus from the tissue, preventing it from adhering to the mucous membrane, unlike cerumen in the external ear canal. The author recommends using a very dilute warm povidone iodine solution in warm tap water for flushing, with the addition of warmed Tris-EDTA in the presence of an identifiable bacterial infection [2].

When there is a need for comprehensive cleaning of the entire external ear canal and possibly the middle ear, ear flushing is the indicated procedure. To ensure safety and effectiveness, it is imperative to conduct this process under general anesthesia, with the placement of an endotracheal tube that is appropriately cuffed. This precaution prevents the inadvertent flow of fluids from the ear into the respiratory tract *via* the eustachian tube.

In cases where the ear canals exhibit hyperplasia, stenosis, or pronounced inflammation, it is advisable to administer systemic glucocorticoid treatment at a dosage of 0.5mg/kg to 1mg/kg once daily for a duration of two to three weeks before initiating the flushing procedure.

The optimal method for ear flushing involves the use of a video otoscope. However, when this equipment is not available, a practical alternative is employing a urinary catheter or a feeding tube connected to a syringe for the delivery of fluids, typically sterile saline. The use of a three-way tap can facilitate the process and enhance its effectiveness.

Video otoscopes offer distinct advantages by providing enhanced visualization of the tympanic membrane and a portion of the middle ear space. Their utility is particularly evident in specialized procedures like polyp extraction and laser therapy, where precision and clarity are essential.

In certain instances, prior to initiating ear flushing, it may be necessary to employ an ear cleansing solution to emulsify and effectively eliminate debris. However, it is crucial to exercise caution when the eardrum is not visible, as virtually all ear cleaning solutions carry the potential for ototoxicity. An exception to this exists in solutions containing only squalene [13].

Myringotomy

In cases where otitis media is either suspected or confirmed through diagnostic imaging methods, the deliberate rupture of the tympanic membrane is a recommended procedure. This intervention serves multiple purposes, including obtaining samples for cytology and culture from the tympanic bulla and facilitating the flushing of the middle ear spaces. The procedure necessitates the use of general anesthesia and should be conducted under direct visualization following the thorough cleansing of the external ear canal, ensuring it is dry prior to the manipulation [13].

Bulla Infusion

The removal of mucus and pus within the tympanic bulla is a pivotal aspect of otitis media treatment. This allows topical medications to permeate the thickened and folded mucoperiosteum. Aqueous formulations of nontoxic topical antibiotics, steroids, or antifungals are placed on the mucoperiosteum to expedite recovery. The medication is infused into the bulla *via* a small catheter until it overflows into the external ear canal. This procedure, involving flushing, suctioning, and bulla infusion, should be repeated weekly during therapy [2].

TOPICAL TREATMENT

Topical Antibiotics

First-line antibiotics commonly include products containing neomycin alone or in combination with other agents and gentamicin. Gentamicin topicals have been associated with ototoxicity. Polymyxin B is also an effective topical antibiotic, particularly against many *Pseudomonas* infections. However, purulent exudates can inactivate polymyxin. Second-line antibiotics consist of tobramycin, injectable amikacin mixed with saline, and ticarcillin-clavulanate potassium. Caution is advised with certain topical aminoglycosides due to the risk of ototoxicity. Third-line antibiotics include mupirocin and fluoroquinolones, ideally chosen based on culture and sensitivity testing. Mupirocin is reserved for multidrug-resistant *Staphylococcus* infections. Injectable formulations may be used against multidrug-resistant infections, such as *Staphylococcus* and *Pseudomonas* [14].

• Fusidic acid is characterized by its bacteriostatic properties, proving effective specifically against Gram-positive cocci. Its mode of action involves interference with bacterial protein synthesis. When combined with framycetin, it demonstrates synergistic activity, notably against Staphylococci and Streptococci.

• Aminoglycosides, on the other hand, exhibit bactericidal attributes with a broad-spectrum application. They operate by disrupting bacterial protein synthesis. It's noteworthy that their efficacy is heightened in an alkaline environment but diminished in an acidic setting, emphasizing the need for concurrent treatment with cleansing agents. However, it is crucial to administer these agents at least one hour before using aminoglycosides. It's important to be cautious when utilizing aminoglycosides topically with a ruptured tympanic membrane, as they carry ototoxic potential.

• Neomycin, a member of the aminoglycoside class, has been associated with topical adverse reactions, including contact/irritant dermatitis.

• Polymyxin B, with its bactericidal qualities, is particularly effective against Gram-negative bacteria. *In vitro* studies have demonstrated its synergistic efficacy when combined with miconazole, especially against multi-resistant staphylococci. Its mechanism of action involves the alteration of cytoplasmic membrane permeability. Polymyxin B is ototoxic and can be inactivated by cellular debris, underscoring the significance of its association with ear cleaning procedures.

• Fluoroquinolones function as bactericidal agents, offering a broad spectrum of action. Their mechanism of action centers on the inhibition of DNA replication, rendering them effective against both Gram-positive and Gram-negative bacteria.

Other Topical Antimicrobials

Silver sulfadiazine exhibits an extensive antibacterial range, demonstrating notable efficacy, particularly against *Pseudomonas aeruginosa*. Remarkably, even at low concentrations of 0.02%, it has displayed complete effectiveness against *P. aeruginosa* and *Staphylococcus* species. This therapeutic agent is typically accessible in cream form and, despite its limited water solubility, a uniform emulsion can be attained through gentle mixing, ensuring its applicability [13].

Antifungal Agents

These are employed in otitis cases associated with yeasts, such as *Malassezia* or *Candida* species. Effective antifungals include clotrimazole, miconazole, thiabendazole, acetic acid, and ketoconazole flush [14].

Topical Glucocorticoids

Glucocorticoids are valued for their multifaceted properties, which encompass anti-inflammatory, anti-pruritic, and anti-proliferative effects. Additionally, they hold the capacity to diminish secretions from sebaceous and ceruminous glands. It's important to note that these substances can be absorbed systemically, leading to the suppression of adrenal gland function, which may persist for a duration exceeding two weeks after the administration of select glucocorticoids for more than a week. Prolonged treatment can potentially result in cutaneous atrophy, the formation of comedones, and the development of demodicosis. The efficacy of glucocorticoids is contingent upon factors such as their intrinsic potency, concentration, and the vehicle used for their administration.

Topical Acaricides

Products without acaricidal properties have proven effective in managing infestations of *Otodectescynotis* in both cats and dogs. Their mechanism of action is believed to involve suffocating the mites. While topical acaricides are an option, it's worth noting that, in the author's perspective, systemic acaricides are often the preferred choice due to their ease of use and their ability to treat the entire body [13].

SYSTEMIC TREATMENT

Systemic Antibiotic

Recommended when there is no otoscopic or radiographic evidence of middle ear cavity fluid or material. Systemic antibiotic therapy is selected based on culture and sensitivity testing of external ear canal exudate. Some antibiotics, such as aminoglycosides, should not be administered for extended periods due to their toxicity. If culture is not attainable, broad-spectrum antibiotics are employed, and if clinical signs do not improve, radiographs of the bullae should be repeated, and surgical management may be considered [5].

Systemic antimicrobial treatment plays a crucial role in managing specific conditions such as otitis media, stenosis, ulcerations, and deep-seated infections in veterinary medicine. The efficacy of systemic antimicrobials in otitis media is attributed to the richly vascularized mucous membrane lining within the middle ear. This unique vascular feature, distinct from the external ear canal, facilitates more effective drug diffusion from the vascular compartment into the bulla space.

When addressing otitis media, the choice of systemic antibiotics should be informed by culture and susceptibility testing. In situations where results are pending, initiating empirical treatment based on the examination of cytological specimens from the bulla content is a prudent course of action. Notably, antibiotics recognized for their effectiveness in treating otitis media include enrofloxacin, marbofloxacin, orbifloxacin, and cefalexin, each administered at specific dosages and frequencies. In cases involving multi-resistant *Pseudomonas* species infections, systemic aminoglycosides may be necessary, though their use warrants careful evaluation due to the potential for severe side effects.

Antimycotics

Systemic antimycotic treatment becomes necessary in cases where patients are afflicted by otitis media attributed to *Malassezia* species or when topical therapy proves impractical. The pharmacological arsenal employed in such instances encompasses itraconazole, fluconazole, and ketoconazole, each administered at specific dosages and frequencies. However, it's noteworthy that in the perspective of the author, ketoconazole should not serve as the primary choice for treating any fungal infection. Instead, preference should be accorded to itraconazole, considering its potential for more effective outcomes [13].

Glucocorticoids

When administered systemically, glucocorticoids offer several valuable benefits, which include the capacity to diminish stenosis, alleviate edema, reduce hyperplasia, facilitate otoscopic examination, and enhance the cleaning process. The initial treatment regimen typically involves a daily dosage ranging from 0.5mg/kg to 1mg/kg, with the specific amount tailored to the severity of the patient's clinical symptoms. As the condition ameliorates, it is advisable to gradually decrease both the dosage and the frequency of administration until the medication is no longer required, ultimately leading to discontinuation [13].

CONCLUSION

Otitis media is most commonly found in dogs with chronic ear diseases in dogs Diagnosis of otitis media is based on clinical history and diagnostic tools to determinie diseases within the bulla. If the integrity of the eardrum cannot be executed, it is, assumed that there is middle ear infection. Precaution should be entertained to avoid the use of potentially ototoxic ear cleaners or topical medications in suspected otitis media cases. Radiological investigation and a CT scan are moderate tool to determine otitis media in dogs. Therapeutic application should be needed by using systemic and topical treatment within the cleaned bulla. Surgical intervention may be required to cure these difficult cases

REFERENCES

[1]   Lundgren B. Otitis media (middle ear infection) in dogs and cats. Vet. Infor. Net. 2021; pp. 1-3.

[2]   Gotthelf LN. Diagnosis and treatment of otitis media in dogs and cats. Vet Clin North Am Small Anim Pract 2004; 34(2): 469-87.
        [http://dx.doi.org/10.1016/j.cvsm.2003.10.007] [PMID: 15062620]

[3]   Gotthelf L. Diagnosis and management of otitis. Dermatology 2008; 60-4.

[4]   Moriello KA. Overview of otitis media and interna. Merck Veterinary Manual 2018.

[5]   Shell LG. Otitis media and otitis lnterna etiology, diagnosis, and medical management. 1988; 18(4): 885–899.

[6]   Sykes JE, Nagle TM, White SD. Canine and feline infectious diseases. Elsevier Health Sciences 2022.

[7]   Cole LK. Otitis media and otitis interna. W.B. Saunders 2006; pp. 593-8.

[8]   Classen J, Bruehschwein A, Meyer-Lindenberg A, Mueller RS. Comparison of ultrasound imaging and video otoscopy with cross-sectional imaging for the diagnosis of canine otitis media. Vet J 2016; 217: 68-71.
        [http://dx.doi.org/10.1016/j.tvjl.2016.09.010] [PMID: 27810214]

[9]   Bischoff MG, Kneller SK. Diagnostic imaging of the canine and feline ear. Vet Clin North Am Small Anim Pract 2004; 34(2): 437-58.
        [http://dx.doi.org/10.1016/j.cvsm.2003.10.013] [PMID: 15062618]

[10]   Garosi LS, Dennis R, Schwarz T. Review of diagnostic imaging of ear diseases in the dog and cat. Vet Radiol Ultrasound 2003; 44(2): 137-46.
        [http://dx.doi.org/10.1111/j.1740-8261.2003.tb01262.x] [PMID: 12718347]

[11]   Belmudes A, Pressanti C, Barthez PY, Castilla-casta E, Cadiergues MC, Fabries L. Computed tomographic findings in 205 dogs with clinical signs compatible with middle ear disease: a retrospective study. Vet Dermatol 2017; 1-8.
        [PMID: 28994490]

[12]   Christina de Oliveira L, Carlos ALL, Raimunda SN. Brilhante, Cibele Barreto M. Carvalho. Etiology of canine otitis media and antimicrobial susceptibility of coagulase-positive staphylococci in Fortaleza City, Brazil. Braz J Microbiol 2006; 37: 144-7.

[13]   Filippo de Bellis. Management and treatment of otitis externa and media. Vet Times [Internet]. Available from: https://www.vettimes.co.uk

[14]   Koch SN, Torres SMF, Kramek B. Patulous Eustachian tube and palatine defect in a Dachshund with chronic unilateral otitis externa and otitis media. Vet Dermatol 2020; 439: 1-6.
        [http://dx.doi.org/10.1111/vde.12829] [PMID: 31908074]

CHAPTER 16

Otitis Interna and its Clinical Management

Bhavanam Sudhakara Reddy[1,*], **Kambala Swetha**[1] and **Sirigireddy Sivajothi**[1]

[1] *College of Veterinary Science-Proddatur, Sri Venkateswara Veterinary University, Andhra Pradesh, India*

Abstract: Otitis interna define as inflammation of inner ear, which will be an extension of infection from the otitis media or secondary to the chronic otitis externa. Improperly treated / untreated cases of otitis media can lead to development of otitis interna by involving the tympanic membrane. Clinical signs in otitis interna were impairment of hearing apparatus *i.e.* deafness and neurological indications such as tilting of the head towards the based on the side of the ear affected, development of the horizontal or rotary nystagmus, unequal legs coordination with diffused strength, circular walking pattern, sudden collapse, and even rolling towards the impacted side. Complication of otitis interna leads to development of life-threatening iotrogenic intracranial infections and meningitis by travelling the infectious organisms to the brainstem. In dogs with severe otitis interna that progressed to an intracranial infection, changes in mentation, ataxic changes, paresis, proprioceptive deficits, and development of seizures. Diagnosis of the otitis interna achieved by detailed history; dermatological, neurological and systemic examination along with the identification of underlying and/or associated factors. Otoscopic examination, cytology, microbial culture, antibiotic sensitivity test, radiography, computerized tomography scan evaluation and magnetic resonance imaging are helpful to differentiate the extent of lesions and severity. Medical management of otitis interna is carried out by identifying the suitable antibiotic by antibiotic sensitivity test followed by the correct dosage and duration approximately ranging from 4 to 8 weeks along with the systemic corticosteroids which have been advised to reduce the stenosis. When there is rupture of tympanic membrane, cautious utilization of topical antibiotic and/or anti-inflammatory preparations are advisable. If medical management fails to respond, surgical intervention are advised with vertical ear canal ablation, lateral ear canal resection, total ear canal ablation with lateral bulla osteotomy.

Keywords: Dogs, LECR, Nervous signs, Otitis interna, TECA, VECA.

INTRODUCTION

The internal ear structures of the dogs consist of three components *i.e.* the cochlea, the vestibule, and the semicircular canals. The cochlea is a spiral-shaped

---

[*] **Corresponding author Bhavanam Sudhakara Reddy:** College of Veterinary Science-Proddatur, Sri Venkateswara Veterinary University, Andhra Pradesh, India; E-mail: bhavanamvet@gmail.com

Tanmoy Rana (Ed.)

osseous tube, reminiscent of a snail's shell. The vestibule contains the utricle and saccule, responsible for detecting linear head movements. The semicircular canals, oriented perpendicular to each other, detect rotational head movements. Fluid movement within the semicircular ducts during head rotation deflects the cupula, leading to bending of the cilia and generation of impulses in the vestibular nerve. Overall, these intricate structures play vital roles in auditory and vestibular function in dogs (Figs. **1** and **2**) [1 - 3].

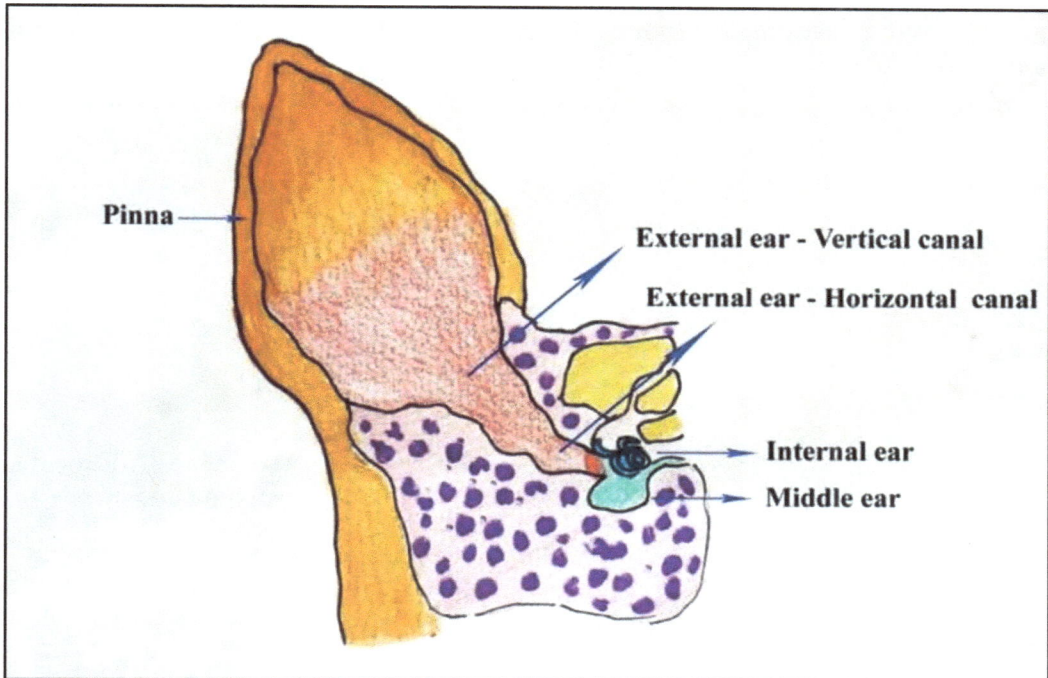

Fig. (1). Schematic diagram of the external, middle and internal ear, dog – Cross-section through skull (Courtesy of Ms. Syed Afreen).

OTITIS INTERNA

Otitis media is considered as an inflammation of middle ear which is a common clinical presentation in dogs and cats. Otitis media damages the tympanic membrane and bulla, and causing the variety of clinical signs ranging from severe pain to development of vestibular sympotoms. Otitis media results from the secondary to the chronic otitis externa that extends through the tympanic membrane and begins of primary factors such as a foreign body and iatrogenic rupture during ear cleaning [4]. Improperly treated / untreated cases of otitis media can lead to development of otitis interna which is considered as an inflammatory disease of inner ear. As a pathological change during the otitis interna can results in impairment of hearing apparatus which leads to deafness and development of neurological signs [5]. In some of the cases it can cause severe otitis interna, a life-threatening iotrogenic intracranial infections and meningitis due to travelling of the infectious organisms from external ear to internal ear and to the brainstem by nerves and vessels located in the internal acoustic meatus. Otitis interna may arise, occasionally accompanied by osteomyelitis of the petrous portion of the temporal bone. As the condition advances in severity over time, lesions may extend retrogradely through the internal acoustic meatus into the cranial cavity, leading to complications such as meningitis, ventriculitis, and encephalitis [6 - 8].

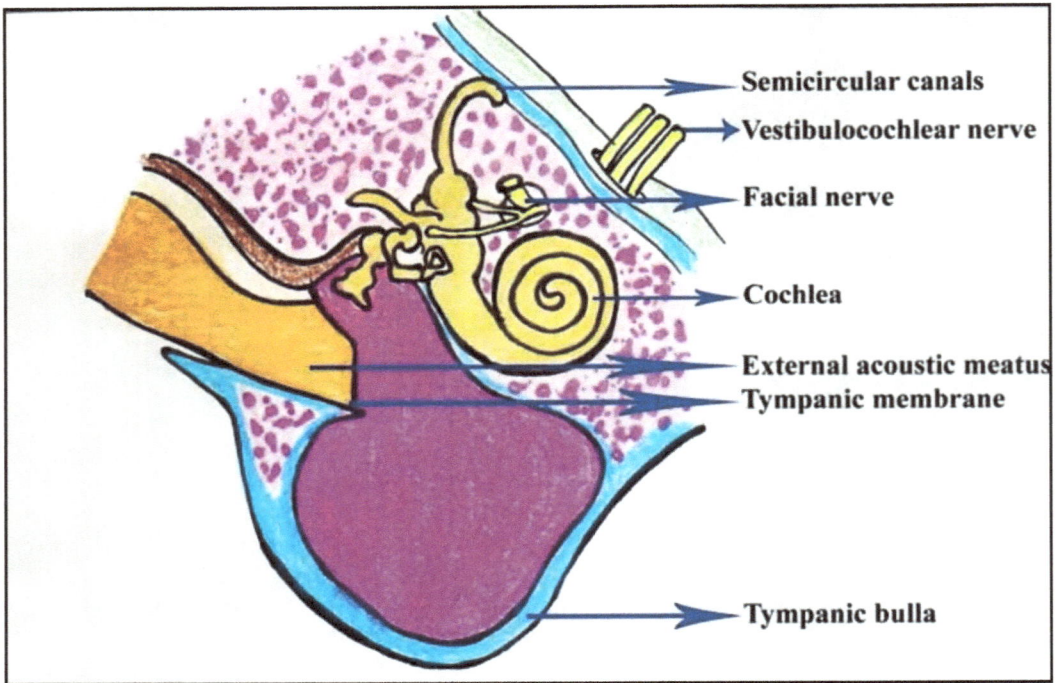

Fig. (2). Schematic diagram of the internal ear, dog – Close up view of the middle ear and internal ear (Courtesy of Ms. Syed Afreen).

Etiology and Pathological Changes

A connection has been observed between otitis externa and otitis interna. Consequently, primary cause for development of otitis interna by involving the diseases progression from external ear infection through the tympanic membrane into the middle ear [9]. Causes of the otitis classified as primary inflammatory origin with in the ear canal, changes in the aural environment and development of secondary complications such as infectious agents like bacterial and fungal organisms [3]. The majority of dogs afflicted with otitis media are at risk of developing otitis interna, which can manifest with or without osteomyelitis of the petrous portion of the temporal bone (Fig. **3**) [10].

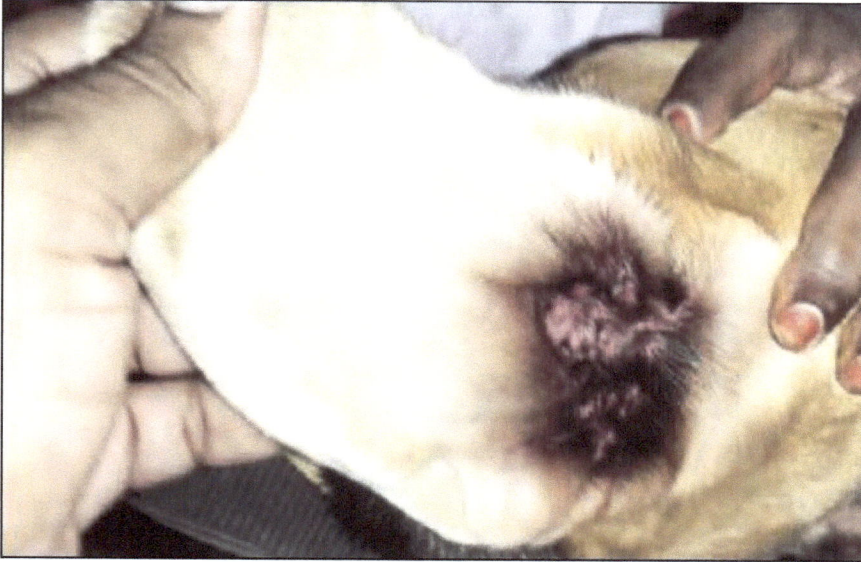

Fig. (3). Dog showing the chronic Otitis.

During the chronic phase of infection, pathological progression involves retrograde spread through the internal acoustic meatus into the cranial cavity, leading to complications such as meningitis, ventriculitis, and encephalitis [11]. The middle ear exudate can vary in macroscopic appearance, ranging from serosanguineous to suppurative and granulomatous. Microscopically, infiltration of neutrophils, macrophages, lymphocytes, and plasma cells occurs in the membranous labyrinth, with neutrophils mixed with fibrin found in the perilymph, and lymphocytes and plasma cells infiltrating the lamina propria of the osseous labyrinth [12 - 15].

Clinical Signs

Most commonly documented clinical findings in dogs with otitis interna were titling of head towards the affected side of ear, development of horizontal or rotary nystagmus, and limb ataxia with abnormal weakness. During the acute stage, dogs may exhibit disorientation, a circling gait, sudden falls, and difficulty in ambulation, sometimes rolling to the affected side. As the condition progresses, clinical findings were less severe and nystagmus also may not be notified. Vomiting may be prominent during the acute stage due to involvement of vestibular connections to the emetic center in the brainstem. In certain bilateral otitis cases, dogs loss the hearing ability [16]. When there is combination of otitis media with otitis interna, it shows the facial nerve paralysis by exhibiting the paralysis of the lips and down drop of commissure on the affected side. While physical examination, head shaking and aural exudate, presence of mucoid discharge in the external ear canal may be noted. Inflammatory lesions around the bulla and temporomandibular joint produces the pain evincing while palpation of the base of the ear and on opening the mouth, respectively. In complicated cases of otitis, neurologic deficits due to inflammation of the nerves which will pass through the bulla will be notified [17]. Due to involvement of the parasympathetic branch of facial nerve causes the damage of innervated lacrimal gland and development of keratoconjunctivitis sicca. In dogs with otitis media and interna results in ipsilateral Horner's Syndrome (*i.e.* miosis, enophthalmos, and ptosis). In dogs with severe otitis interna that progressed to an intracranial infection, changes in mentation, ataxic changes, paresis, proprioceptive deficits, and development of seizures [18, 19].

Diagnosis

History

Complete detailed history about the dermatological signs, previous episodes of otitis is very essential along with the presence of underlying and associated factors to obtain comprehensive information about otitis.

Otic Examination

Preliminary ear examinations are done by visualization of exudate and amount of inflammation, to record the hyperplasia by visualization of horizontal and vertical ear canals, presence of any visible masses/ any foreign bodies; and determine the intactness of tympanic membrane to determine the medical management or surgery. Dogs with severe lesions requires the general anesthesia or sedation for through otoscopic evaluation [20]. Two types of otoscopes are available *i.e.* regular handled otoscopes which should have a strong light source and second one video-otoscope. Visualization with help of otoscope helps the physician to determine the diagnosis of extent of lesions with fine details and determination of disease extent. Further Otitis interna may also be diagnosed *via* imaging, including radiography to detect osseous changes to the bulla (Figs. **4** and **5**) [21, 22].

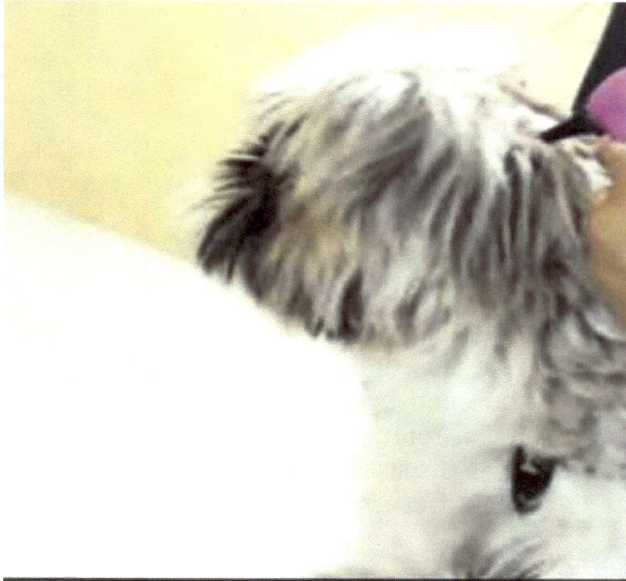

Fig. (4). Otoscopic examination (Courtesy of Dr.S.Rajyalaxmi).

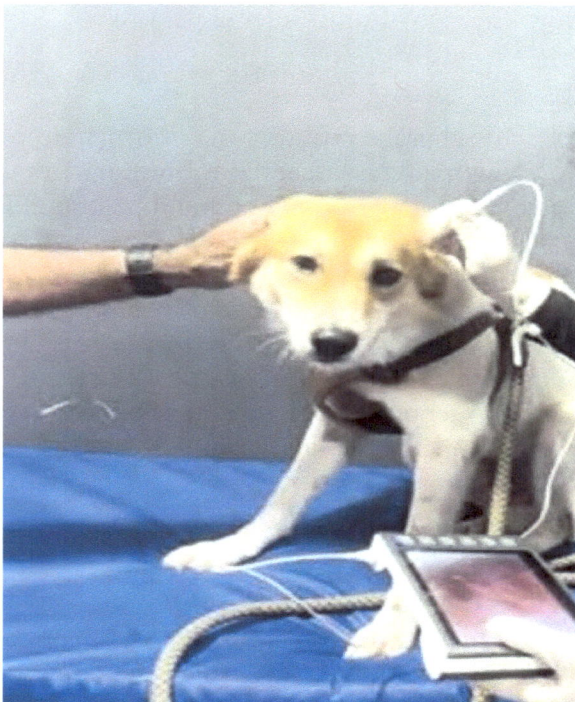

Fig. (5). Video otoscopic examination of ears.

Physical Examination

Dermatological Examination

In dogs with otitis interna, performing complete physical examination is required which includes detailed dermatological examination for identification of underlying or preputing factors.

Neurological Examination

Detailed neurological examination of the nervous system is essential for identification of concurrent neurological abnormalities including facial nerve paralysis, nystagmus, ataxia and head tilt. Dogs exhibiting signs of vestibular origin should be carefully distinguished from those with peripheral vestibular disease or central vestibular disease. Most of the dogs with otitis interna may develop peripheral vestibular diseases due to vestibulocochlear nerve injury.

Systemic Examination

In some of the systemic disease including pharyngitis, temporo-mandibular joint inflammation can show the sigs of otitis interna [23].

Otic cytology

Examination of the otic discharges provides the information of types of exudates and etiology for otitis which is very essential to formulate the topical therapy. In dogs with otitis interna, cytological samples should be obtain from the horizontal canal of the ear. Most commonly noticeable microorganisms in the otic discharges were coccoid bacteria namely *Staphylococcus pseudintermedius*, while the most common type of rod bacteria was *Pseudomonas aeruginosa*. *Malassezia* species were the common yeast organisms along with mite infestation [24]. Another important way to describe the intensity of otitis is by the demonstration of inflammatory cells and /or neoplastic cells for their quantity under the each field. Recording the presence of leukocytes provides the information about the reactivity of the host to the active infection (Fig. **6**) [25, 26].

Bacterial Culture and Sensitivity

Carrying out the culture test and antibiotic sensitivity tests are essential while carrying out the medical management of otitis interna. It is useful in identifying the specific otic pathogens and modulation of therapeutic regimens. Selection of topical antimicrobial agents based on the culture sensitivity is essential to prevent development of antimicrobial resistance [27]. In cases of chronic otitis which is associated with combination of *cocci* and /or rod bacteria which can be noticed on cytology. In dogs with intact tympanic membranes, sample should be collected from the different parts of the ear separately to record the various microbial pathogens that are involved. Due to presence of anatomical variations, recovered microorganisms also varies with the location and sensitivity patterns also differ from isolates (Figs. **7** and **8**) [28, 29].

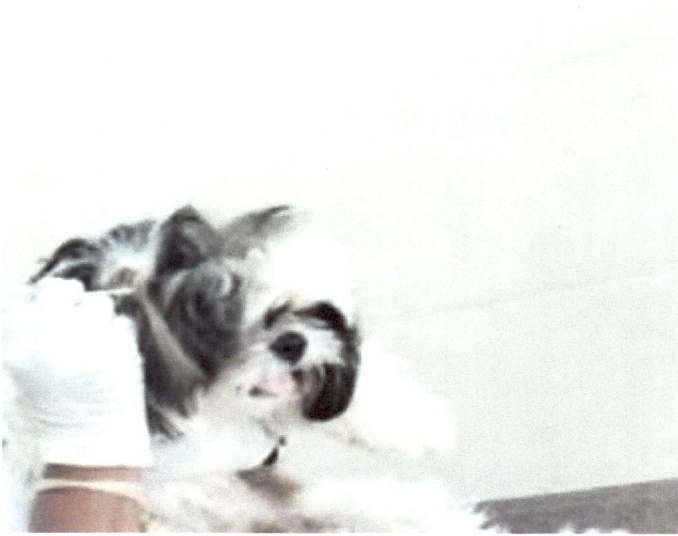

Fig. (6). Collection of the ear swab for microbial culture.

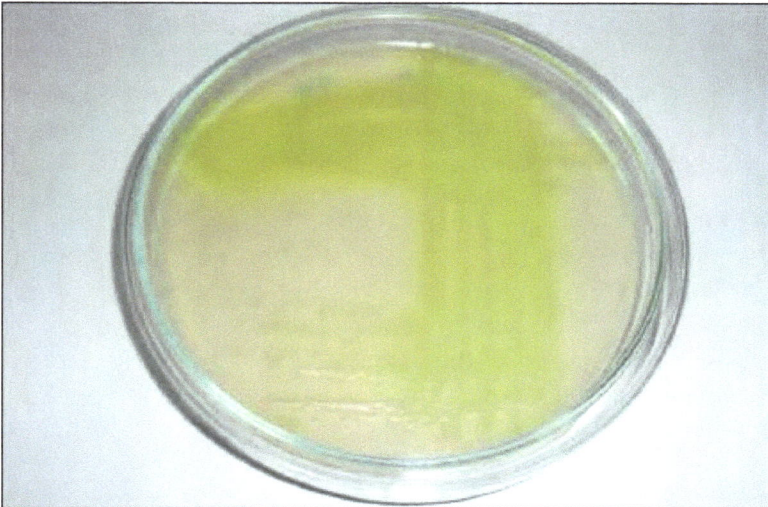

Fig. (7). Microbial isolation and culture in dogs with recurrent otitis.

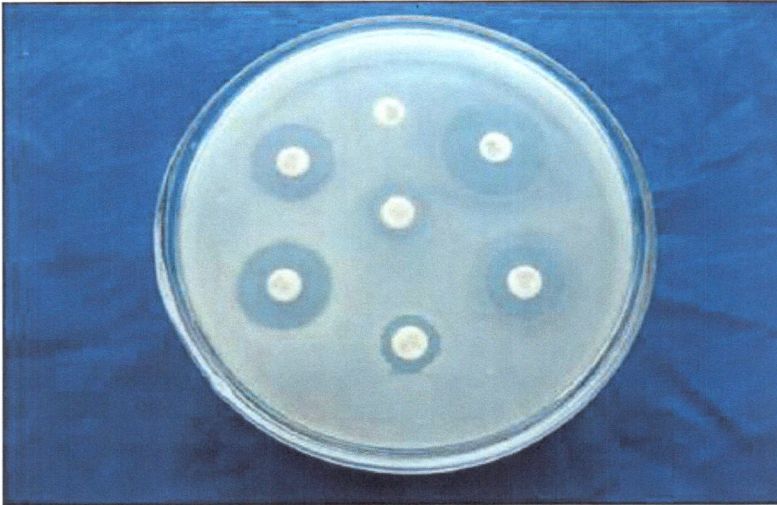

Fig. (8). Antibiotic sensitivity test for selection of antibiotic.

Diagnostic Imaging Techniques

Dogs with chronic otitis and recurrent otitis or otitis associated with neurological signs *i.e.* vestibular signs or facial nerve paralysis, para-aural swelling, or pain on opening the mouth usually require diagnostic imaging techniques (Table **1**). Radiography is highly essential to diagnose the neoplasia and/or otitis interna. Radiographic examination of the tympanic bullae is very essential when suspected for otitis interna. It also is needed to determine the causative obvious vestibular signs to differentiate from other conditions [30]. Most of the dogs affected with otitis interna will not show specific radiographic abnormalities. CT scan evaluations are crucial for assessing otitis media, as they provide more detailed information compared to plain radiography.

MRI is advised in dogs with vestibular signs and it is not possible to differentiate between a central and peripheral vestibular syndrome. It is also advised to evaluate possible caudal fossa parenchyma brain lesions and middle ear pathology [31]. CT and MRI are more sensitive diagnostic testing options in dogs with neurologic signs in association with previous history of otitis. After carrying out the MRI, assessment of cerebrospinal fluid is essential to carry out the differential diagnosis between the meningitis and otitis interna [31].

Deep Ear Flushing

Ear flushing is useful as the diagnostic tool as well as therapeutic regimen. It is recommended that use of anti-inflammatory drugs for 2 to 3 weeks period along with the topical glucocorticoids reduces the narrowing of ear canals (Fig. **9**). This method, requires general anesthesia for complete cleaning and examination of tympanic membrane [32, 33].

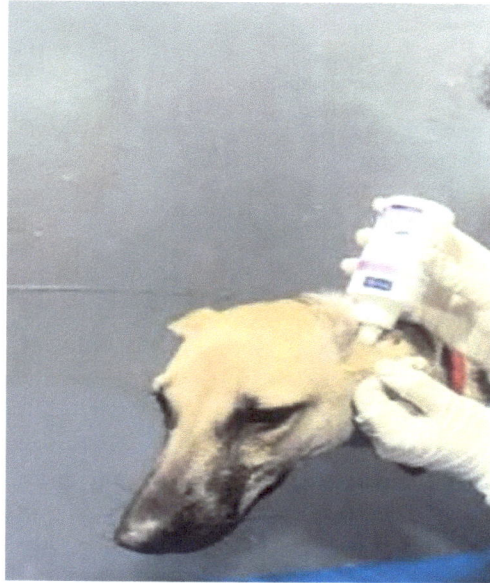

Fig. (9). Regular application of ear cleaners.

Table 1. Pros and cons of different diagnostic imaging techniques.

Diagnostic Imaging Techniques	Pros	Cons
Radiography	1. To detect the mineralization and neoplasia of the ear canal and bony changes in the bulla wall 2. Sedation not required	1. Not useful to detect soft tissue changes 2. Not useful to rule out otitis media 3. Not sensitive as CT and MRI for detection of otitis media
Ultrasonography	1. Relatively quick and noninvasive 2. Useful to detect the thickening and fluid in tympanic bulla 3. Sedation not required	1. Cannot distinguish between fluid and tissue in the middle ear
CT	1. Good imaging for diagnosis of bony changes in bullae from soft tissue reactions. 2. Can detect presence of fluid in tympanic bulla 3. Can detect otitis interna, tumors, and meningitis	1. It requires general anesthesia 2. Requires administration of intravenous contrast material 3. Not as sensitive for identifying otitis interna, tumors, and meningitis compared with MRI 4. Expensive

(Table 1) cont.....

Diagnostic Imaging Techniques	Pros	Cons
MRI	1. Good for assessing soft tissue structures of external ear, inner ear, adjacent neural structures, and brain 2. To detect tumors and their specific location 3. To detect meningitis	1. Not useful to detect the mineralization of the external canal 2. It requires general anesthesia 3. Requires administration of intravenous contrast material 4. Expensive

Treatment

Medical management: General rules for management of otitis interna includes: 1. Making relief from discomfort and pain. 2. Frequent removal of the debris and discharges from ear canal. 3. Frequent visits for elimination of microbial agents in both external and middle ears. 4. Reversing the patho-physiological alterations if addressable. 5. Accurate identification of the primary causes of otitis is essential for effective treatment. If otoscopic examination and tympanic bullae radiographs do not reveal evidence of fluid within the middle ear cavity, systemic antibiotics are continued for a duration of 6 to 8 weeks. However, the selection of antibiotics should always be based on cytological examination or antibiotic sensitivity tests of the exudate obtained from the ear canal. In cases involving inflammation of the vestibulocochlear and facial nerves, systemic corticosteroids may be recommended to reduce stenosis [34, 35]. If any dog exhibits the emesis, antiemetic medication should be administered. Exercise caution while using topical antibiotic and/or anti-inflammatory preparations if the tympanic membrane is ruptured. In cases where intracranial involvement accompanies otitis interna, antibiotic therapy should be continued for at least three months [36 - 39].

Surgical Management

Most of the cases of otitis interna successfully recovered with medical management. However, it fails sometimes and then there is chance for development of secondary facial paresis/paralysis, head tilt and may be permanent deafness. If medical management fails to respond, surgical intervention advised with vertical ear canal ablation (VECA), lateral ear canal resection (LECR), total ear canal ablation with lateral bulla osteotomy (TECA/LBO) [40, 41].

Lateral Ear Canal Resection

Lateral ear canal resection (LECR) entails resection of lateral wall of the vertical canal in dogs with recurrent otitis. The success rate of LECR varies based on the severity and extent of inflammation. Certain breeds may exhibit a higher recovery rate, especially if LECR is performed early in the disease progression. However, in dogs with mineralizing changes affecting different parts of internal ear may have the poor success rate in recovery. LECR is particularly recommended for dogs with stenotic vertical ear canals or cases where improved drainage and easier topical application of medications are needed. Conversely, the procedure is not suitable to dogs which were suffering with severe proliferative diseases and mineralization of the cartilage, narrowing of the horizontal ear canals (Fig. **10**) [42, 43].

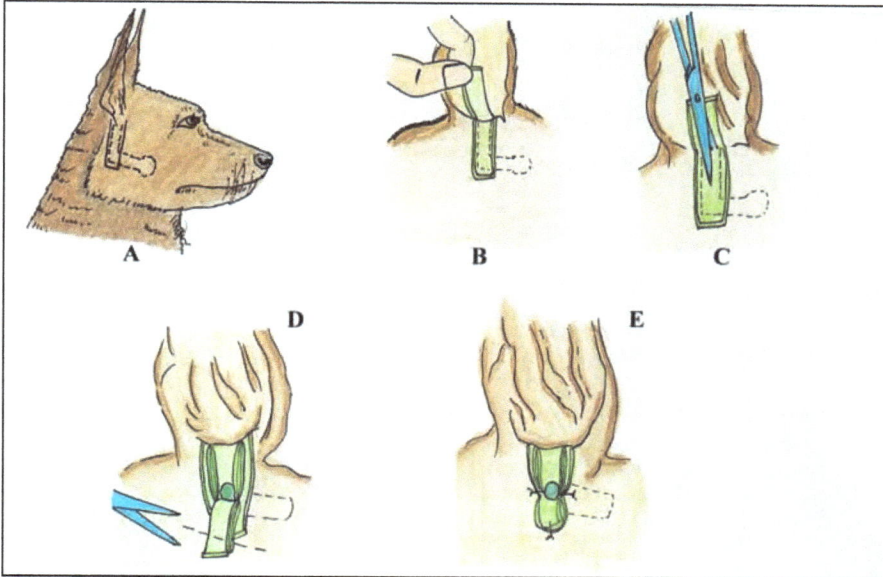

Fig. (10). Illustrated picture showing the procedure of lateral ear canal resection. **A.** drawing the line at site one-half the length of the vertical ear canal below the horizontal ear canal. **B.** Making two parallel incisions lateral to the vertical canal. **C.** Exposing the lateral cartilages by reflecting the skin flap dorsally. **D.** Reflect the cartilage flap distally and resect the distal half to drain. **E.** Placing sutures (Courtesy of Ms. Syed Afreen).

Total Ear Canal Ablation with Lateral Bulla Osteotomy (TECA/LBO)

Total Ear Canal Ablation and Lateral Bulla Osteotomy (TECA/LBO) is recommended for dogs with visible masses which cannot be eliminated through medical management, as well as for cases involving tumor growth in the ear canal and severe end stage otitis which was failed to respond to the conservative medical management. However, it's crucial to note that successful outcomes are contingent upon effectively managing or controlling underlying skin diseases, as failure rates may increase otherwise. The incidence of complications associated with this procedure varies, with approximately 24% of patients experiencing side effects, and 10% encountering long-term deficits (Fig. **11**) [44 - 46].

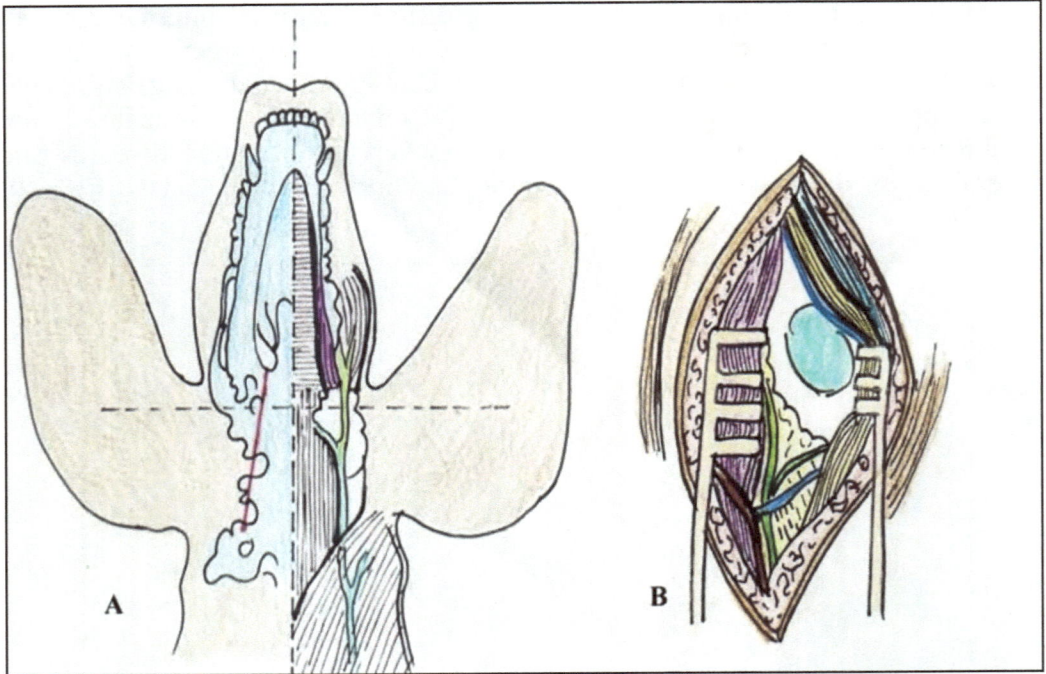

Fig. (11). Ventral bulla osteotomy. **A.** Making the two line one from mandibular rami and a second imaginary line long axis of the ventral aspect of the head. Midline of the neck incision should be made parallel with the midline of the neck **B.** Incise the platysma muscle and deepen the incision by bluntly dissecting the digastricus muscle from the hypoglossal and styloglossal muscles (Courtesy of Ms. Syed Afreen).

Vertical Ear Canal Ablation (VECA)

Vertical ear canal ablation is utilized to preserve a functional horizontal canal in cases where the vertical canal is severely diseased. Although vertical ear canal ablation may not be as potent as total ear canal ablation due to the possibility of active infection in the horizontal canal and the potential for recurring infections in the remaining ear canal, it is considered less invasive. If the horizontal ear canal remains unaffected, preserving healthy tissue can maintain functionality. Vertical ear canal ablation offers advantages over lateral resection as it more effectively removes diseased tissues, with less interference with cartilage, resulting in reduced pain and improved healing. This procedure combines the benefits of lateral wall resection, such as drainage, ventilation, and preservation of hearing, with those of total ear canal ablation (Fig. **12**) [47, 48].

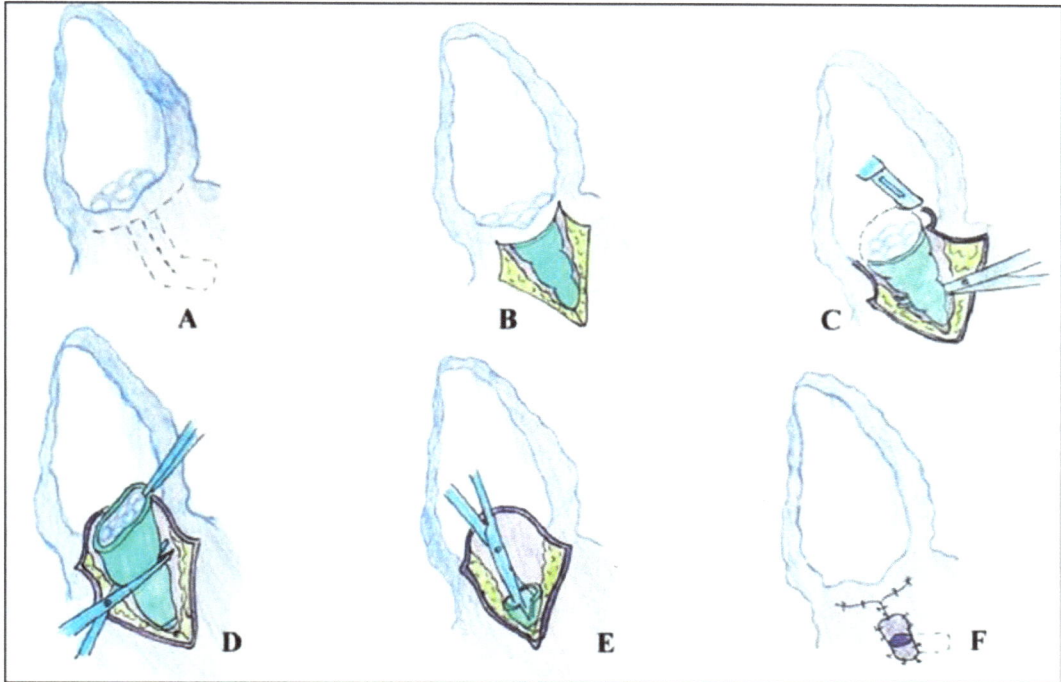

Fig. (12). Vertical ear canal ablation. **A.** T shape incision below the upper edge of the tragus. **B.** Retraction of skin flaps to expose the lateral aspects of the vertical canal. **C.** Continuation of the horizontal incision through the cartilage around the external auditory meatus **D.** Making the transaction of canal vertically 1 cm dorsal to the horizontal canal. **E.** Incise the vertical canal cranially and caudally to create the dorsal and ventral flops. **F.** Reflection of the ventral flap to downward and fix to skin (Courtesy of Ms. Syed Afreen).

Laser Surgery Options

The CO_2 laser is a valuable tool for removing or ablating certain ear canal cysts, polyps, and tumors. CO_2 laser at a 10,600 nm wavelength, the CO_2 laser is highly absorbed by water and it shows the photothermal interaction. This interaction leads to tissue vaporization with low tissue damage, low penetration with limited surrounding tissue damage [49].

Advantages of Surgical Considerations

In healthy dogs, ears naturally clean themselves by shedding epithelial cells and removing debris. However, in cases of inflammation, proliferative conditions, obstruction, or neoplastic diseases, the ear's self-cleaning function can be compromised. Surgical interventions can help restore the ear's ability to self-clean by creating a suitable environment for this natural process (Table **2**).

Disadvantages of Surgical Considerations

Surgical interventions for treatment of otitis interna are reported to be seldom in controlling of underlying factors. It is highly recommended in tumor excision and polyp removal. Any surgical intervention preliminary addressed the primary diseases, adverse food reactions and atopic dermatitis should be eliminated [50].

Table 2. Different surgical techniques for management of chronic Otitis.

Type of Surgery	Indications	Diagnostic Methods
Lateral ear canal resection	Presence of stenotic vertical ear canals Presence of vertical canal infection alone	Video Otoscopy CT Scan
Vertical ear canal ablation	Presence of stenotic vertical ear canals Involvement of medial wall of the vertical canal	Video Otoscopy CT Scan
Total ear canal ablation+ lateral bulla osteotomy	Failure to remove physical masses by medical management Tumors in ear canal End stage otitis media which is not responded to medical therapy	Video Otoscopy CT Scan MRI

PROGNOSIS

Early identification of otitis, coupled with the selection of suitable antibiotics and appropriate duration of therapy or surgery, typically leads to a favorable prognosis for recovery. However, presence of vestibular deficits which includes tilting of head, ataxia may persist as complications to the otitis. In cases of osteomyelitis involving the osseous bulla and petrous temporal bone, long-term medication may be necessary. In rare instances, the infection may ascend the vestibulocochlear and facial nerves to the brain stem, potentially resulting in a brain stem abscess or meningitis and the development of central vestibular signs.

CONCLUSION

Inflammation of the middle ear can lead to inflammation of the inner ear structures (otitis interna) turning into loss of balance and deafness. Otitis interna can be diagnosed based on similar signs of otitis media with loss of balance. Otoscopic and x-rays examination are important tool for the inner ear inflammation.Long-term antibiotic therapy for 3 to 6 weeks is usually necessary to eradicate the infection. The animal should be examined periodically during the treatment period to evaluate recovery as well as to monitor for the side effects of long-term antibiotic treatment.

REFERENCES

[1] Grono LR. Studies of the microclimate of the external auditory canal in the dog. I. Aural temperature. Res Vet Sci 1970; 11(4): 307-11.
[http://dx.doi.org/10.1016/S0034-5288(18)34293-0] [PMID: 5499312]

[2] Cole LK. Anatomy and physiology of the canine ear. Vet Dermatol 2010; 21(2): 221-31.
[PMID: 20230592]

[3] Njaa BL, Cole LK, Tabacca N. Practical otic anatomy and physiology of the dog and cat. Vet Clin North Am Small Anim Pract 2012; 42(6): 1109-26.
[http://dx.doi.org/10.1016/j.cvsm.2012.08.011] [PMID: 23122171]

[4] Hill P. Small Animal Dermatology: A practical guide to the diagnosis and management of skin diseases in dogs and cats. Oxford, UK: Butterworth-Heinemann 2002; pp. 143-7.

[5] Scott DW, Miller WH, Griffin CE. Muller and Kirk's small animal dermatology. 6th ed., Philadelphia: W.B. Saunders 2001.

[6] Moriella KA. Overview of otitis media and interna. Merck Veterinary Manual 2018.

[7] Paterson S. Topical ear treatment – options, indications and limitations of current therapy. J Small Anim Pract 2016; 57(12): 1-11.
[http://dx.doi.org/10.1111/jsap.12583] [PMID: 27747880]

[8] Jaeger K, Linek M, Power HT, et al. Breed and site predispositions of dogs with atopic dermatitis: a comparison of five locations in three continents. Vet Dermatol 2010; 21(1): 119-23.
[http://dx.doi.org/10.1111/j.1365-3164.2009.00845.x] [PMID: 20187918]

[9] Hnilca KA. Small animal dermatology: a color atlas and therapeutic Guide. 3rd ed. Elsevier Saunders 2011; pp. 83-4.

[10] Harvey RG, Harari J, Delauche AJ. Etiopathogenesis and classification of otitis externa. 2001: 81-122.

[11] Campbell KL. Other external parasites. In: Ettinger SJ, Feldman EC, Eds. Textbook of veterinary internal medicine. 6th ed. St. Louis, Missouri: Saunders Elsevier 2005; Vol. 1: pp. 66-7.

[12] Hill PB, Lo A, Eden CAN, et al. Survey of the prevalence, diagnosis and treatment of dermatological conditions in small animals in general practice. Vet Rec 2006; 158(16): 533-9.
[http://dx.doi.org/10.1136/vr.158.16.533] [PMID: 16632525]

[13] Koch SN, Torres MF, Plumb DC. Canine and Feline Dermatology Drug Handbook. Ames, IA: Wiley-Blackwell 2012.
[http://dx.doi.org/10.1002/9781118704745]

[14] Saridomichelakis MN, Farmaki R, Leontides LS, Koutinas AF. Aetiology of canine otitis externa: a retrospective study of 100 cases. Vet Dermatol 2007; 18(5): 341-7.
[http://dx.doi.org/10.1111/j.1365-3164.2007.00619.x] [PMID: 17845622]

[15] Zur G, Lifshitz B, Bdolah-Abram T. The association between the signalment, common causes of canine otitis externa and pathogens. J Small Anim Pract 2011; 52(5): 254-8.
[http://dx.doi.org/10.1111/j.1748-5827.2011.01058.x] [PMID: 21539570]

[16] Radlinsky MG, Mason DE. Diseases of the ear. In: Ettinger SJ, Feldman EC, Eds. Textbook of veterinary internal medicine. 6th ed. St. Louis, Missouri: Saunders Elsevier 2005; Vol. 2: pp. 1171-4.

[17] Rosenkrantz WS, Mendelsohn CL. Dermatologic therapy. In: Miller W, Griffin CE, Campbell K, Eds. Muller and Kirk's Small Animal Dermatology. 7th ed. St. Louis: Elsevier 2013; pp. 109-83.

[18] Rosy CR. Challenges in otitis. Proceedings of the Seventh World Congress of Veterinary Dermatology. Vancouver, BC, Canada. 2012; pp. 24-8.

[19] Rosser EJ Jr. Causes of otitis externa. Vet Clin North Am Small Anim Pract 2004; 34(2): 459-68.
[http://dx.doi.org/10.1016/j.cvsm.2003.10.006] [PMID: 15062619]

[20] Miller WH, Griffin CE, Campbell KL. Muller & Kirk's Small Animal Dermatology. 7th ed. St. Louis, Missouri: Elsevier 2013; pp. 243-9.

[21] Picco F, Zini E, Nett C, *et al.* A prospective study on canine atopic dermatitis and food-induced allergic dermatitis in Switzerland. Vet Dermatol 2008; 19(3): 150-5.
[http://dx.doi.org/10.1111/j.1365-3164.2008.00669.x] [PMID: 18477331]

[22] Angus JC, Lichtensteiger C, Campbell KL, Schaeffer DJ. Breed variations in histopathologic features of chronic severe otitis externa in dogs: 80 cases (1995–2001). J Am Vet Med Assoc 2002; 221(7): 1000-6.
[http://dx.doi.org/10.2460/javma.2002.221.1000] [PMID: 12369678]

[23] Gotthelf LN. Diagnosis and treatment of otitis media in dogs and cats. Vet Clin North Am Small Anim Pract 2004; 34(2): 469-87.
[http://dx.doi.org/10.1016/j.cvsm.2003.10.007] [PMID: 15062620]

[24] Defalque V, Rosser EJ Jr, Peterson AD. Aerobic and anaerobic bacterial microflora of the middle ear cavity in normal dogs. 20th Proc North Am Vet Dermatol Forum 2005: 159.

[25] Ginel PJ, Lucena R, Rodriguez JC, Ortega J. A semiquantitative cytological evaluation of normal and pathological samples from the external ear canal of dogs and cats. Vet Dermatol 2002; 13(3): 151-6.
[http://dx.doi.org/10.1046/j.1365-3164.2002.00288.x] [PMID: 12074704]

[26] Angus JC. Otic cytology in health and disease. Vet Clin North Am Small Anim Pract 2004; 34(2): 411-24.
[http://dx.doi.org/10.1016/j.cvsm.2003.10.005] [PMID: 15062616]

[27] Graham-Mize CA, Rosser EJ Jr. Comparison of microbial isolates and susceptibility patterns from the external ear canal of dogs with otitis externa. J Am Anim Hosp Assoc 2004; 40(2): 102-8.
[http://dx.doi.org/10.5326/0400102] [PMID: 15007044]

[28] Lyskova P, Vydrzalova M, Mazurova J. Identification and antimicrobial susceptibility of bacteria and yeasts isolated from healthy dogs and dogs with otitis externa. J Vet Med A Physiol Pathol Clin Med 2007; 54(10): 559-63.
[http://dx.doi.org/10.1111/j.1439-0442.2007.00996.x] [PMID: 18045339]

[29] Greene CE. Otitis externa. In: Greene CE, Ed. Infectious diseases of the dog and cat. 3rd ed. St. Louis, Missouri: Saunders Elsevier 2006; pp. 815-7.

[30] Remedios AM, Fowler JD, Pharr JW. A comparison of radiographic *versus* surgical diagnosis of otitis media. J Am Anim Hosp Assoc 1991; 27: 183-8.

[31] Dvir E, Kirberger RM, Terblanche AG. Magnetic resonance imaging of otitis media in a dog. Vet Radiol Ultrasound 2000; 41(1): 46-9.
[http://dx.doi.org/10.1111/j.1740-8261.2000.tb00426.x] [PMID: 10695880]

[32] Zamankhan Malayeri H, Jamshidi S, Zahraei Salehi T. Identification and antimicrobial susceptibility patterns of bacteria causing otitis externa in dogs. Vet Res Commun 2010; 34(5): 435-44.
[http://dx.doi.org/10.1007/s11259-010-9417-y] [PMID: 20526674]

[34] King SB, Doucette KP, Seewald W, Forster SL. A randomized, controlled, single-blinded, multicenter evaluation of the efficacy and safety of a once weekly two dose otic gel containing florfenicol, terbinafine and betamethasone administered for the treatment of canine otitis externa. BMC Vet Res 2018; 14(1): 307.
[http://dx.doi.org/10.1186/s12917-018-1627-5] [PMID: 30305092]

[35] Di Cerbo A, Morales-Medina JC, Palmieri B, *et al.* Functional foods in pet nutrition: Focus on dogs and cats. Res Vet Sci 2017; 112: 161-6.
[http://dx.doi.org/10.1016/j.rvsc.2017.03.020] [PMID: 28433933]

[36] Guillot J, Bensignor E, Jankowski F, Seewald W, Chermette R, Steffan J. Comparative efficacies of oral ketoconazole and terbinafine for reducing *Malassezia* population sizes on the skin of Basset

Hounds. Vet Dermatol 2003; 14(3): 153-7.
[http://dx.doi.org/10.1046/j.1365-3164.2003.00334.x] [PMID: 12791049]

[37]   Chesney CJ. Food sensitivity in the dog: a quantitative study. J Small Anim Pract 2002; 43(5): 203-7.
[http://dx.doi.org/10.1111/j.1748-5827.2002.tb00058.x] [PMID: 12038852]

[38]   Cavana P, Peano A, Petit JY, *et al.* A pilot study of the efficacy of wipes containing chlorhexidine
0.3%, climbazole 0.5% and Tris- EDTA to reduce *Malassezia pachydermatis* populations on canine
skin. Vet Dermatol 2015; 26(4): 278-e61.
[http://dx.doi.org/10.1111/vde.12220] [PMID: 26083147]

[39]   Mueller RS, Fieseler KV, Fettman MJ, *et al.* Effect of omega-3 fatty acids on canine atopic dermatitis.
J Small Anim Pract 2004; 45(6): 293-7.
[http://dx.doi.org/10.1111/j.1748-5827.2004.tb00238.x] [PMID: 15206474]

[40]   Patterson S, Tobias KM. Atlas of Ear Diseases of the Dog and Cat. Ames, IA: Wiley-Blackwell 2012.
[http://dx.doi.org/10.1002/9781118702710]

[41]   Murphy KM. A review of techniques for the investigation of otitis externa and otitis media. Clin Tech
Small Anim Pract 2001; 16(4): 236-41.
[http://dx.doi.org/10.1053/svms.2001.27601] [PMID: 11793879]

[42]   Layton CE. The role of lateral ear resection in managing chronic otitis externa. Semin Vet Med Surg
(Small Anim) 1993; 8(1): 24-9.
[PMID: 8456200]

[43]   Sylvestre AM. Potential factors affecting the outcome of dogs with a resection of the lateral wall of the
vertical ear canal. Can Vet J 1998; 39(3): 157-60.
[PMID: 9524720]

[44]   Beckman SL, Henry WB Jr, Cechner P. Total ear canal ablation combining bulla osteotomy and
curettage in dogs with chronic otitis externa and media. J Am Vet Med Assoc 1990; 196(1): 84-90.
[http://dx.doi.org/10.2460/javma.1990.196.01.84] [PMID: 2295558]

[45]   Devitt CM, Seim HB III, Willer R, McPherron M, Neely M. Passive drainage *versus* primary closure
after total ear canal ablation-lateral bulla osteotomy in dogs: 59 dogs (1985-1995). Vet Surg 1997;
26(3): 210-6.
[http://dx.doi.org/10.1111/j.1532-950X.1997.tb01486.x] [PMID: 9150559]

[46]   Krahwinkel DJ, Pardo AD, Sims MH, Bubb WJ. Effect of total ablation of the external acoustic
meatus and bulla osteotomy on auditory function in dogs. J Am Vet Med Assoc 1993; 202(6): 949-52.
[http://dx.doi.org/10.2460/javma.1993.202.06.949] [PMID: 8468221]

[47]   Mathews KG, Hardie EM, Murphy KM. Subtotal ear canal ablation in 18 dogs and one cat with
minimal distal ear canal pathology. J Am Anim Hosp Assoc 2006; 42(5): 371-80.
[http://dx.doi.org/10.5326/0420371] [PMID: 16960041]

[48]   Smeak DD. Lateral approach to subtotal bulla osteotomy in dogs: Pertinent anatomy and procedural
details. Compend Contin Educ Pract Vet 2005; 27(5): 377-85.

[49]   Aslan J, Shipstone MA, Mackie JT. Carbon dioxide laser surgery for chronic proliferative and
obstructive otitis externa in 26 dogs. Vet Dermatol 2021; 32(3): 262-e72.
[http://dx.doi.org/10.1111/vde.12960] [PMID: 33830550]

[50]   Nesbitt GH, Freeman LM, Hannah SS. Correlations of fatty acid supplementation, aeroallergens,
shampoo, and ear cleanser with multiple parameters in pruritic dogs. J Am Anim Hosp Assoc 2004;
40(4): 270-84.
[http://dx.doi.org/10.5326/0400270] [PMID: 15238557]

CHAPTER 17

Paradigm of Ear Canal Ablation (ECA) and Clinical Results of Bulla Osteotomy

K. Manoj Kumar[1,*], **D. Sai Bhavani**[2] and **B. Prakash Kumar**[3]

[1] *Department of Veterinary Clinical Complex, CVSc, Garividi, Vizianagaram District, Andhra Pradesh-535101, India*

[2] *State Institute of Animal Health, Tanuku, West Godavari District, Andhra Pradesh-534211, India*

[3] *Department of Veterinary Surgery and Radiology, CVSc, Garividi, Vizianagaram District, Andhra Pradesh-535101, India*

Abstract: Total Ear Canal Ablation (TECA) and Bulla Osteotomy are surgical procedures in veterinary medicine utilized to address various ear-related conditions, primarily in dogs and cats. TECA is indicated for chronic inflammatory ear diseases, trauma, neoplasia, cholesteatoma, congenital malformations, and failed prior surgeries. It involves the complete removal of the ear canal, often coupled with Lateral Bulla Osteotomy (LBO) for middle ear issues. LBO is essential for conditions like otitis media. Preoperative evaluations encompass physical exams, otoscopy, and imaging, with antibiotic and analgesic administration. Surgical equipment includes specialized instruments like rongeurs, curettes, and retractors. The surgical procedures require meticulous technique to ensure patient safety and involve incisions, dissection, and removal of affected tissue, with a focus on preserving vital structures like the facial nerve. Postoperative care includes pain management, bandaging, swelling control, antibiotic therapy, and drain/suture management. Potential complications include nerve damage and hearing loss. TECA and Bulla Osteotomy are crucial interventions for alleviating chronic ear problems in animals, enhancing their overall quality of life.

Keywords: Bulla osteotomy, Cholesteatoma, Ear canal, Otitis externa, Otitis media, Tympanic bulla, Total ear canal ablation.

INTRODUCTION

Ear infections in dogs are a prevalent issue that can inflict considerable distress and suffering on our beloved canine companions. These infections, scientifically referred to as otitis, commonly occur in the external ear canal due to the warm, moist environment that provides a breeding ground for bacteria, yeast, and other

* **Corresponding author K. Manoj Kumar:** Department of Veterinary Clinical Complex, CVSc, Garividi, Vizianagaram District, Andhra Pradesh-535101, India; E-mail: manojvety12@gmail.com

Tanmoy Rana (Ed.)

pathogens [1, 2]. The symptoms of ear infections in dogs can vary in severity but often include telltale signs such as persistent scratching or pawing at the affected ear, head shaking, redness or inflammation of the ear canal, odorous discharge, and evident discomfort or pain, sometimes manifested through vocalization or aggression when the ear is touched. Bacteria and debris can accumulate in the horizontal ear canal over time, leading to a middle ear infection when they access the tympanic cavity [3]. As the infection progresses, the tympanic membrane and ear canal lining thicken, and calcification can occur in the cartilage. In severe cases of middle ear infection, the ear canal lining may undergo metaplasia, and new bone can form within the tympanic bulla, a condition known as bulla osteitis, which becomes a persistent source of infection. Cholesteatomas, an unusual and aggressive consequence of chronic inflammatory middle ear disease, can develop from a displaced portion of the tympanic membrane that adheres to the inflamed mucosa in the tympanic cavity [4]. These cholesteatomas result from the shedding of cells from the keratinized membrane, forming a cystic structure that causes extensive bone resorption and remodeling in the bulla. Surgical intervention becomes necessary when medical therapy is ineffective or unlikely to succeed, particularly in cases of chronic and end-stage changes or the presence of cholesteatoma as revealed by radiographic imaging. Chronic otitis externa is the primary cause of middle ear disease, and the most common surgical procedure for accessing the tympanic cavity is the total ear canal ablation (TECA) combined with lateral bulla osteotomy (LBO) of the tympanic bulla (Smeak, 1988). This approach allows for the complete removal of chronically diseased ear canal tissue and exposure of the tympanic cavity through a single incision. In cases where epithelium and debris are not entirely removed from the tympanic cavity, or secondary infections are not effectively treated after TECA and LBO, severe deep-seated infections can occur. This complication can be more painful for the patient than the original ear condition and is challenging and costly to address [5]. Therefore, it is crucial to avoid this complication. Although some surgeons may be cautious about aggressive LBO due to concerns about potential complications like facial nerve or inner ear damage or excessive bleeding, it remains essential to ensure thorough debridement in the tympanic cavity. Achieving complete debridement is a critical aspect of the successful TECA and LBO procedure, and this article offers a detailed description of the relevant anatomy, a step-by-step surgical procedure with illustrations, and guidelines for safe debridement within the tympanic cavity, with a focus on minimizing risks.

PREOPERATIVE CONSIDERATIONS

Owner Education

Owners should be thoroughly informed about the purpose and expectations after TECA LBO, including the potential for serious postoperative complications. The primary goal of the surgery is to improve the pet's comfort by completely removing the source of chronic infection, eliminating the need for further ear cleaning, and alleviating the malodorous discharge (Beckman *et al.,* 1990). While some concerns about post-surgery appearance and potential hearing loss exist, TECA LBO is generally well-received by owners, especially when their pets experience relief from chronic ear problems (Book author).

Physical Examination

During the physical examination, the external ear, deeper ear canals, and regional lymph nodes are assessed. Blood-tinged ear discharge may raise suspicion of neoplasia [6]. A cranial nerve examination is performed to evaluate for facial nerve dysfunction, inner ear involvement, and Horner's syndrome, which may affect about 15% of dogs considered for TECA [7]. A dermatologic examination is essential in cases where chronic ear problems are linked to a systemic skin disorder [8]. Staging is performed in cases of suspected neoplastic ear disease, including palpation of local lymph nodes and fine-needle aspirates for cytology.

Otoscopic Examination

A thorough otoscopic examination is best performed under anesthesia. The ear canal is cleaned, examined, and samples are collected for bacterial culture, susceptibility testing, and cytologic examination [9]. Special attention is given to identifying tumors, growths, and assessing the degree of stenosis in the horizontal ear canal. Fine-needle aspirates of suspicious masses can aid in distinguishing between benign and malignant ear diseases [10].

Imaging Evaluation

Radiographic imaging, such as plain film radiography or positive-contrast ear canalography, is used to examine the external, middle, and internal ear [11]. Chest radiographs may be taken to assess for metastatic disease or other conditions in older patients. Imaging, such as computed tomography (CT) or magnetic resonance imaging (MRI), can help evaluate the external ear canal, tympanic membrane, and tympanic bulla. CT is recommended before surgery, particularly in dogs with neurologic deficits or signs of upper airway obstruction. CT has been found to be more sensitive than plain film radiography for evaluating otitis media

[12]. MRI is recommended when there is uncertainty between central and peripheral vestibular syndromes [13]. However, if the suspicion of otitis media is high based on clinical signs, surgical exploration is indicated despite equivocal imaging results [14].

Preoperative Antibiotic and Analgesia Regimens

Given the difficulty of achieving asepsis in the proliferative and stenotic ear canal, contamination is inevitable during surgery [15]. Prophylactic intravenous antibiotic therapy should be initiated before surgery. Antibiotics effective against likely bacterial contaminants, such as amoxicillin–clavulanate, aminoglycosides, or ticarcillin, are chosen based on culture data when available. TECA LBO is a highly painful procedure in small animals [16]. Therefore, preoperative analgesia is crucial to reduce postoperative pain and prevent the establishment of chronic pain states. Local nerve blockade and continuous local infusion of anesthetics have been explored for intraoperative analgesia, although their efficacy remains debated. Continuous incisional lidocaine delivery has shown promise in providing postoperative analgesia [17].

Patient Preparation

Patient preparation for procedures involving wide surgical clipping, such as lateral wall resection, total ear canal ablation with bulla osteotomy, and vertical canal ablation, is essential. When performing a unilateral procedure, it is recommended to clip the hair from the top of the skull, between the ears, down to the lower edge of the jaw on the same side. Additionally, clip from the level of the outer corner of the eye to the ear's opening, extending backward for a similar distance. For the surrounding skin, standard presurgical skin preparation methods suffice. However, for the often inflamed and damaged epithelium in the inner ear and vertical canal, it is more appropriate to use a diluted iodine solution.

Patient Positioning

In nearly all cases of aural surgery, the patient is placed in a lateral recumbent position, with their nose aligned parallel to the surgical table. Achieving this position can be made more comfortable by using a sandbag or a towel placed beneath the neck and the side of the lower jaw that's closest to the table. Additionally, the patient's head should be rotated so that both sides of the lower jaw are positioned vertically above one another, creating a perpendicular alignment with the table. To ensure a clear operating area and better access to the surgical site, it's often beneficial to gently pull back and secure the front limbs in a caudal direction, away from the head of the table.

Anesthetic Considerations

In the realm of veterinary medicine, the anesthesia and pain management considerations for animals undergoing ear surgery are of paramount importance. Ear surgeries, including Total Ear Canal Ablation (TECA) and Bulla Osteotomy often involve significant pain and discomfort for the animals. To address this, various anesthetic protocols are employed, with the choice of protocol dependent on the patient's health status. While it is common to use premedications like butorphanol and buprenorphine in dogs, it has been observed that hydromorphone and morphine provide more effective analgesia for both dogs and cats undergoing ear surgery. Local anesthesia, typically bupivacaine hydrochloride, plays a crucial role in mitigating pain during and immediately after the procedure. Adequate time for the local anesthetic to take effect, approximately 15 to 20 minutes, is vital, and care must be taken to ensure a relatively blood-free surgical site during this period [18]. However, it is essential to emphasize that local anesthesia should not be the sole method of pain control and must be used in conjunction with other analgesics. Ketamine infusions, both as boluses and constant rate infusions, are another strategy to enhance intraoperative management and postoperative pain control in animals with chronically painful ears. In specific combinations, such as fentanyl, lidocaine, ketamine (FLK), or morphine, lidocaine, ketamine (MLK) CRIs, these drugs provide effective analgesia and play a crucial role in alleviating pain. In addition to intraoperative pain management, postoperative analgesics must be administered to ensure the animal's comfort and recovery [19]. By customizing anesthetic and analgesic protocols to the individual patient's needs, veterinarians can provide the highest standard of care, effectively manage pain, and facilitate a smooth recovery process for their animal patients undergoing ear surgery.

Surgical Equipment and Suture Materials

In TECA LBO (Lateral Bulla Osteotomy), specialized surgical equipment is indispensable in addition to the standard instruments found in a general surgery pack. Bone rongeurs, such as the preferred Cleveland or Zaufal rongeurs, play a critical role in removing the thicker bone of the lateral tympanic bulla and osseous external auditory meatus. For larger breed dogs with extensive bulla bone proliferation, a double-action Ruskin rongeur may be necessary. The Kerrison Down-Bite Laminectomy Punch is a valuable tool for safely removing bone from the caudal aspect of the external auditory meatus [20]. Delicate Lempert or Beyer rongeurs are employed to refine the surgical site by eliminating rough edges, while some surgeons opt for air-driven burrs for efficient bone removal. Freer periosteal elevators come in handy for soft tissue reflection around the ventrolateral bulla face. When deeper tissue retraction and exposure are required, delicate Senn retractors or larger Army-Navy retractors are employed. However, caution is advised against using Gelpi retractors during deep dissection to avoid potential harm to the facial nerve and nearby vascular structures. Angled Daubenspeck bone curettes and malleable Halle bone curettes are instrumental for reaching the deep recesses of the tympanic cavity [21]. Monofilament suture (*i.e.,* polydioxanone, polyglyconate, poliglecaprone 25, polypropylene, or nylon) should be used to suture the epithelial tissue of the canal to the skin. Absorbable suture should be used for subcutaneous sutures.

TOTAL EAR CANAL ABLATION (TECA)

TECA is most commonly performed in dogs with irreversible inflammatory ear canal disease. This condition is characterized by proliferative epithelial hyperplasia, ear canal stenosis, and, in some cases, calcified periauricular tissue [22, 23]. It is often coupled with chronic otitis media (inflammation of the middle ear). Owners may opt for TECA when other treatment modalities have failed or when they are unable to provide ongoing medical therapy. Other indications for TECA in dogs include severe ear trauma, invasive neoplasia (abnormal tissue growth), acquired aural cholesteatoma (a cyst within the ear), congenital ear canal malformations or atresia (closure or absence of the ear canal), failed prior ear surgeries, and ear canal avulsion (tearing away) [24]. In cats, TECA is primarily performed for neoplastic (cancerous) invasion of the ear canal or global polypoid inflammatory disease [25].

Surgical Procedure

This intricate procedure begins with careful patient positioning, where the animal is placed in lateral recumbency with its head elevated, creating an optimal surgical field for the impending operation. Preoperative steps involve thorough aseptic preparation of the pinna and surrounding skin to minimize the risk of postoperative infection. The key incision takes the form of a T-shape, with the horizontal component running parallel to and just below the upper edge of the tragus. From the midpoint of the horizontal incision, a vertical incision is carefully extended just past the level of the horizontal canal (Fig. **1A**). This incision reveals the lateral aspect of the vertical ear canal. The horizontal incision is then continued around the opening of the vertical ear canal using a scalpel blade (Fig. **1B**) and the proximal and medial aspects of the vertical canal are dissected using curved Mayo scissors while maintaining proximity to the ear canal cartilage to avoid damaging critical structures (Fig. **1C**). Special attention is given to the protection of the facial nerve and the great auricular artery during this dissection process, with the facial nerve, in particular, requiring careful identification as it courses caudoventrally to the horizontal canal. If necessary, the nerve is gently retracted to ensure its safety. In cases where the facial nerve becomes entrapped within thickened, calcified horizontal canal tissue, a meticulous dissection is carried out to free the nerve. The dissection then proceeds to the level of the external acoustic meatus, (Fig. **1D**) where the attachment of the horizontal canal is excised with precision, using instruments such as a scalpel blade, rongeur, or Mayo scissors, while being exceedingly cautious to avoid facial nerve damage (Fig. **1E**). Subsequently, the entire ear canal is removed, and deep cultures are sampled for diagnostic purposes, with the excised ear being submitted for histologic examination. To prevent chronic fistulation, a curette is employed to thoroughly eliminate any adherent secretory tissue from the rim of the external acoustic meatus. Depending on the specific case, a lateral bulla osteotomy may be performed to access and address issues within the tympanic cavity [26]. The surgical site is then meticulously flushed with sterile saline solution before proceeding to closure. The subcutaneous tissue is sutured with absorbable materials, typically using 2-0 or 3-0 sutures, and the skin is closed in a T-shaped pattern. Drainage may be required, and this can be achieved by inserting a Penrose drain or soft rubber tubing ventral to the incision in a dependent area through a separate stab incision, or alternatively, closed suction drainage methods may be employed (Fig. **1F**). To secure the drain near the tympanic cavity, a single suture of chromic catgut (4-0 or 5-0) is utilized, and the drain is secured to the skin at the exit site. This comprehensive surgical procedure demands precision and meticulous care at every step, with particular emphasis on safeguarding critical structures, such as the facial nerve and the great auricular artery, and adhering to stringent aseptic techniques to ensure optimal postoperative outcomes for the patient. The excised ear canal is submitted for histologic evaluation, and middle ear tissue samples are collected for culture and susceptibility testing. In conclusion, Total Ear Canal Ablation is a complex surgical procedure that demands precision, specialized equipment, and careful technique to achieve successful outcomes while prioritizing patient safety. This comprehensive guide serves as a valuable resource for veterinary surgeons, highlighting the significance of equipment selection and surgical skill in TECA procedures.

Sub Total Ear Canal Ablation

In cases involving dogs with erect ears, a modification of this technique has been described to preserve the ear's natural shape [26]. This modification includes an inverted L-shaped skin incision over the vertical canal, sparing the distal portion of the vertical canal, which results in a stoma just ventral to the external orifice. This procedure has been performed in dogs with chronic otitis externa/media without apparent problems reported at a 1-year follow-up. It's essential to discuss methods to prevent ear droop with owners before surgery. Subtotal ear canal ablation is suitable for animals with erect ears, while a subset of dogs with pendulous ears can also benefit from it when the medial surface of the pinna and the distal auricular cavity is minimally affected by the disease process. However, animals with masses or severe changes in the vertical ear canal due to otitis externa, especially pendulous-eared breeds, are not suitable candidates for subtotal ear canal ablation, as the risk of recurrent disease in the remaining vertical canal would be too high to warrant these tissue sparing techniques

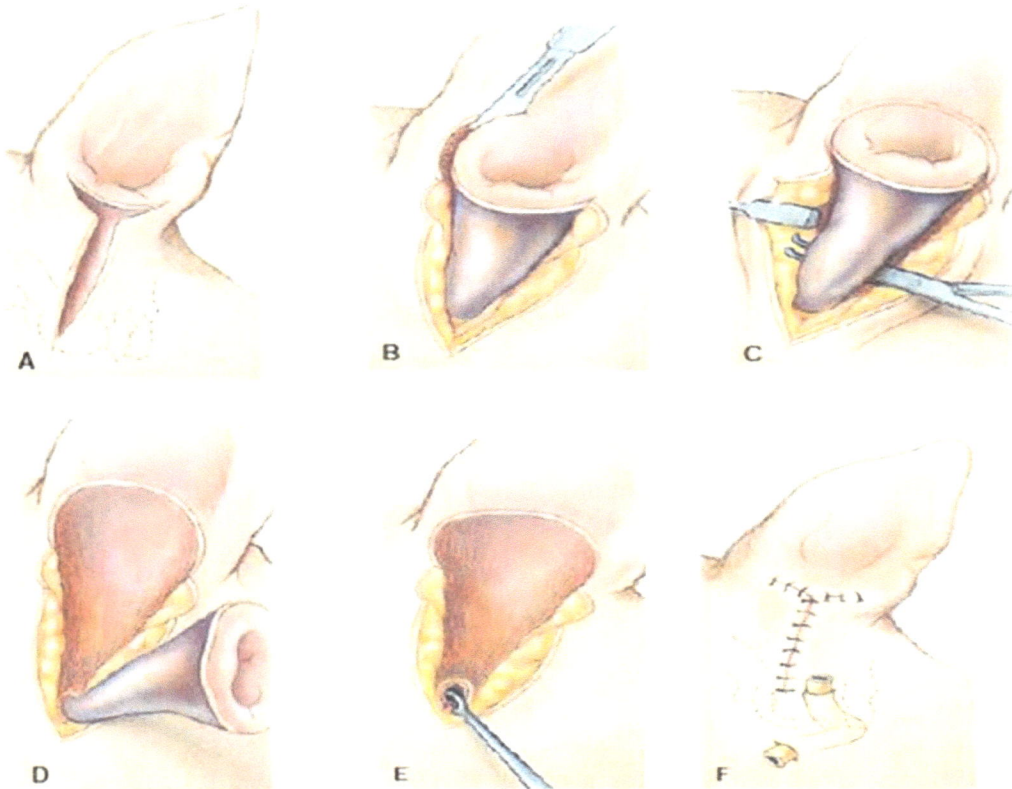

Fig. (1). Total ear canal ablation. (A) Make a T-shaped incision where the horizontal part runs parallel and is positioned just below the upper border of the tragus. Starting from the midpoint of the horizontal incision, make a vertical cut that continues until it reaches slightly beyond the level of the horizontal ear canal. (B) Lift the skin flaps, uncover the loose connective tissue, and reveal the lateral side of the vertical ear canal and proceed to extend the horizontal incision around the entrance of the vertical ear canal using a scalpel blade. (C) Carefully separate the tissues surrounding the upper and inner portions of the vertical ear canal. (D) Continue the dissection to the level of the external acoustic meatus. (E), Using a scalpel blade, rongeur, or Mayo scissors, remove the attachment of the horizontal canal to the external acoustic meatus. Then, employ a curette to delicately eliminate any secretory tissue adhering to the rim of the external acoustic meatus. (F) If desired, place a Penrose drain.

Surgical Procedure

In the described surgical procedure, a single vertical incision is meticulously made along the external ear canal, beginning just ventral to the midpoint of the external orifice and extending down to the ventral region of the horizontal ear canal (Fig. **2A**). This incision provides access to the ear canal for further manipulation. Using retractors to hold the tissue aside, the central section of the vertical ear canal is carefully separated from its soft-tissue attachments through a combination of blunt and sharp dissection techniques (Fig. **2B**). Once freed, this central portion is then transected, effectively removing it (Fig. **2C**). Subsequently, the proximal part of the vertical canal and the horizontal canal are excised, following the standard Total Ear Canal Ablation (TECA) procedure (Fig. **2D**). After this removal, a lateral bulla osteotomy and curettage are performed to address issues within the bulla. The cut end of the distal vertical ear canal is grasped and elevated, allowing for the medial and lateral vertical ear canal cartilages to be aligned and joined together using multiple simple interrupted or cruciate sutures. It's crucial to ensure that these sutures do not penetrate the epithelium of the vertical canal to prevent any complications. Once the cartilages are securely sutured, the surgical site is closed with subcutaneous and skin closures in a routine manner. This entire procedure results in the creation of a shallow, blind-ended auricular cavity while preserving the entire circumference of the annular cartilage surrounding the external orifice.

Modified Total Ear Canal Ablation in Cats

In some cases, postoperative pinna deformity following Total Ear Canal Ablation (TECA) in cats can lead to dissatisfaction among pet owners. However, a recently reported surgical technique offers a potential solution to enhance the cosmetic outcome and ultimately improve owner satisfaction. This innovative method involves the use of a single-pedicle advancement flap situated at the base of the pinna during a modified TECA procedure. The process begins with a vertical incision at both the cranial and caudal ends of an elliptic incision, centered around the external auditory meatus (Fig. **3A**). The single-pedicle advancement flap is then dissected ventrally, providing access to the subcutaneous tissue over the vertical ear canal (Fig. **3B**). Following lateral bulla osteotomy and ear canal excision, the top of the advancement flap is pulled down to the base of the pinna to assess whether further release of the flap is necessary to minimize tension on the pinna (Fig. **3C**). Once the optimal positioning is determined, the flap is sutured securely to the base of the pinna, contributing to more upright ear carriage (Fig. **3D**) and an improved aesthetic outcome, which can significantly enhance owner satisfaction with the procedure.

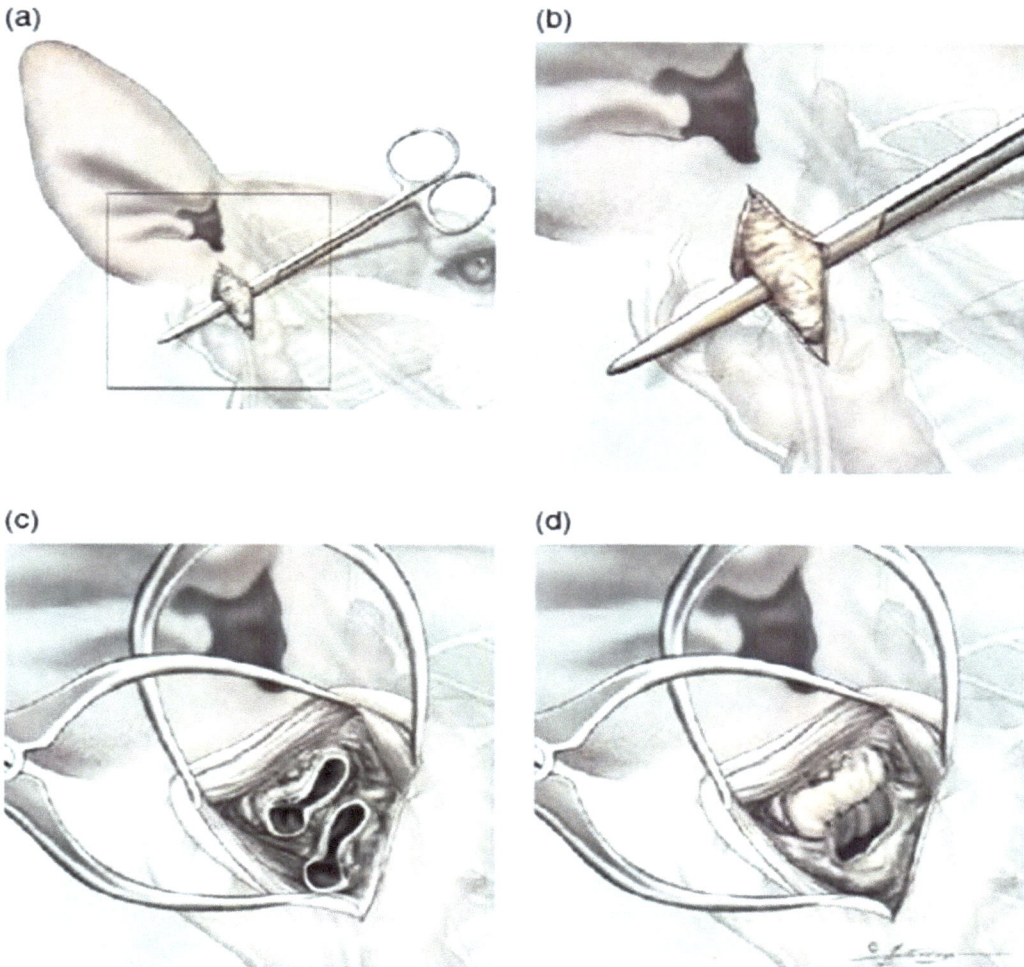

Fig. (2). (**A**) Line drawing showing the location of the skin incision parallel to, and directly over, the vertical ear canal. (**B**) The vertical canal is dissected free of its attachments and elevated by passing an instrument (Metzenbaum scissors) behind the canal. (**C**) The canal is transected and the distal portion closed with cruciate sutures placed in the cut edges of the cartilage while avoiding the epithelium. (**D**) Following closure of the distal canal, the proximal vertical canal and horizontal canal are followed down to the tympanic bulla as with a standard total ear canal ablation. (From Eric Monnet, editor: Small Animal Soft Tissue Surgery, 1st ed. St Louis, 2013, Mosby.) © D. Giddings.

BULLA OSTEOTOMY

Bulla osteotomy, a surgical procedure commonly employed in veterinary medicine, plays a pivotal role in addressing a spectrum of middle ear disorders afflicting dogs and cats. This procedure, named after the bony bulla encompassing the middle ear, is a vital solution for conditions like chronic ear infections, tumors, and foreign body obstructions. Its diverse techniques, including subtotal, ventral, and lateral approaches, offer veterinarians precise means to access and treat these issues. Following surgery, diligent post-operative care, including pain management and antibiotics, is essential for a successful recovery. Bulla osteotomy often leads to a significant improvement in the quality of life for our cherished animal companions, offering them relief from the pain and discomfort associated with middle ear disorders while underlining the importance of skilled veterinary professionals in ensuring their well-being.

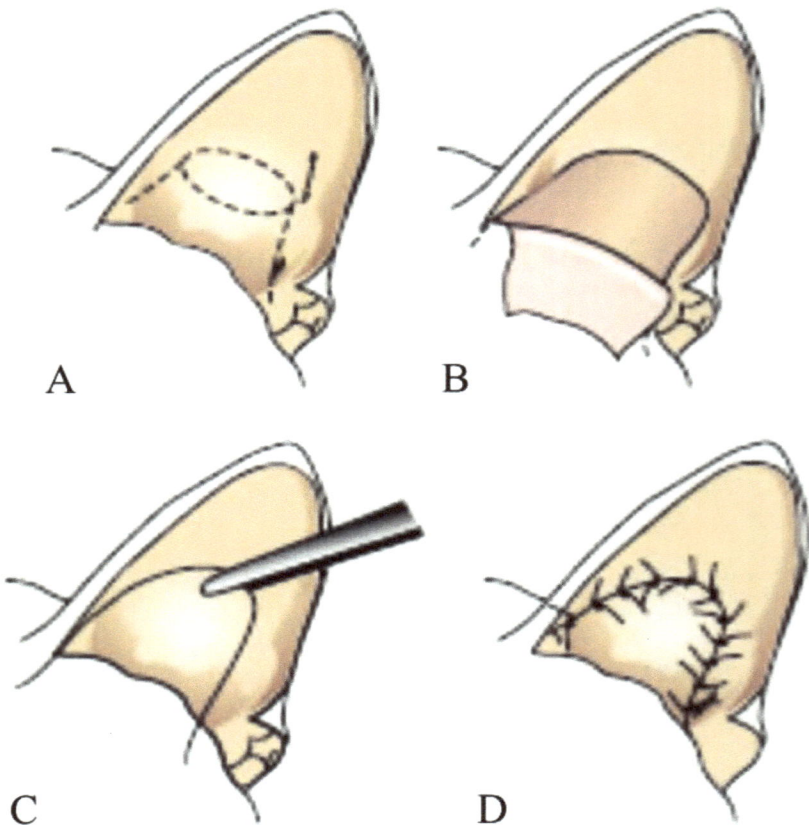

Fig. (3). To perform a modified total ear canal ablation (TECA) in a cat (**A**), make a vertical incision at the cranial and caudal ends of an elliptic incision centered around the external auditory meatus. (**B**) Dissect the single pedicle advancement flap ventrally, allowing exposure of the subcutaneous tissue over the vertical ear canal. (**C**) After lateral bulla osteotomy and excision of the ear canal, pull the top of the advancement flap to the base of the pinna to determine whether further release of the flap is necessary to reduce tension on the pinna. (**D**) Suture the flap to the base of the pinna. (From Fossum TW, editor: Small animal surgery, 4th ed. St Louis, 2013, Mosby.)

Lateral Bulla Osteotomy (LBO)

Lateral bulla osteotomy is often performed in conjunction with TECA, particularly in dogs. This approach allows for the exploration of the middle ear, which is frequently affected by long-standing otitis externa (external ear inflammation) in these animals [27]. During otitis externa, debris and secretory epithelium may accumulate within the tympanic bulla (a bony structure in the middle ear), potentially leading to complications. Therefore, LBO is a crucial part of the surgical procedure. Over time, the technique for LBO has evolved. Initially, TECA was performed without bulla osteotomy, resulting in a high rate of infection-related complications [28, 29]. Later, when curettage of the tympanic bulla lining was added following LBO, the complication rate decreased considerably [28]. More recently, an aggressive bulla osteotomy, involving the lateral bulla and floor, has been advocated to ensure complete debris removal and improve drug delivery and immune defense [30]. However, combining the ventral approach to the tympanic cavity with TECA has shown a high rate of complications, including facial nerve damage and recurrent deep infection, with no clear advantage over the standard TECA LBO technique (Sharp, 1990). One notable advantage of lateral bulla osteotomy is that it does not require repositioning of the animal during surgery. This can be particularly advantageous in cases where the pet's health condition or the surgical environment makes repositioning challenging or risky.

Surgical Procedure

The procedure begins with the surgeon making a precise incision and carefully dissecting the tissue from the lateral aspect of the bulla, a bony structure within the ear, using a small periosteal elevator. Great care is taken to avoid damaging vital structures such as the external carotid artery and the maxillary vein, which are located just ventral to the bulla. Once the tissue is dissected, the lateral and ventral aspects of the bulla are removed using a specialized surgical tool called a rongeur. This bony excision provides access to the caudal aspect, the rear portion of the middle ear canal (Fig. **4**). The extent of bony excision may be adjusted based on the surgeon's judgment and the specific requirements of the case to fully visualize and access the contents of the tympanic cavity. With access established, a curette is used to meticulously remove any infected material within the tympanic cavity. Care must be taken to avoid sharp dissection and curettage in the rostral or rostromedial areas of the cavity to prevent damage to the auditory ossicles or inner ear structures. Finally, the surgeon gently irrigates the tympanic cavity with saline to ensure a thorough cleaning, removing any remaining debris or contaminants. This step creates a clean and infection-free environment conducive to optimal healing. Lateral bulla osteotomy, often performed in conjunction with Total Ear Canal Ablation (TECA), is preferred when repositioning the animal is not necessary and contributes to the resolution of ear problems and overall well-being of the animal patient.

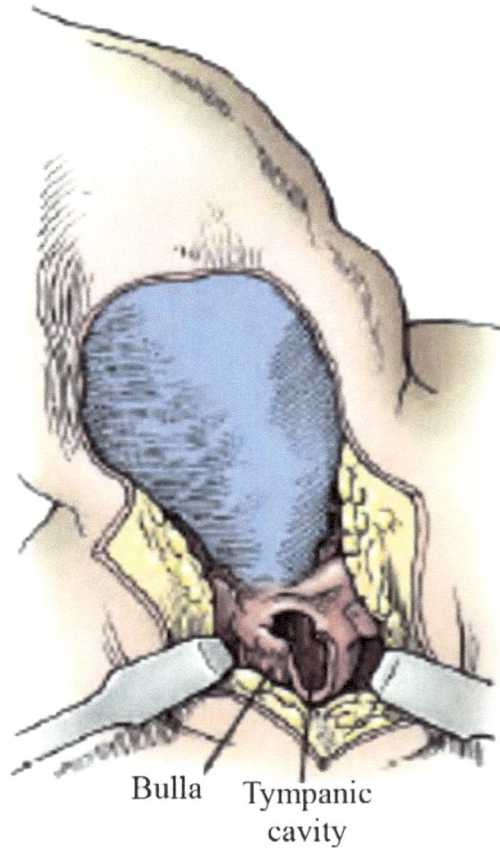

Fig. (4). Lateral Bulla Osteotomy **(From Fossum TW, editor:** *Small animal surgery***, ed 4, St Louis, 2013, Mosby.)**

Ventral Bulla Osteotomy

Ventral bulla osteotomy is a surgical procedure in veterinary medicine used to gain increased access to the tympanic cavity. It can be performed alone or alongside lateral ear resection and is particularly beneficial when middle ear neoplasia is suspected, especially in cats with nasopharyngeal polyps. Ventral bulla osteotomy offers superior drainage of the bulla compared to lateral bulla osteotomy and eliminates the need to reposition the animal during the procedure.

Surgical Procedure

In this surgical procedure, the patient is positioned in dorsal recumbency to ensure stability and comfort. Aseptic surgical techniques are employed, and a generous surgical area around the angle of the mandible is prepared. The bulla, which is located immediately caudal and medial to the vertical ramus of the mandible, is identified using two imaginary lines: one connecting the mandibular rami and the other along the long axis of the ventral aspect of the head (Fig. **5A**). An incision is made, with its size varying between dogs (7 to 10 cm) and cats (3 to 5 cm). The incision is centered 2 cm toward the affected side from the intersection of the imaginary lines (Fig. **5A**). The platysma muscle is incised, and the linguofacial vein, if present, is retracted. Further dissection is performed by bluntly dissecting the digastricus muscle (lateral) from the hyoglossus and styloglossus muscles (medial). Care must be taken to avoid damaging the hypoglossal nerve, located on the lateral aspect of the hypoglossus muscle. Self-retaining retractors like Gelpi or Weitlaner are used to spread and retract the digastric and glossal muscles, exposing the bulla (Fig. **5B**). Access to the bulla is achieved by confirming its location, which is craniomedial to the cornu process of the hyoid bone and caudomedial to the angle of the mandible. A hole is initially created in the ventral aspect of the bulla using a Steinmann pin, and it is then enlarged with a small rongeur (*e.g.,* Lempert). The interior of the bulla is meticulously examined for signs of inflammation, neoplastic tissue, or foreign bodies. Samples are collected for culture, sensitivity, and histopathologic examination. If signs of infection are present or if continued drainage is anticipated, a small, fenestrated drain tube is placed in the cavity and exits through a separate stab incision. The fenestrated part of the drain tube is sutured to the bulla using small chromic gut sutures (4-0 to 6-0). Depending on the amount of exudation, the drain is typically removed within 3 to 7 days following the surgery.

Subtotal Bulla Osteotomy

Subtotal bulla osteotomy is a surgical intervention used to treat conditions such as bulla osteitis (inflammation of the bulla) and expanding cholesteatoma (a benign growth of keratinized squamous epithelium). The procedure involves the removal of a portion of the bulla's bony structure to access and address these conditions effectively.

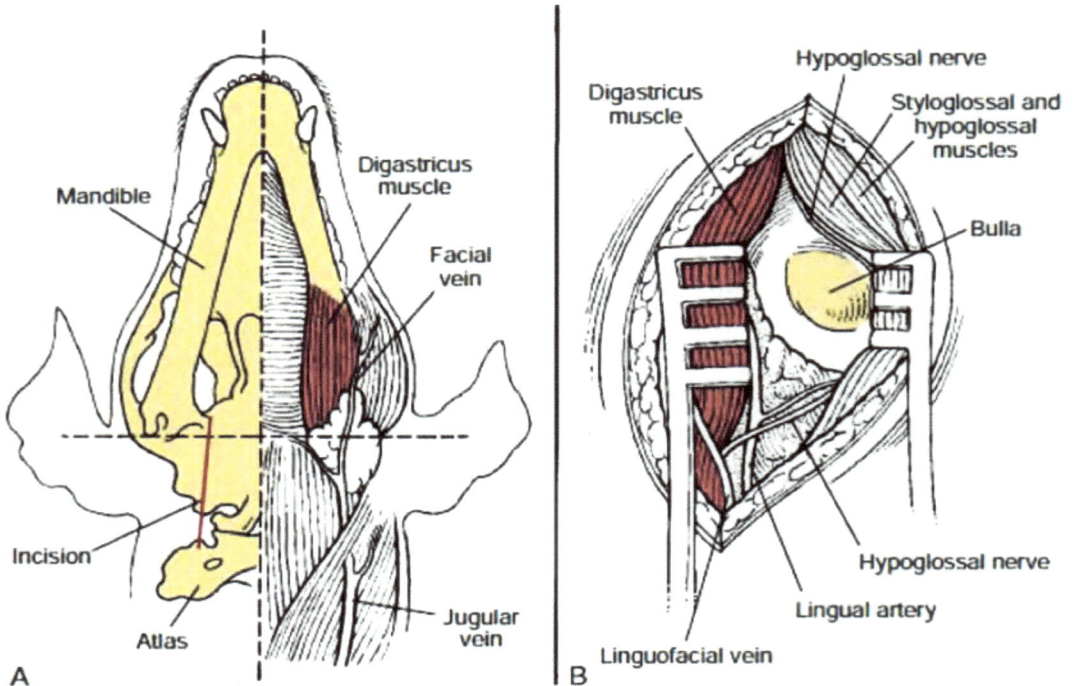

Fig. (5). Ventral bulla osteotomy. (**A**) For ventral bulla osteotomy, draw an imaginary line connecting the mandibular rami and a second imaginary line along the long axis of the ventral aspect of the head. Make a 7 to 10 cm incision parallel with the midline of the neck and centered 2 cm toward the affected side from where these imaginary lines intersect. (**B**) Incise the platysma muscle, retract the linguofacial vein if necessary, and deepen the incision by bluntly dissecting the digastricus muscle (lateral) from the hypoglossal and styloglossal muscles (medial). Confirm the location of the bulla; use self-retaining retractors. to spread the digastricus and glossal muscles and retract them from the bulla. (From Fossum TW, editor: Small animal surgery, 4th ed., St Louis, 2013, Mosby.)

Surgical Approach

Before delving into the surgical steps, it's essential to highlight the importance of a cautious approach. The bulla may be extensively remodeled due to underlying conditions, which can complicate the surgery. Additionally, vital neurovascular structures are closely adhered to the ventral aspect of the tympanic bone, with the facial nerve being of utmost concern (Fig. **6A**). Therefore, the surgeon must avoid direct tension on the facial nerve during the procedure. The surgical approach begins with the careful elevation of soft tissue from the ventral and lateral aspects of the bulla. This initial step is crucial for exposing the deeper structures within the bulla. It's essential to avoid sharp dissection near the external auditory meatus to prevent damage to the retroarticular vein. Once soft tissue has been gently retracted, the surgeon proceeds to remove the ventral aspect of the osseous ear canal using rongeurs. During this step, it's imperative to remove all epithelium and the tympanic membrane. The malleus is often removed along with the tympanic membrane (Fig. **6B-C**). Subsequently, the lateral aspect of the bulla is removed using rongeurs as well. In subtotal bulla osteotomy, the entire lateral face and ventral bulla bone are excised. It's worth noting that in some cases, a greenish-brown epithelialized pouch may be found on the bulla's face, traveling ventrally from the external auditory meatus (Fig. **6D**). This pouch is typically adhered to structures under the bulla floor, and careful separation is required to prevent profuse hemorrhage. After removing the lateral bulla bone, the interior aspect of the tympanic bulla is thoroughly inspected following irrigation with tepid sterile saline. Any debris and abnormal epithelium, often appearing as greenish-brown thickened tissue, must be removed from the rostral, ventral, and caudal aspects of the tympanic cavity. However, it's important to note that the remaining ossicles are not removed unless abnormal soft tissue is adhered to them in the epitympanic recess [31]. This approach is critical to avoid damage to the delicate inner ear structures. One of the primary goals during this procedure is the complete removal of any epithelial remnants. These remnants can serve as a source of recurrent deep infection post-surgery [30, 31]. Therefore, meticulous attention is paid to ensure all remnants are eliminated. In cases where the dorsal surface of the tympanic cavity requires attention, care is exercised not to curette this area aggressively, as it could result in damage to the promontory area and subsequent inner ear damage (Fig. **6E-F**). Instead, attached soft tissue is gently teased from this area using hemostatic forceps. The medial aspect of the tympanic bone requires special care, as the internal carotid artery may be at risk of damage, especially when imaging indicates erosion of the bone. The use of a video-otoscope during surgery is recommended, as it provides excellent visualization of the inner tympanic cavity and aids in identifying debris and epithelial remnants [32].

POSTOPERATIVE CARE AND ASSESSMENT IN EAR CANAL RESECTION OR ABLATION

Postoperative care and assessment are vital aspects of ensuring the successful recovery of animals undergoing these surgical interventions. This essay delves into the key components of postoperative care and assessment, including pain management, bandaging, swelling control, antibiotic therapy, and the removal of drains and sutures. Pain management is a fundamental aspect of postoperative care. It not only addresses the ethical responsibility of ensuring the animal's comfort but also plays a critical role in promoting faster healing and reducing stress. Appropriate postoperative analgesics should be administered, taking into consideration the specific guidelines for dosing and administration outlined in anesthetic protocols. Additionally, tranquilizers may be considered if the animal displays signs of dysphoria or anxiety, further enhancing postoperative comfort. Bandaging and collar use are essential elements of postoperative care for ear canal resection or ablation. A bandage is applied over the surgical site to protect the wound, prevent hematomas, and maintain the integrity of the surgical area. To ensure that the bandage remains undisturbed, veterinarians use Elizabethan collars or sidebar collars (cone collars) that restrict the animal from removing the bandage or causing self-inflicted harm. These collars are indispensable in facilitating proper wound healing. If head-encircling bandages are used, be sure to avoid applying them too tightly, since respiratory difficulty from airway obstruction can be encountered [30]. Excessive swelling can pose a challenge in the aftermath of these surgeries. To address this concern, cold packs are applied to the side of the face multiple times a day during the initial 24 to 36 hours following surgery. These cold packs aid in reducing inflammation, alleviating pain, and minimizing swelling around the surgical area. Proper care must be taken to ensure that the cold pack is not applied directly to the skin, which could potentially lead to frostbite or tissue damage. Antibiotic therapy is another crucial element of postoperative care. It is vital for preventing and managing postoperative infections. The choice of antibiotics should be based on culture results to tailor the treatment to the specific pathogen involved. Typically, antibiotics are administered for an extended period, ranging from 3 to 4 weeks, to ensure the prevention of recurrent infections and to support complete healing [1, 10]. Drain and suture management is also integral to the postoperative care plan. Penrose drains are often placed during surgery to aid in the drainage of fluids and prevent the accumulation of postoperative fluid collections [12, 24]. The timing for the removal of these drains typically falls within 3 to 7 days post-surgery, depending on the patient's progress and the surgeon's assessment. Sutures used to close surgical incisions are usually removed after a designated healing period, typically around 10 to 14 days post-surgery. Suture removal should be performed with care to avoid causing any damage or discomfort to the patient.

COMPLICATIONS

Ear canal surgery, particularly procedures such as total ear canal ablation with bulla osteotomy, can have various complications that veterinarians and pet owners need to be aware of. These complications can impact the pet's overall health and quality of life. In this essay, we will discuss some of the significant complications associated with ear canal surgery in dogs and cats.

Nerve Damage and Horner Syndrome

One potential complication of ear canal surgery is nerve damage, specifically damage to the postganglionic sympathetic fibers running through the middle ear (Cook, 2004). This can result in a condition known as Horner's syndrome. Horner's syndrome is characterized by clinical signs such as enophthalmos (a sunken appearance of the eye), elevation of the third eyelid, miosis (constricted pupil), and ptosis (drooping of the upper eyelid). These symptoms occur due to decreased innervation to the smooth muscles responsible for various eye movements. Horner's syndrome can occur in both dogs and cats but appears to have a higher risk in cats, possibly due to anatomical differences. The incidence of this complication can be as high as 27% to 42% in cats after total ear canal ablation and may be permanent in some cases (Bacon *et al.,* 2003).

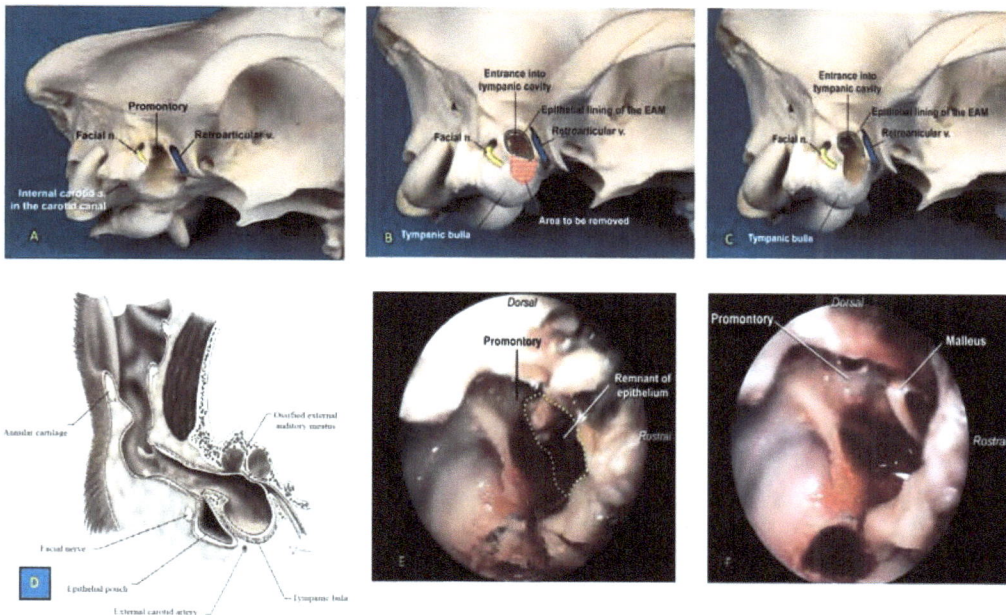

Fig. (6). Sub Total Bulla Osteotomy. (**A**) Close-up, oblique ventrolateral view of important deep structures surrounding the tympanic bulla of the skull. A distinct bony rim separates the osseous EAM from the stylomastoid foramen (*i.e.,* exit site for the facial nerve). (n = nerve; v = vein). (**B**) The notch to be created in the ventral floor of the osseous ear canal. The epithelial tissue lining the ear canal is also indicated. (**C**) While the freed edge is grasped, the epithelial "cuff" is elevated both rostrally and caudally (the epithelium is shown elevated partially on the caudal aspect) from the osseous ear canal beginning at the notched area.The ridge of bone separating the EAM from the stylomastoid foramen is now well exposed.. (**D**) Transverse section through the head showing horizontal canal and tympanic bulla. A pouch of secretory epithelium often forms between the annular cartilage and the tympanic bulla extending into the external auditory meatus. Soft tissues are carefully dissected from the pouch and ventral aspect of the tympanic bulla. (**E**) A greenish epithelial remnant in the rostral compartment of the cavity must be removed entirely without damaging the malleus. (**F**) Excellent exposure of the completely evacuated tympanic cavity is achieved with the described subtotal bulla osteotomy technique. (From Compendium on Continuing Education for the Practicing Veterinarian (2005) - Lateral Approach).

Facial Nerve Damage

Another critical concern in ear canal surgery is the potential for damage to the facial nerve. The facial nerve has a vulnerable path around the ventral half of the ear canal, making it susceptible to swelling, inflammation, and trauma. Facial nerve injury can result in facial palsy, which includes symptoms like a droopy lip, lack of a blink reflex in the affected eye, and a dropped ear on the same side [3, 18]. The incidence of postoperative facial nerve injury can vary, with up to 39% in dogs and as high as 56% in cats. Permanent damage can occur in a percentage of these cases, affecting the pet's facial expressions [4].

Hemorrhage

While not common, major hemorrhage can occur during ear canal surgery, with reported incidence rates ranging from 3% to 14% [24, 26]. Hemorrhage is typically a result of damage to the retroglenoid vein and can be life-threatening. The vein's retraction into the retroglenoid foramen can make direct ligation challenging (Smeak *et al.,* 1998). Managing hemorrhage in this context often involves packing the foramen with bone wax. Proper surgical technique and careful handling can help minimize the risk of hemorrhage [12].

Wound Dehiscence

Wound dehiscence, the separation of surgical incisions or wounds, can occur as a complication of ear canal surgery. In dogs, it is more common after lateral wall resection and may result from factors like poor patient selection, inadequate surgical technique, self-inflicted trauma, or issues with local wound healing. Suturing in a bloody field, excessive use of local cautery, or inadvertently suturing the surrounding skin to cartilage instead of integument can contribute to wound dehiscence. This complication can also be observed in up to 25% of cases following total ear canal ablation. In some instances, wound infection or discharge may occur even without dehiscence [18].

Auditory Function

Postoperative deafness is a concern for pet owners after total ear canal ablation with bulla osteotomy. Pets with chronic otitis externa may already have reduced hearing abilities, and surgery may further impact their auditory function. However, some dogs are still able to respond to high-pitched or very loud noises after surgery [22, 31]. Brainstem auditory-evoked responses to air-conducted stimulation may be lost, but the ability to hear through acoustic bone conduction, if present before surgery, should remain permanently [27].

CONCLUSION

Total ear canal ablation (TECA) is the complete removal of the vertical and horizontal ear canals with the associated secretory epithelium. This important salvage procedure is often performed for the irreversible inflammatory ear canal disease in dogs. In addition, a lateral bulla osteotomy (LBO) is normally performed with TECA where otitis media is often associated with long-standing otitis externa in dogs as well as the exploration of the tympanic cavity with best surgical approach. A perfect and complete preoperative procedure including blood and physical work-up is needed to determine the extent and nature of the chronic ear disease progress with a good prediction of surgical or anaesthetic complications. Otoscopic examination is the most efficient procedure to be performed while the dog is anesthetized. TECA LBO is considered as very painful procedure in small animals. Pre-emptive analgesia should be considered for the pain management associated with TECA LBO.

REFERENCES

[1]   Bacon NJ, Gilbert RL, Bostock DE, White RAS. Total ear canal ablation in the cat: indications, morbidity and long-term survival. J Small Anim Pract 2003; 44(10): 430-4.
[http://dx.doi.org/10.1111/j.1748-5827.2003.tb00101.x] [PMID: 14582656]

[2]   Beckman SL, Henry WB Jr, Cechner P. Total ear canal ablation combining bulla osteotomy and curettage in dogs with chronic otitis externa and media. J Am Vet Med Assoc 1990; 196(1): 84-90.
[http://dx.doi.org/10.2460/javma.1990.196.01.84] [PMID: 2295558]

[3]   Cole LK. Otoscopic evaluation of the ear canal. Vet Clin North Am Small Anim Pract 2004; 34(2): 397-410.
[http://dx.doi.org/10.1016/j.cvsm.2003.10.004] [PMID: 15062615]

[4]   Cook LB. Neurologic evaluation of the ear. Vet Clin North Am Small Anim Pract 2004; 34(2): 425-35.
[http://dx.doi.org/10.1016/j.cvsm.2003.12.001] [PMID: 15062617]

[5]   De Lorenzi D, Bonfanti U, Masserdotti C, Tranquillo M. Fine-needle biopsy of external ear canal masses in the cat: cytologic results and histologic correlations in 27 cases. Vet Clin Pathol 2005; 34(2): 100-5.
[http://dx.doi.org/10.1111/j.1939-165X.2005.tb00020.x] [PMID: 15902659]

[6]   Devitt CM, Seim HB III, Willer R, McPherron M, Neely M. Passive drainage *versus* primary closure after total ear canal ablation-lateral bulla osteotomy in dogs: 59 dogs (1985-1995). Vet Surg 1997; 26(3): 210-6.
[http://dx.doi.org/10.1111/j.1532-950X.1997.tb01486.x] [PMID: 9150559]

[7]   Dvir E, Kirberger RM, Terblanche AG. Magnetic resonance imaging of otitis media in a dog. Vet Radiol Ultrasound 2000; 41(1): 46-9.
[http://dx.doi.org/10.1111/j.1740-8261.2000.tb00426.x] [PMID: 10695880]

[8]   Eom KD, Lee HC, Yoon J. Canalographic evaluation of the external ear canal in dogs. Vet Radiol Ultrasound 2000; 41(3): 231-4.
[http://dx.doi.org/10.1111/j.1740-8261.2000.tb01484.x] [PMID: 10850873]

[9]   Fossum TW. Surgery of the ear. In: Fossum TW, Ed. Small Animal Surgery. St. Louis: Mosby 2002; pp. 229-53.

[10]   Guillaumot P, Poncet C, Bouvy B. Outcome after total ear canal ablation and subtotal bulla osteotomy (TECASBO) in 23 dogs. Wien Tierarztl Monatsschr 2011; 98(5-6): 106-13.

[11]   Hardie EM, Linder K, Pease AP. Aural cholesteatoma in twenty dogs. Vet Surg 2008; 37(8): 763-70.
[http://dx.doi.org/10.1111/j.1532-950X.2008.00455.x] [PMID: 19121172]

[12]   Haudiquet PH, Gauthier O, Renard E. Total ear canal ablation associated with lateral bulla osteotomy with the help of otoscopy in dogs and cats: retrospective study of 47 cases. Vet Surg 2006; 35: E1-E20.

[13]   Krahwinkel DJ. In: Slatter D, editor. Textbook of Small Animal Surgery. 3rd ed. Philadelphia: Saunders; 2003. External ear canal; pp. 1746-1757.

[14]   Little C, Lane J, Pearson G. Inflammatory middle ear disease of the dog: the pathology of otitis media. Vet Rec 1991; 128(13): 293-6.
[http://dx.doi.org/10.1136/vr.128.13.293] [PMID: 2035227]

[15]   Marino DJ, MacDonald JM, Matthiesen DT, *et al.* Results of surgery in cats with ceruminous gland adenocarcinoma. J Am Anim Hosp Assoc 1994; 30: 54-8.

[16]   Matthiesen DT, Scavelli T. Total ear canal ablation and lateral bulla osteotomy in 38 dogs. J Am Anim Hosp Assoc 1990; 26: 257-67.

[17]   McAnulty JF, Hattel A, Harvey CE. Wound healing and brain stem auditory evoked potentials after experimental total ear canal ablation with lateral tympanic bulla osteotomy in dogs. Vet Surg 1995; 24(1): 1-8.
[http://dx.doi.org/10.1111/j.1532-950X.1995.tb01285.x] [PMID: 7701765]

[18]   Okamoto Y, Miyatake K, Inoue T, Minami S. Total ear-canal ablation preserving the auricular annular cartilage. Nippon Juishikai Zasshi 2001; 54(10): 791-4.
[http://dx.doi.org/10.12935/jvma1951.54.791]

[19]   Petersen AD, Walker RD, Bowman MM, Schott HC II, Rosser EJ Jr. Frequency of isolation and antimicrobial susceptibility patterns of *Staphylococcus intermedius* and *Pseudomonas aeruginosa* isolates from canine skin and ear samples over a 6-year period (1992-1997). J Am Anim Hosp Assoc 2002; 38(5): 407-13.
[http://dx.doi.org/10.5326/0380407] [PMID: 12220023]

[20]   Pomianowski A, Adamiak Z. Bone-conducted brainstem auditory evoked response in a dog with total bilateral ear canal ablation: a case report. Vet Med (Praha) 2010; 55(1): 39-41.
[http://dx.doi.org/10.17221/20/2010-VETMED]

[21]   Remedios AM, Fowler JD, Pharr JW. A comparison of radiographic *versus* surgical diagnosis of otitis media. J Am Anim Hosp Assoc 1991; 27: 183-8.

[22]   Rohleder JJ, Jones JC, Duncan RB, Larson MM, Waldron DL, Tromblee T. Comparative performance of radiography and computed tomography in the diagnosis of middle ear disease in 31 dogs. Vet Radiol Ultrasound 2006; 47(1): 45-52.
[http://dx.doi.org/10.1111/j.1740-8261.2005.00104.x] [PMID: 16429984]

[23]   Smeak DD, Crocker CB, Birchard SJ. Treatment of recurrent otitis media that developed after total ear canal ablation and lateral bulla osteotomy in dogs: nine cases (1986–1994). J Am Vet Med Assoc 1996; 209(5): 937-42.
[http://dx.doi.org/10.2460/javma.1996.209.05.937] [PMID: 8790545]

[24]   Smeak DD, Dehoff WD. Total ear canal ablation. Clinical results in the dog and cat. Vet Surg 1986; 15(2): 161-70.
[http://dx.doi.org/10.1111/j.1532-950X.1986.tb00197.x]

[25]   Smeak DD, Inpanbutr N. Lateral approach to subtotal bulla osteotomy in dogs. Compend Contin Educ Pract Vet 2005; 27: 377-84.

[26]   Smeak DD, Kerpsack SJ. Total ear canal ablation and lateral bulla osteotomy for management of end-stage otitis. Semin Vet Med Surg (Small Anim) 1993; 8(1): 30-41.
[PMID: 8456202]

[27]   Smeak DD. Total ear canal ablation and lateral bulla osteotomy. In: Bojrab MJ, Ed. Current Techniques in Small Animal Surgery. Baltimore: Williams & Wilkins 1988; pp. 102-9.

[28] Tranquilli WJ, Grimm KA, Lamont LA. Pain Management for the Small Animal Practitioner. 2nd ed. Jackson, WY: Teton NewMedia 2004; pp. 101-3.

[29] Vogel PL, Komtebedde J, Hirsh DC, Kass PH. Wound contamination and antimicrobial susceptibility of bacteria cultured during total ear canal ablation and lateral bulla osteotomy in dogs. J Am Vet Med Assoc 1999; 214(11): 1641-3.
[http://dx.doi.org/10.2460/javma.1999.214.11.1641] [PMID: 10363095]

[30] White RAS, Pomeroy CJ. Total ear canal ablation and lateral bulla osteotomy in the dog. J Small Anim Pract 1990; 31(11): 547-53.
[http://dx.doi.org/10.1111/j.1748-5827.1990.tb00683.x]

[31] Williams JM, White RAS. Total ear canal ablation combined with lateral bulla osteotorny in J the cat. J Small Anim Pract 1992; 33(5): 225-7.
[http://dx.doi.org/10.1111/j.1748-5827.1992.tb01121.x]

[32] Wolfe TM, Bateman SW, Cole LK, Smeak DD. Evaluation of a local anesthetic delivery system for the postoperative analgesic management of canine total ear canal ablation – a randomized, controlled, double-blinded study. Vet Anaesth Analg 2006; 33(5): 328-39.
[http://dx.doi.org/10.1111/j.1467-2995.2005.00272.x] [PMID: 16916355]

CHAPTER 18

Neurological Disturbances

Chinmoy Maji[1,*]**, Kruti Debnath Mondal**[2] **and Arkaprabha Shee**[3]

[1] *Subject Matter Specialist (Animal Health), North 24 Parganas Krishi Vigyan Kendra, Ashokenagar, West Bengal University of Animal and Fishery Sciences, West Bengal, India*

[2] *Teaching Veterinary Clinical Complex, Faculty of Veterinary and Animal Sciences, I. Ag. SC., BHU, Mirzapur, UP, India*

[3] *Subject Matter Specialist (Vet. & Ani. Sc.), Dhaanyaganga Krishi Vigyan Kendra, RKMVERI, Sargachi, Murshidabad, West Bengal, India*

Abstract: Canine ear consists of external pinna, external ear canal, middle ear and inner ear. External ear with its cartilage structure catches the sound while middle ear through its three unique ossicle structures and tympanic membrane transmits the wave to internal ear. The bony labyrinth and associated structures of inner ear along with different nerve innervations in inner and middle ear acts as sensory organ for hearing and balance. The complex nerve structure which passes part of its course through middle or internal ear structures also innervates the surrounding facial, lip, ear, nose, eye, neck regions. Thus, a little obstacle or infection (otitis media or interna) in middle or inner ear affects the nerve function and creates different muscular or nueurogenic abnormality presented through different clinical symptoms. Among various canine ear problems, the most common vestibular diseases (peripheral and central), namely horner's syndrome, hemifacial spasm, deafness, facial nerve paralysis are discussed briefly in this chapter.

Keywords: Cranial nerves, Facial paralysis, Horner's syndrome, Otitis media, Vestibular disease.

INTRODUCTION

A large portion of animal communication depends on the auditory system, which is built to detect and analyze sound in the surroundings. With specific frequencies and amplitudes, sounds are pressure waves in the atmosphere. The auditory system interprets a sound's frequency as its pitch and its amplitude as its loudness. Having at least one ear is necessary for hearing, but having two allows the auditory system to detect differences in the timing or strength of sound waves impinging on the two ears. Animals' capacity to move their ears around to search

---

* **Corresponding author Chinmoy Maji:** Subject Matter Specialist (Animal Health), North 24 Parganas Krishi Vigyan Kendra, Ashokenagar, West Bengal University of Animal and Fishery Sciences, West Bengal, India; E-mail: chinmoy_19@rediffmail.com

the surroundings for various sounds and determine where the sound is coming from, improves their hearing as well. The cerebral cortex is responsible for hearing, but the brainstem mediates auditory reflexes like tilting the head in reaction to sound. The auditory system, which includes the external, middle, and inner ears, includes the organ of Corti, a sensory receptor. The cochlear nerve transmits auditory impulses to the cochlear nuclei in the medulla oblongata and innervates the organ of Corti in the inner ear. The medial geniculate nucleus of the thalamus, which in turn projects to the auditory cerebral cortex, receives axons from the organ of Corti as they ascend the brainstem (Fig. **1**).

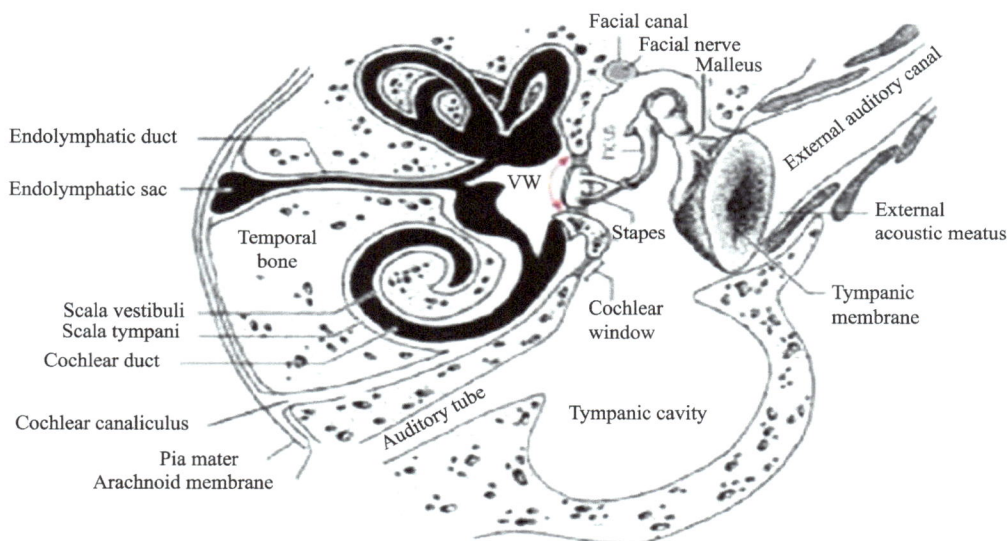

Fig. (1). The auditory system [22].

NEURO ANATOMY AND NEUROLOGICAL PATHWAYS RELATED TO EAR DISEASES

Anatomically ear comprises of external auditory canal, middle ear and inner ear (Fig. **1**). The external auditory meatus collects the sound and direct towards tympanic membrane. Middle ear starts with three small ossicles or bones named as malleus, incus, stapes and Eustachian tube. Malleus is attached with tympanic membrane and the incoming sound waves are amplified by the series of small ossicles and transfer to inner ear through stapes to oval window of inner ear. Eustachian tube maintains the air pressure in middle ear there by helps in proper transmission of sound waves. The bony labyrinth of the inner ear is made up of semicircular canals, vestibule and cochlea. The membranous labyrinth underlies the bony labyrinth. The semicircular canal and vestibules take care of vestibular function whereas cochlea is associated with auditory functions [1, 2].

The three semicircular canals are oriented perpendicular to each other representing the three planes in space and thus can detect movement in all planes. One end of theses canals is dilated to form ampulla and are attached with vestibule. The ampulla houses a structure called as crista ampullaris in the membranous labyrinth. They carry the receptors cells named hair cells that form synapsis with the vestibulocochlear nerve of CNS system and thus are responsible for detection of rotational head movement in different planes. The membranous labyrinth of vestibules, semicircular canal and Scala media of cochlea are filled with a fluid called endolymph. The rotation of head and eyeball is due to hydrodynamics of endolymph. The cilia of hair cells are extended into the cupula. The cupula is gelatinous poly saccharide mound [3]. The rotation of head creates a motion in endolymph deflecting cupula from its place, thereby creating a nerve impulse. The utricles and saccules are the two structures take care of the static position and linear acceleration of head. The saccule and utricle are attached to vestibules and placed in a vertical plane and horizontal plane respectively. The dilatation on these structures is called macula and lined by hair cells with the cilia extending into a gelatinous structure called otolithic membrane. There are calcium carbonate crystals called otoliths or statoconia [4]. The otoliths move faster due to its inertia when body starts moving in linear direction and thereby creating a sensation or nerve impulse in the hair cells and in turn stimulate the vestibulochoclear nerve. The axons of vestibular nerve after joining with cochlear branch of cranial nerve VIII runs through internal acoustic meatus to rostral medulla oblangata of brain stem. A mainstream of neurons joins with four vestibular nuclei but a few directly connect with the cerebellum by caudal cerebellar peduncle. The neural impulse acts through extensors muscles innervated by neurons. Suppose the head of an animal tilt towards right then the right extensor muscles are stimulated and the left extensor muscles inhibited, thereby preventing falling down to left.

The vestibular neurons also pass through the nuclei of cranial nerves III, IV and VI. These three neurons innervate different muscles of eyeball and are responsible for eyeball movement. The vestibular system in this way coordinates the changes required in eyeball movement with varied position of head and thereby keep the image stable in retina. These important neuroanatomy of ear plays a mainstream role in vestibular function of body [5].

The trigeminal, facial, vagus and second cervical nerves, in particular, are in charge of the sensory innervation of the pinna. The skin of the skull and the mucosa of the intraosseous portion of the external ear canal are sensory organs of the trigeminal nerve (mandibular branch). The mandibular nerve is released at the oval foramen by the auriculotemporal nerve, which then exits between the auricular cartilage on the caudal side and the base of the masseter muscle on the cranial side. The external acoustic meatus nerve, which is sensory to the external acoustic meatus and a ramus to the tympanic membrane, is released close to the tympanic membrane.

The rostral auricular nerves, which are released by the auriculotemporal nerve, link the skin over the lateral side of the tragus, a tiny amount of the rostroventral region of the pinna's concave surface, and the rostral border of the pinna. On the other hand, the rostrodorsal side of the pinna, which is released by the dorsal branch of the second cervical nerve, is connected to the convex surface of the pinna, including the pinna's apex, *via* the cutaneous branches. Its cutaneous region wraps around the pinna's cranial border and along its medial side (concave surface) rostrally.

The cranial boundary of the cutaneous region of the auricular branches of the facial nerve overlaps ventrally and rostrally with that of the auriculotemporal branch of the mandibular branch of the trigeminal nerve as well as the cutaneous area of the second cervical nerve. On the convex surface of the pinna, the dorsal branch of the second cervical nerve overlaps laterally with the greater auricular nerve from the ventral branch of the second cervical nerve and dorsomedially with the dorsal cutaneous branch of the third cervical nerve. The second cervical nerve's ventral branch's greater auricular nerve, which is the bigger of its two terminal branches, travels dorsocranially to the base of the pinna before splitting into two branches that proceed in the direction of the ear's apex. The greater auricular nerve's cutaneous region covers the convex and concave surfaces of the pinna. The greater auricular nerve overlaps the cutaneous sections of the greater occipital nerve dorsally on the convex surface of the pinna and the auricular branches of the seventh cranial nerve on the concave side of the pinna. The external ear receives motor innervation from the facial nerve (Fig. **2**).

The facial nerve also innervates the platysma of the neck, the caudal belly of the digastricus, the stylohyoid, and the superficial muscles of the head and face. The ventral side of the medulla oblongata is where the facial nerve emerges, leaving ventro laterally through the trapezoid bodies. Through the internal acoustic meatus, the face nerve, as well as the vestibular and cochlear nerves, escapes the cranial cavity. The facial canal enters the middle ear cavity close to the vestibular (oval) window. After travelling a short distance in the internal acoustic meatus, the facial nerve reaches the facial canal of the petrous temporal bone. From there, the facial nerve branches into the chorda tympani and stapedial nerves.

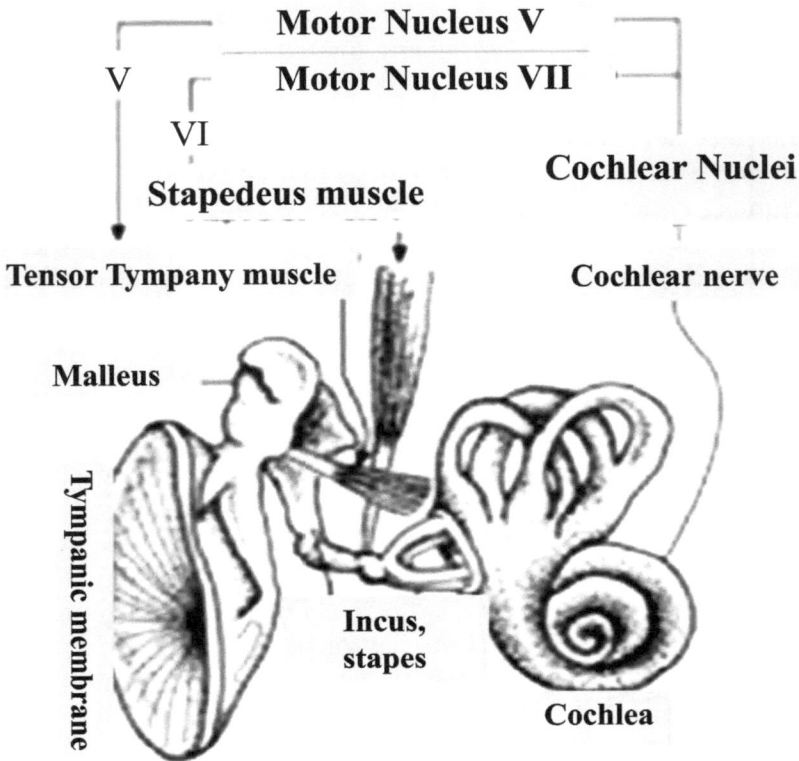

Fig. (2). The neurological pathway of ear.

The nerve crosses the medial surface of the handle of the malleus as the chorda tympani proceeds into the middle ear cavity. The tympanic membrane's medial surface is then traversed. After that, it emerges through the tympanic bulla's rostrodorsal wall through the petrotympanic fissure and connects to the mandibular nerve's lingual branch.

The stylomastoid foramen is the skull's outlet for the facial nerve. The face nerve's lateral internal auricular branches extend out into the external ear canal. The caudal auricular nerve and muscles are both served by muscular branches that the facial nerve sends after emerging between muscles at the base of the ear. A digastric branch emerges from the facial nerve as it bends ventrally and rostrally around the annular cartilage. The caudal internal auricular nerve serves as a sensory nerve and nourishes the caudal surface of the pinna. The lateral internal auricular nerve, which provides the nonosseous external ear canal, and the middle internal auricular nerve, which supplies the skin of the rostral part of the concave region of the pinna, are both produced by the facial nerve. The facial nerve wraps itself around the caudal edge of the jaw on the surface of the masseter muscle before splitting into the cervical, buccal, and auriculopalpebral branches. The auriculopalpebral nerve ascends from the base of the ear and splits into rostral auricular branches that innervate the superficial and deep scutuloauricularis muscles, and palpebral branches that create a rostral auricular plexus between the eye and ear.

DEVELOPMENT OF NEUROLOGICAL DISTURBANCES

Otitis media is the most common precursor of about all neurological disturbances in dog. The primary cause of otitis media is the expansion of otitis externa. If left untreated, otitis media frequently develops into otitis interna, an infection of the inner ear. Both otitis externa and otitis media are often characterised by ear drainage and ear canal irritation. Antibiotics must be used correctly to treat these illnesses. Antibiotics known as aminoglycosides, such as amikacin, kanamycin, tobramycin, and neomycin, may produce ototoxic effects and they may induce degeneration of the sensory hair cells of the organ of Corti. The facial nerve that travels through the facial canal in the petrosal bone may be affected by otitis media. The tympanic bulla and a tiny piece of the facial canal are separated from one another by no bony wall (Fig. **1**). The only connective tissue separating the facial nerve from the tympanic cavity at this point in the canal is basic squamous epithelium-lined loose connective tissue. Due to its proximity to the facial nerve in the inner ear, the vestibulocochlear nerve may also be affected by an infection of the facial nerve. Thus, vestibular symptoms and facial palsy are frequently linked. When the postganglionic axons in the middle ear are infected, otitis media can also result in Horner's syndrome. Due to their placement in the inner ear, the facial and vestibulocochlear nerves are frequently both impacted by otitis media interna.

THE MICROBIAL ENVIRONMENT OF THE EAR CANAL IN RELATION TO HEALTH AND DISEASE

Otitis externa's pathophysiology is still not fully understood. The presence of hair and polyps in the ear canal, the kind of pinnae, allergies, seborrhea, nutritional and hormonal variables, and neoplastic illnesses are some of the conditions that may make an animal more susceptible to ear infections. Infections may be a primary or a subsequent consequence of the afore mentioned risk factors. These elements may work together or separately to create an environment where the ear canal is more likely to become infected.

Moisture buildup causes the epithelial lining to become macerated, which raises the risk of infection. Entrapment of carbon dioxide may be linked to a tendency to specific illnesses, particularly fungal infections, even if its role in ear infections has not been confirmed. It has been demonstrated that a buildup of carbon dioxide and moisture increases the likelihood of fungal infections. The chance of infection may be increased by the fatty exudates of the ear canal.

The lipid milieu of the ear canal may encourage the lipophilic yeast, growth of *Malassezia conis* Lipid-rich surroundings may encourage the organism even if they may not be necessary for *M. conis* to develop. The fatty acids produced by the glands lining the ear canal or those released by commensal bacteria as they break down more complex secretions may irritate the lining of the canal, providing an ideal environment for microbial growth.

The accuracy of the diagnosis, elimination of the underlying risk factors, and identification of any potential microorganism involvement are all necessary for a successful treatment outcome. To identify and cure ear infections, one needs take the following actions:

1. An assessment of the animal's general health.

2. Amount, consistency, and colour of ear exudates are assessed.

3. Gathering and analysing stained ear exudate smears.

4. Exudates from aberrant ears can be cultured to check for the presence of harmful organisms.

5. Making use of susceptibility data.

Small amounts of yellowish ceruminous discharge should be present in a healthy ear canal, but the epidermal lining shouldn't be inflamed or ulcerated. Increased amounts of a yellowish, more fluid discharge from infected ears are a sign of infections brought on by bacteria, particularly gram-negative bacteria like *Pseudomonas aeruginosa* and/or *Proteus*. Infections with the ear mite *Otodectes cynotis, Microsporum conis*, or a combination of *M. canis* and bacteria, typically coagulase-positive staphylococci, are typically linked to brownish-black discharge in the ear wax. When *M. canis* is present in some ears, the wax may be yellowish, especially if other organisms are also present [6].

VESTIBULAR DISEASE

Ear, though an organ of hearing is important for maintenance of balance and positioning of eyeballs. The maintenance of body balance with head preventing falling down is called proprioception. The vestibular system is responsible for this action. The vestibular system coordinates the head movement along the line of eye, trunk and limb movement, maintaining balance and posture of animal. It has two components: central and peripheral system. The central component consists of motor and proprioceptive neurons passing through brain stem and located in central nervous system. The vestibular nuclei are located in brain stem. The peripheral component resides in inner ear. The vestibulo cochlear nerves and its receptors plays a major role in vestibular function. Plethora of clinical signs manifests in vestibular dysfunction. Ataxia, proprioceptive deficit, head tilting, nystagmus, strabismus and vomiting are noticed in vestibular dysfunctions. An important aspect for treatment of vestibular dysfunction or disease is to pin down the causative component. This can be achieved by correctly identifying the differentiating clinical signs between peripheral and central vestibular disease and help from diagnostic modalities. In this section we will focus on the involvement of ear infections or other causes that lead to peripheral vestibular disease, differentiation from central nervous system related vestibular dysfunction and prevailing treatment approach for the condition. To understand the peripheral vestibular dysfunction, we need to know about neuroanatomy of ear.

RISK FACTORS

The association of disease prevalence with various factor like breed, age, body weight, pure breed *vs.* cross breed *etc.* are essential to know the epidemiology of the disease.

Breed

Pure breed dogs are more often reported in referral hospitals with clinical signs of vestibular disease than the cross-breed. Among the pure breeds, French Bull dogs and Bull dogs are at higher risk as compared to cross breeds. Otitis interna and otitis media are common in Bull dogs and thus increase prevalence rate of peripheral vestibular disease rate. Adding to it, the higher incidence rate of gliomas in the brachycephalic dogs upsurge the vestibular dysfunction cases. The Spaniel breeds like king Charles spaniels and Cavalier king Charles spaniels are also at higher risk against the cross breeds. CKSC are more predisposed to neurological diseases like occipital hypoplasia or syringomyelia, granulomatous meningo-encephalomyelitis showing similar clinicals signs as vestibular dysfunction [7].

Age

The older dogs of more than 9 years are at high risk of developing the vestibular dysfunction. This might be due to the higher incidence rate of brain tumor or idiopathic peripheral vestibular diseases in older dogs.

Body Weight

The vestibular dysfunction complains are rare in smaller breeds like Shih-Tzu, West highland white terrier, Yorkshire terrier. The breeds under 10 kg are at lower risk of developing vestibular disease. The genetic make-up of the smaller breeds might play a role in it.

Sex

the male and females are equally susceptible to acquire the diseases.

CLINICAL SIGNS

The ear diseases of inner ear and middle ear can manifest vestibular syndromes. The affection of the vestibular receptors or vestibulocochlear nerve develops peripheral vestibular disease. Apart from this facial paralysis, Horner's syndrome may be associated along with the vestibular signs. This is because of the cranial nerve VII (facial nerve) and occulosympathetic nerve passes though the petrous temporal bone that houses inner ear. The clinical signs are generally ipsilateral to the ear disease and rarely manifest as bi-lateral. Sometimes the peripheral infection or toxicity may extend into central nervous system and show progression of clinical signs related to central system.

Peripheral Vestibular Disease

The most common clinical signs of vestibular disease are nausea, vomiting, head tilt, ataxia, falling, leaning, nystagmus, horizontal or positional strabismus.

Vomiting is most common signs noticed regardless of cause of VD in dogs. the connection of vestibular nuclei axons and vomiting center of brain stem seems to be the cause of it. Frequent vomiting becomes worrisome for the owner and grown into well fare issue [7].

The rotation of median plane of head along the body axis is defined as head tilt. In this case one of the ears remains in lower plane than other. The head is tilted to ipsilateral side of affected ear in peripheral vestibular disease. It is because of the weak extensor muscle activity in ipsilateral side as compared to normal (contralateral side). In case of limbs, the affected animal on flexion may show decreased extensor tone in affected side of ear disease than the opposite side. If the head turn is associated with circling motion or body twist then it indicates a forebrain lesion rather than peripheral vestibular lesion [1].

Nystagmus is process of spontaneous eyeball movement in the opposite direction of head turn to keep the vision stationary. This is called positive "doll's eye" movement. As soon as the head come to stationary the eyeball returns to middle or normal position. This is named vestibulo-occular reflex. The nystagmus has two phases. One is the slow phase which slowly turns the eye ball into the opposite direction of the head rotation. Other one is the fast phase that occurs faster (jerky movement) and turns the eyeball back to normal position in the direction of rotation. By practice the nystagmus is named after the fast phase. For an example, if the direction of fast phase is left, then it is called left nystagmus. However, if it is a pathological nystagmus, then the lesion is present opposite to the direction of fast phase (in left nystagmus vestibular lesion of ear is present on right side). This is because in peripheral vestibular disease, the affection of side of semicircular canal releases low intensity base line impulses than the normal side [8]. So, the eyeball muscle retracts the eye ball to normal side.

In the absence of head turn or rotation, no nystagmus is observed in normal animals. The pathological nystagmus is divided into two types; one is spontaneous and other one is positional. In the former one, the nystagmus is observed without any head rotation whereas in later one, it develops only after turning the head to either side or dorsally or by placing the animal on its back over ground. According to direction of fast phase it may be horizontal, vertical or rotatory. In the peripheral vestibular disease, the observed nystagmus is of horizontal, rotatory or positional type. In chronic cases of otitis interna, there may be presence of positional nystagmus. In this cases, spontaneous nystagmus may be present at the beginning of infection. Later on, the lost vestibular impulses may get compensated by central preprogramming of eye movement and postural response and other sensory impulses. In these animals with time the spontaneous nystagmus disappears but can be elicited by changing the position of head or animal body due to loss of compensation process.

Strabismus is a condition in which both the eyes don't look into same place at same time. That means eyeball of one eye might be laterally deviated whereas the other eyeball is centrally paced at the same time. This is also called as crossed eye. In peripheral vestibular disease the affected animal may exhibit ventral or venterolateral strabismus. Ataxia or wobble walking, falling, leaning and rolling are seen in vestibular disorder. These are due to inferior impulses generated from the affected side of ear. The falling or leaning occurs towards ipsilateral side of lesion. The signs are of unilateral origin. In bilateral affections, the head sway side to side with and a symmetrical ataxia noticed for both sides. The sign like head tilting is not noticed. The physiological nystagmus cannot be provoked by moving head.

Sometimes, the ear infections or neoplasia spreads into CNS and causes predominant clinical signs of central origin vestibular disease (Fig. **3**).

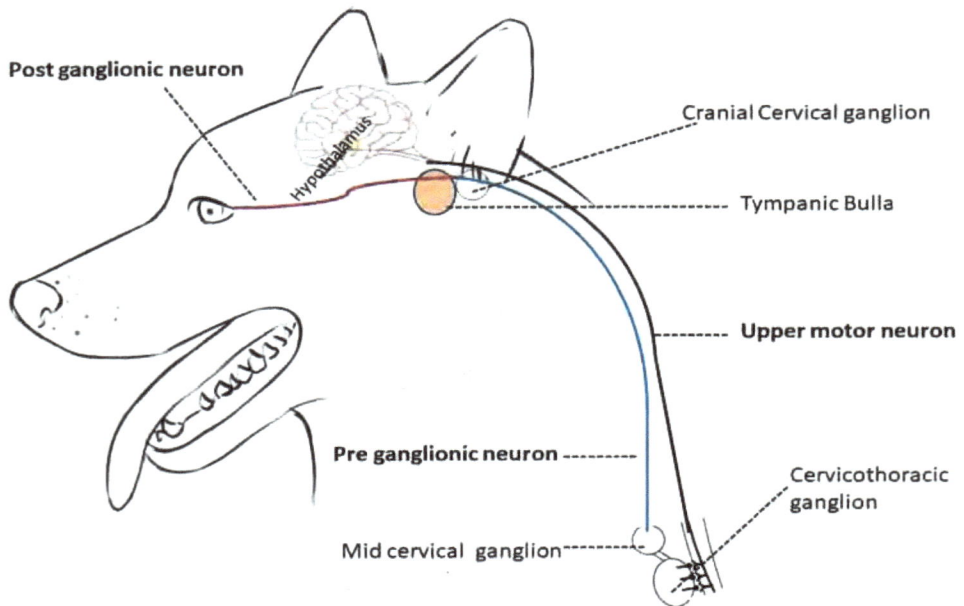

Fig. (3). Cranical Nerve Vestibular syndrome.

Difference of Clinical Signs between Peripheral Vestibular Disease *vs.* Central Vestibular Disease

The prognosis of central vestibular disease is always guarded as compared to peripheral Vestibular Disease. The proper identification of clinical signs is important to identify the origin of vestibular disease. In central origin, animal will have weak proprioception and falling down or hemi paresis or paresis are common clinical signs. When vestibular nuclei of brain stem regions are affected, the descending motor pathway and ascending proprioceptive pathways cannot transmit the impulses. This result in paresis to the ipsilateral side of damage. However, head tilting without proprioceptive deficit is characteristic signs of peripheral vestibular disease. Paradoxical head tilt is seen in central origin vestibular disease [9]. In this condition, the head tilt is noticed away from the side of lesion. It is identified by presence of paresis in one side (ipsilateral side to lesion) and presence of head tilt in opposite side. horizontal, central, rotatory and positional nystagmus are possible in central vestibular disease. But in general, ventral nystagmus is not noticed in peripheral VD. The stupor or comatose demeanor is noticed in central VD but not in peripheral VD. The alert state is facilitated by activation of reticular nucleus located in brain stem and thus damage to the nucleus may develop signs of comatose or stupor. The Horner's syndrome or facial nerve paralysis are noticed in peripheral VD as theses nerve have close proximity with inner ear. The otitis interna or neoplasia may hamper the nerve passing by and develops nerve deficit syndromes. However, in Central VD, all cranial nerve related deficit syndrome may observe (Table **1**). In the following table, the difference of clinical signs that separates the two origins of vestibular diseases is described-

Table 1. Clinical diseaaes, peripheral vestibular disease and central vestibular disease.

Clinical signs	Peripheral Vestibular Disease	Central Vestibular Disease
Head tilt	Ipsilateral to lesion	Ipsilateral or paradoxical
Spontaneous/ positional nystagmus	Horizontal, rotatory or positional	Horizontal, rotatory, ventral or positional
Conscious Proprioception deficit	Not present	hemiparesis or paresis present on the side of lesion
Demeanor	Normal	Stupor or Comatose
Horner's Syndrome	Commonly Present in the same side of the lesion	Rarely found
Cranial nerve deficit	Facial nerve deficit	Cranial nerves V, VII, IX, X, XII deficit

Causes of Peripheral Vestibular Dysfunction

The commonly identified etiologies of peripheral VD are otitis interna, otitis media, neoplasm, ototoxicity due to drugs, naso-ostopharyngeal polyps or idiopathic peripheral vestibular disease.

Otitis Interna or Media

More than 50% of cases of vestibular disease have the origin from infections or inflammations of the inner ear. In this case the inner ear infection may be accompanied by neurological signs of peripheral vestibular disease and non-neurological signs like head shaking, otitis discharge, ear etching and ear ache (bulla pain and temeporomandibular pain).

The treatment of otitis externa or media includes flushing and clearing of ear canal and removing the debris. The antibiotics, anti-inflammatory and sometime steroids are used for about 3–4-week period until recovery. Sometime during these procedures, the debris or flushing fluid may enter the inner ear and cause inflammation and thus possible cause of vestibular signs. One must be cautious not to use potential ototoxic agents or drugs in flushing or instillation process of otitis treatment.

Neoplasia

The neoplasm of auditory canals can directly put pressure on the vestibulochochlear nerves or semicircular tubes of inner ear. The neoplasm may extend into the neuronal component or spread out to central nervous system. Ceruminous adenoma, Ceruminous adenocarcinoma, Sebaceous adenoma, Sebaceous adenocarcinoma, squamous cell carcinoma and feline lymphoma are the common types of cancerous growth noticed in ear. In rare occasions vestibular neuron origin tumor called vestibular neuro fibroma may be identified [8].

Nasopharyngeal polyps and aural/otic polyps

In cats the inflammatory polyps are the prevailing neoplasia that affects the nasopharynx. However, the occurrence of otic polyps and nasopharyngeal polyps are rare in dogs, but the presentation of clinical manifestations is same. In both the species theses may lead to peripheral vestibular symptoms.

Ototoxicity

The ototoxic substances like aminoglycosides, furosemide, platinum based anti-neoplastic agents, salicylic acid, chlorhexidine, 10% fipronil and detergents, if used topically in ear with damaged tympanic membrane or systemically, are harmful for the hair cells (vestibular receptor cells).

Hypothyroidism

Peripheral cranial nerve mono/poly neuropathy develops in hypothyroidism. Some authors believe, myxomatous compression of cranial nerve VIII and Cranial nerve VII while passing through skull foramina impairs the impulse transmission in hypothyroidism [8]. One recent report [10] showed that a Rottweiler dog diagnosed with hypothyroidism suddenly developed disorientation, bilateral convergent strabismus and enophthalmos. This is a case of hypothyroid associated neuropathy resulting in vestibular disease symptoms.

Congenital Vestibular Disease

Congenital Vestibular Disease is reported in Doberman, Cocker, Akitas breed of dogs. Similarly, Siamese, Tonkinese and Burmese breeds of cats reported for this condition. Bilateral affection is rare in comparison to unilateral affections. Generally, the dysfunction is ostensible from the birth and sometimes recovers spontaneously. But, in some cases, animal's tilt head may remain permanent or partial as residual effect. No treatment is prescribed to such patients.

Idiopathic Vestibular Disease

It is the second most common cause of vestibular disease in dogs. The disease is also recorded in cats. It is otherwise called "old dog vestibular diseases" because of high incidence rate in geriatric dogs. Unlike dogs, it is seen in all age groups of cats. The head tilt, ataxia, nystagmus are the clinical signs noticed without involvement of cranial nerve deficit or Horner's syndrome. The etiology of this condition is unknown and only diagnosed by method of exclusion for all other etiology.

DIAGNOSIS

The process of identifying the peripheral vestibular disease largely depends upon the correct identification of clinical signs and proper history of animal. The neurological examination can be divided into six components. Mental state assessment, gait evaluation, postural reactions, spinal reflexes, cranial nerve, and sensory examination are to be evaluated serially during physical examination. This is important as the vestibular function is the result of a broad neuroanatomical function. However, we need the help of different diagnostic modalities to ascertain the pathology of peripheral vestibular disease in the inner canal affections. Some are listed below;

Otoscopy

The external ear canal of dog has two components; vertical and horizontal canals. Otoscopy is an instrument with which we can directly visualize the auditory canal up to tympanic membrane by inserting a long nose or tube with a light source into ear canal. The commonly used otoscope in clinical practices named "Gowllands otoscope set for pet animals". This otoscope set has longer nose and can adjust the angle with horizontal canal as well. The external ear canal and middle ear disorders can be evaluated by the help of otoscopy. However, the stenosis or blockage of auditory canals due to inflammation or neoplasm many a time limit its usefulness.

Endoscopy

It a technique which combines otoscopy and videography. It includes a flexible tube that carries a video camera for recording the aural canals, tympanic membrane. The mid ear through damaged tympanic membrane can peep into by it.

Myringotomy

It is surgical technique applied on tympanic membrane. In this technique, a small incision is made on the tympanic membrane with the help of myringotomy knife to make an access to the middle ear. In this process the secretion or exudation fluids are removed to outside. The culture swab might be collected during the procedure to ascertain the type of bacterial infection or population at infection site. The culture and sensitivity testing of collected sample can be performed. Generally, *Staphylococcus, Pseudomonas, Streptococcus, Proteus, Malassezia* and *Candida* are the major organisms isolated from middle ear infections [8].

Radiography

The use of radiation (X ray) to see bone, organs and tissue is called radiography. It is a noninvasive technique and provides the images in white to black and gray shadows. Bones looks white whereas soft tissues seems gray and air as black. The water muffles the image formation and forms gray shadow. With the help of radiograph sometimes the aural polyps can be identified in the middle ear. The tympanic bulla cavity of dogs and cats are located in middle ear and with the help of radiograph the anomalies or pathological conditions can be ascertained. Moreover, the radiographic view enables the comparison between left and right view of middle ear. So, it helps in detections of unilateral affections.

Canalography

When the rupture of tympanic membrane is not ascertained by radiography, water soluble iodide agent is instilled in external ear and the radiograph is taken in dorsoventral and rostro caudal (open mouth) view. The damaged membrane will allow seepage of contrast material in middle ear and will be captured by radiograph [11].

CT

Computed tomography scan is an imaging technique that uses the same technology as radiograph for recoding internal structures of body. It utilizes a rotatory X-ray tube and a row of detectors placed in gantry (that holds both X ray tube and detectors). The X-ray tube and detectors move in circular motion around the patient in the gantry to get a three-dimensional X-ray images of the patient. The tomograph prepared by computer assisted program (cross-section of body image) of a body region does not allow overlaps of surrounding structures and thus help to study better as compared to simple radiograph. The CT scan of the ears is generally taken on transverse plane with thin contiguous slice of 1.5 mm and high-resolution construction algorithm. The sedated patients are kept in sternal recumbency with head pads to support the head and scanning is completed in about one minutes. As X-ray easily differentiates between air and bones, the CT becomes the perfect choice to examine the middle ear. If the disease is in soft tissue, then contrast iodide agents can be injected in veins. The agents tend to localize in vascular structures at point of damage if blood brain barrier is damaged. In CT scan, nasopharyngeal polyps, middle ear infections with presence of fluid or tissue, bulla thickening, otitis interna and meningitis due to ear infections are easily identified.

Ultrasonography

It is noninvasive technique just like radiography to view the internal organs and the structures. Instead of X-ray here ultrasound frequencies (more than 20,0000 Hz) sound waves are sent through transducers and the differential reflection property of different tissues makes a sonogram. The differential reflection property of tissue is expressed as echogenicity. In the sonogram the bone tissue will appear hyper echoic due to higher reflection rate whereas liver tissue will appear anechoic. In animals the presence of air in the ear canals prevents sonogram formation because of maximum reflection of sound waves by tissue to air interface. Unlike other tissues air don't absorb sound waves rather reflect the most. So, no image is formed. This difficulty can be overcome in ultrasound examination of ear by deliberately filling the external auditory canal with normal saline or if middle ear is filled with fluid or solids as an outcome of disease the sound can be transmitted and form the sonogram. The examination of external ear can be conducted by placing the transducer in lateral aspect of head. But for examining bulla of middle ear animal may be placed in sternal or lateral recumbency and transducer is placed on ventral aspect of head. The normal bulla appears as a hyperechoic reflecting line with convexity towards the transducer. An acoustic shadowing and reverberating artifacts are produced as a result of passing of sound waves in air filled cavity. The bulla wall thickening, fluid filled bulla and any tumor mass in bulla can be identified by ultrasound technique [4].

MRI

Magnetic resonance imaging is technique that detects the activity of hydrogen ion in the body or tissue that is under strong influence of a magnetic field. It is suitable for the imaging of soft tissues of middle or inner ear structures. The cortical bone and air in the middle or inner ear cavity have very less hydrogen present. Thus, it produces black indistinguishable image of bones and ear canals. Thus, structures of bulla or paranasal sinus are challenging to study in MRI. MRI is the most potent technique to diagnose the otitis interna as compared to radiograph, ultrasound and CT scan [11]. It can study the inner ear and its associated neuronal structures. The conditions like otitis interna, nasopharyngeal polyps, detecting bulla thickening are easily detected by the MRI scan.

TREATMENT AND MANAGEMENT

Antiemetics, antibiotics and systemic antibiotics are most commonly used therapy in peripheral vestibular diseases. The antiemetics drug commonly used in United Kingdom is Maropitant. Maropitant is used orally @2 mg/kg daily until vomiting or nausea stopped. In antibiotics, amoxicillin with clavulanate and fluoroquinolones group of antibiotics are commonly used for otitis media or externa. However, in otitis externa or media, culture and sensitivity testing increase the chance of quick recovery and prevent ototoxicity. The use of systemic glucocorticoids as inflammatory is although controversial used in most of the positive cases of vestibular disease with good success rate [7]. Oral prednisolone @ 0.5 to 1 mg/kg can be given for a longer period. Other supportive therapies like Vitamin B complex, Methyl cyanocobalamin, thiamine is also used in these patients and helpful in recovery of neuritis.

In specific conditions like hypothyroidism, levothyroxine tablets are given to maintain optimum thyroxine level and thus preventing secondary hypothyroid related neuropathy. In nasopharyngeal polyps, otoscopic endoscopy guided surgical recession, followed by antibiotics and anti-inflammatory therapy is indicated.

In otitis media, if medicinal treatment is ineffective, then bulla osteotomy may be considered. In this process the vestibular disease symptoms mostly recovers but the facial paralysis may be permanent as a complication of surgery.

The ear canal must be routinely cleaned with vet recommended ear cleanser. The most commonly available, nontoxic option is the normal saline. The potential ototoxic drugs instillation should be avoided during routine cleaning or treatment of otitis externa. Metronidazole commonly used as systemic antidiarrheal therapy that act against gram negative gut bacteria and protozoans. Sometimes, its toxicity also has central origin vestibular symptoms.

Meningitis

Bacterial meningitis or meningoencephalitis may be caused by the transfer of causative agents from otitis media or interna infection through hematogenous route or direct extension of the lesions. The first report in veterinary medicine was claimed to be reported by Spangler and Dewey [12] of a dog with vestibular signs and chronic otitis externa and media. The dog was presented with head tilt to left side, proprioceptive deficit, rotatory nystagmus and lateral recumbency. The left ear tympanic membrane was found damaged. On examination, they found some bacilli and cocci from CSF and also isolated some bacilli from mid ear fluid of left side. They also noted thrombocytopenia and neutrophilia in complete blood count and suspected concurrent infection of Ehrlichiosis. However, after continuous treatment with antibiotics like sulpha-trimethoprim and metronidazole along with doxycycline and other supportive treatment the patient showed improvement.

The link between neurological dysfunction and ear infection was again accentuated by Struge *et al.* [13]. The different neurological dysfunction such as lethargy, obtundation, cranial nerve V deficit, cranial nerve VII deficit and cervical pain were recorded in cats. The presence of fluids in tympanic bulla and presence of nasopharynx polyps in some cases confirms the otitis in these patients. Dog was presented with seizures, stupor and inability to walk. One cat and dog with clinical signs were euthanized and the PM examination of the nervous tissue revealed pyogranulomatous otitis media with osteomyelitis, pyogranulomatous meningoencephalitis indicating extension of organisms from otitis. Martin-Vaquero *et al.* [14] reported the possible transmission of *Streptococcus equi* subspecies *zooepidemicus* from otitis media or interna in a cat causing meningoencephalitis. Although rare, but there is always a possibility of meningitis from secondary infection to otitis media or interna in dogs and cats.

HORNER'S SYNDROME

As the name indicates the syndrome word is used here to define a group of clinical signs related to the loss of sympathetic innervation to the eye which is believed to be first identified in 1869 by a Swiss ophthalmologist Johann Friedrich Horner. The cardinal diagnostic sign of Horner's syndrome is miosis (the pupil of the affected eye becomes constricted or small), ptosis(drooping of the eye lids on the affected side), apparent enopthalmos (the affected eye appears sunken) and prolapse of third eyelid often with redness.

Usually, it may appear as eye related disease as the symptoms shows but the underlying causes may include the connection with ear more particularly the middle and inner portion. The ocular sympathetic innervation is divided into three stages- central, preganglionic and postganglionic. The cell consisting the first order neurones are located in the hypothalamus and rostral midbrain. The axons part of these neurones are elongated through the lateral tectotegmentospinal tract up to the level of T1 to T3. Here the central neurones synapse with preganglionic nerves in the intermediolateral cell column of the first three thoracic segments (T1-T3). These preganglionic neurones leaves the spinal cord, first met the cervicothoracic ganglia, and then the mid cervical ganglia to join the vago sympathetic trunk which lies in the carotid sheath.

Then the preganglionic nerves continue its course rostrally up to the synapse point with post ganglionic neurones *i.e.* cranial cervical ganglia which is situated ventromedial to tympanic bullae. The involvement of ear related etiological factor may be started from here. The post ganglionic neurones, originated from cranial cervical ganglion, run close to middle ear cavity to enter the calvarium. Later the nerves join with ophthalmic branches of trigeminal nerve. Then together these nerves are distributed to the orbit supplying periorbital smooth muscle, muscles of eyelids and iris. Problems arises due to sympathetic supply of these muscles are responsible for Horner's Syndrome (Fig. **3**).

Generally, it has been seen from the cases presented so far and literature concerned that Golden retriever shows higher tendency to develop horner's syndrome. In case of dog, mostly the cause are idiopathic and the prognosis is good as it resolves spontaneously within six months. In some cases it may be permanent. The most important part of treating the disease is to locate the underlying causes and its source in the nerve pathway.

As miosis is the cardinal sign of the disease, it is usually detected by anisocoria (unequal pupil size). There are two types of muscle in the iris to control the amount of light entering the eye- parasympathetic system controlled constrictor pupillae muscle (responsible for miosis) and sympathetic system controlled dilator pupillae muscle (responsible for mydriasis). Anisocoria is minimum in bright light but more obvious in dim light. In eye examination, the pupillary reactions to drugs are usually measured. Ptosis and prolapse of the third eyelid are important additional signs. Dogs presented with these symptoms should undergo several diagnostic tests like normal blood examination, otoscopic examination and thoracic radiograph including neck region.

HEMIFACIAL SPASM

Hemifacial spasm is a classic form of myoclonus and may be associated with the affection of middle ear diseases. Usually, it occurs with the cause of facial nerve (cranial nerve VII) deficits of dog.

The facial nerve of dog is originated from the rostral medulla oblongata of the brain stem. Then the cranial nerve exits the brain stem near the vestibulocochlear nerve, course through the facial canal of the petrous temporal bone followed by stylomastoid foramen through which it exit the skull and split into 3 branches namely- auricular, palpebral and buccal branches. Any inflammation related to middle ear area which affects the facial nerve course, may interrupt the nerve muscle interaction in facial muscle. As a result, there is a spontaneous, unilateral, irregular twitching of the muscles of the affected side. The affected muscle become hypertonic resulting the face and nose portion to be pulled caudally. Ipsilateral deviation of the philtrum of the nose, an ipsilateral smaller palpebral fissure resembling blepharospasm and ipsilateral caudal displacement of the ear are frequently encountered clinical signs [15]. The condition is classified as myoclonus and clearly distinguished from tremor by its asynchronous frequency and "shock-like" character. Usually, this short of myoclonus is seen only for a short period but recurs frequently throughout the day. In case of dog a persistent contraction is seen which is distinctive in nature. Palpebral fissure may be narrowed caused by partial closure of the eyelids, elevation of the ear, and wrinkling of the face. Hemifacial spasm is attributed to facial nerve compression near its entry zone most commonly due to the presence of an aberrant vessel compressing or encircling the nerve. Sometimes hemifacial spasm are seen just before the onset of facial paralysis [16, 17]. Hemifacial spasms are mostly idiopathic in nature in case of dog [18] though may occur secondary to intracranial lesion [15]. The differential diagnosis should be clearly understood with other nerve problems exhibiting similar clinical features like denervation resulting from chronic facial nerve paralysis where palpebral reflexes are not seen usually [15]. Some researchers based on electromyography termed the condition as 'hemifacial tetany' observing the difference pattern of the disease with human [19].

Diagnosis is based upon the history of specific clinical signs, CT scan of cranial portion, Analysis of cerebrospinal fluid (CSF) for any neoplastic involvement, Electrophysiological assessment by electromyography of the facial muscles and facial motor nerve stimulation test *etc.* may be beneficial. The treatment mainly based on the removal of underlying cause along with classification of myoclonus involved. Antiepileptic drugs like valproate, levetiracetum and piracetum are effective in cortical myoclonus within which levetiracetum is the most commonly used drug (Fig. **4**)

FACIAL NERVE PARESIS OR PARALYSIS-

Facial nerve paralysis is another common neurological disturbance commonly seen in dog and cat, involving problems in the course of facial nerve (cranial nerve VII) and commonly associated with the affection of middle or inner ear especially otitis media. As the facial nerve during its course (previously explained) run through facial canal which is adjacent to tympanic cavity lacking any bony wall separation, it is totally exposed at the cavity for a very short length (Fig. **4**) [20]. The lesion at this level causes paralysis of facial muscular activity including eyelid, lip, ear and nose portion where the branches of facial nerves innervates. Motor dysfunction of CN VII produces ipsilateral drooping and inability to move the ear and lip, a widened palpebral fissure and absent spontaneous and provoked blinking, absent abduction of the nostril during inspiration, and deviation of the nose toward the normal side due to the unopposed muscle tone on the unaffected side [9, 21]. Facial spasm is not uncommon with narrowing of palpebral fissure. The most common sign is related to loss of palpebral reflex and menace response with inability to blink. If the buccal branch is affected paralysis of lips and nostrils are seen. Likewise lesion in palpebral branch causes paresis or paralysis of eyelids only, lesion in auriculopalpebral branch causes paresis or paralysis of eyelids with ear.

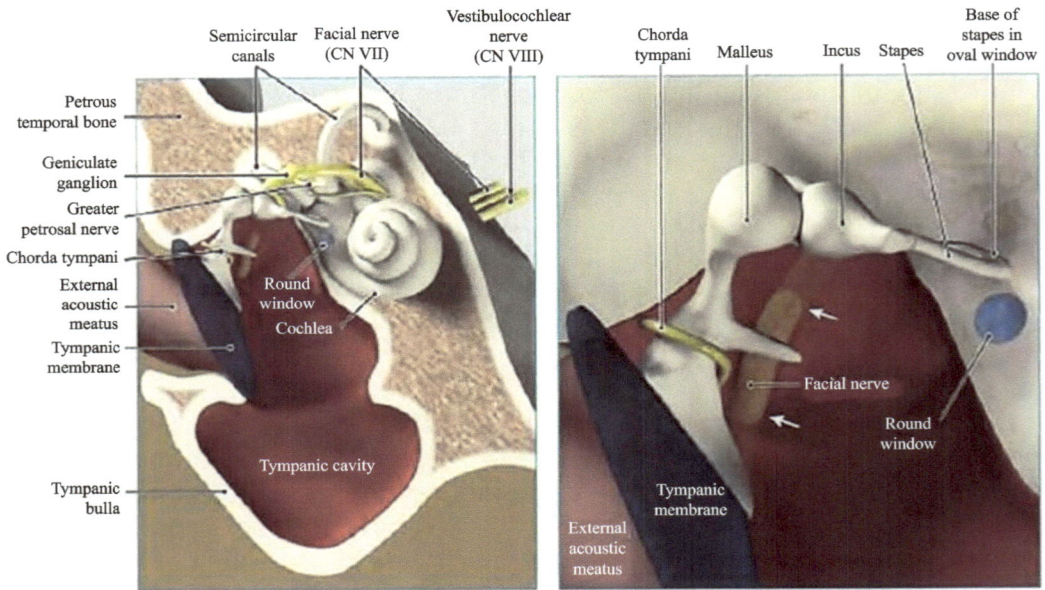

Fig. (4). Hemifacial syndrome in ear diseases [22].

Facial nerve paralysis should be differentially diagnosed with other conditions. Sometimes other clinical disease conditions like any infection or abnormal growth in middle ear, trauma in temporal region or trauma originated from peripheral nerve, intracranial neoplasm like meningioma, hypothyroidism or sulfonamide hyper sensitivity may show similar neuropathic symptoms. Idiopathic causes are the most common in case of facial nerve paralysis. The diagnosis of idiopathic facial nerve paralysis is made by exclusion of other possible causes. Total ear canal ablation lateral bulla osteotomy (TECA LBO) is very much linked with the incidence of facial nerve paralysis in dog.

Diagnosis is mainly based on history of clinical signs with otoscopic examination with cytology and culture. Motor function of facial nerve may be assessed through palpebral reflex, corneal reflex, menace response, and pinching of the face. Thyroid test is also important as hypothyroidism can affect cranial nerves. A skull radiographs, CT or MRI test is helpful to determine the extent of the lesion if surgery is needed. A Schirmer tear test is indicated in case of less tear production leading to corneal ulceration as parasympathetic portion of the facial nerve causes reduced tear and saliva production on the side of the lesion. Prognosis is variable depending on etiology. Infectious, thyroid related or neoplasm is curable in first stage if detected. Prognosis is uncertain if the cause is idiopathic and does not respond with drugs for a longer period.

Deafness

There are two types of origin for deafness- one is hearing loss through conductive impairment and another through sensorineural impairment. If there is impedance to transmission of external sound waves to the inner ear and CNS, then conductive deafness occurs. If there is any congenital or acquired abnormalities in middle or inner ear, cochlear nerve and auditory nervous system, then it is called sensorineural deafness. Stenosis or obstruction of the ear canal from chronic otitis externa, foreign bodies, ceruminoliths, aural neoplasms, ototoxicity from drugs or chemicals that damage hair cells, the stria vascularis, the organ of Corti, or cochlear neurons may be the reasons of acquired deafness. Clinical findings like loss of spiral ganglion cells, atrophy of the organ of Corti, atrophy of the stria vascularis, thickening of the basilar membrane, lipofuscin accumulation within cochlear hair cells, and nerve cell loss and gliosis within the cochlear nuclei. Are believed to be the outcome when the deafness occurs through aging ototoxic drugs. It has been observed after brain stem auditory evoked response (BAER) testing in many studies that removal of obstructive debris by cleaning had potentially increased the hearing abilities of dog. Damage in the middle ear particularly rupture of the tympanic membrane, damage to the ossicular chain, or fluid accumulation within the middle ear may cause conductive hearing loss. Congenital sensorineural deafness is common in many breeds of dogs and cats with a predilection for white coat colors, and there is a strong association of deafness with blue irises. The most commonly affected canine breeds include Dalmatians, English Setters, Australian Shepherds, Border Collies, and Shetland Sheepdogs, although there are many others. Absence of melanocyte results degeneration of stria vascularis followed by collapse of Reissner's membrane and the cochlear duct and degeneration of the hair cells of the organ of Corti and ultimately leading to deafness [11, 12, 22] (Fig. **5**).

Antibiotics
- All aminoglycosides
- Chloramphenicol
- Polymyxin B
- Tetracyclin
- Vancomycin
- Bacitracin
- Minocyclin

Antineoplastic agents
- Cisplatin

Antifungal
- Amphoterecin B
- Griseofalvin

Antiseptics
- Acetic Acid
- Benzalkonium chloride
- Chlorhexidine
- Ethanol
- Iodophore
- Methiolate

Diuretics
- Furosemide
- Bumetanide

Other agents
- DSS
- Propylene Glycol
- Toluene
- Mercury
- Detergents

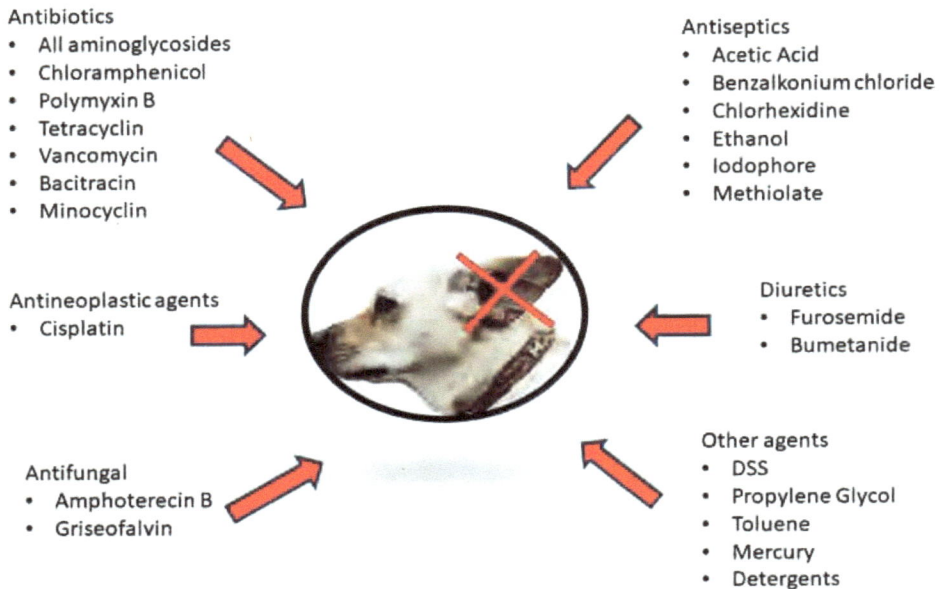

Fig. (5). Drug contraindication in ear diseases.

DRUG INTERACTION RELATED TO EAR DISEASES

Numerous substances have been classified as ototoxic, and several of them harm the Corti organ permanently (Fig. **5**). The aminoglycoside antibiotics, including gentamicin and streptomycin, are an excellent example of drugs with a history of ototoxicity. The potential risks of using certain disinfectants, including chlorhexidine, during ear surgery should not be understated because they are also recognised for their ototoxic effects. Similarly, before using chlorhexidine for ear cleaning and flushing, animals should be checked for otitis externa, or infection of the external ear canal. Ototoxic substances must enter the inner ear to cause harm.

For instance, a ruptured tympanum may allow chlorhexidine solution to enter the middle ear of an animal suffering from otitis externa and otitis media (infection of the middle ear). Chlorhexidine is one of several substances that may enter the inner ear through the round window, including germs, poisons, and medications. When chlorhexidine from the inner ear enters the cochlea fluid and travels to the vestibular and organ of Corti, it damages the sensory cells in those organs. The dog experiences ataxia (uncoordinated movement) and nystagmus (oscillation of the eyes) as aberrant vestibular signals after waking up from anesthesia following an ear cleaning.

CONCLUSION

There are four major neuroanatomical structures (facial nerve, the ocular sympathetic tract, the vestibular receptors, and the cochlea) correlated with the ear. In addition, ear infection can be broadly divided into inflammatory and non-inflammatory conditions The infection of ears leads to different neurologic clinical signs. Facial nerve paralysis and/or Horner syndrome (HS) may occur on the same side as middle ear disease. On the other hand, the clinical signs of inner ear disease accompanies peripheral vestibular syndrome that reflects injury to the vestibular nerve or receptor organs.

REFERENCES

[1]   Cook LB. Neurologic evaluation of the ear. Vet Clin North Am Small Anim Pract 2004; 34(2): 425-35.
        [http://dx.doi.org/10.1016/j.cvsm.2003.12.001] [PMID: 15062617]

[2]   Reece WO, Erickson HH, Goff JP, Uemura EE, Eds. Dukes' physiology of domestic animals. John Wiley & Sons 2015.

[3]   Jenkins TW. The Ear-hearing and Equilibrium Functional Mammalian Neuroanatomy. 2nd ed., Philadelphia: Lea & Febiger 1978.

[4]   Kent M, Platt SR, Schatzberg SJ. The neurology of balance: Function and dysfunction of the vestibular system in dogs and cats. Vet J 2010; 185(3): 247-58.
        [http://dx.doi.org/10.1016/j.tvjl.2009.10.029] [PMID: 19944632]

[5]   Cole LK. Anatomy and physiology of the canine ear. Vet Dermatol 2009; 20(5-6): 412-21.
        [http://dx.doi.org/10.1111/j.1365-3164.2009.00849.x] [PMID: 20178478]

[6]   Kowalski JJ. The microbial environment of the ear canal in health and disease. Vet Clin North Am Small Anim Pract 1988; 18(4): 743-54.
        [http://dx.doi.org/10.1016/S0195-5616(88)50077-3] [PMID: 3062878]

[7]   Radulescu SM, Humm K, Eramanis LM, *et al.* Vestibular disease in dogs under UK primary veterinary care: Epidemiology and clinical management. J Vet Intern Med 2020; 34(5): 1993-2004.
        [http://dx.doi.org/10.1111/jvim.15869] [PMID: 32776616]

[8]   Rossmeisl JH Jr. Vestibular disease in dogs and cats. Vet Clin North Am Small Anim Pract 2010; 40(1): 81-100.
        [http://dx.doi.org/10.1016/j.cvsm.2009.09.007] [PMID: 19942058]

[9]   Garosi LS, Lowrie ML, Swinbourne NF. Neurological manifestations of ear disease in dogs and cats. Vet Clin North Am Small Anim Pract 2012; 42(6): 1143-60.
        [http://dx.doi.org/10.1016/j.cvsm.2012.08.006] [PMID: 23122174]

[10]   Rushton JO, Leschnik M, Nell B. Suspected hypothyroid-associated neuropathy in a female rottweiler dog. Can Vet J 2013; 54(4): 368-72.
        [PMID: 24082164]

[11]   Benigni L, Lamb C. Diagnostic imaging of ear disease in the dog and cat. In Pract 2006; 28(3): 122-30.
        [http://dx.doi.org/10.1136/inpract.28.3.122]

[12]   Spangler EA, Dewey CW. Meningoencephalitis secondary to bacterial otitis media/interna in a dog. J Am Anim Hosp Assoc 2000; 36(3): 239-43.
        [http://dx.doi.org/10.5326/15473317-36-3-239] [PMID: 10825096]

[13]　Sturges BK, Dickinson PJ, Kortz GD, *et al.* Clinical signs, magnetic resonance imaging features, and outcome after surgical and medical treatment of otogenic intracranial infection in 11 cats and 4 dogs. J Vet Intern Med 2006; 20(3): 648-56.
[http://dx.doi.org/10.1111/j.1939-1676.2006.tb02910.x] [PMID: 16734103]

[14]　Martin-Vaquero P, da Costa RC, Daniels JB. Presumptive meningoencephalitis secondary to extension of otitis media/interna caused by *Streptococcus equi* subspecies *zooepidemicus* in a cat. J Feline Med Surg 2011; 13(8): 606-9.
[http://dx.doi.org/10.1016/j.jfms.2011.04.002] [PMID: 21640625]

[15]　Van Meervenne SAE, Bhatti SFM, Martlé V, *et al.* Hemifacial spasm associated with an intracranial mass in two dogs. J Small Anim Pract 2008; 49(9): 472-5.
[http://dx.doi.org/10.1111/j.1748-5827.2008.00565.x] [PMID: 18631227]

[16]　Roberts SR, Vainisi SJ. Hemifacial spasm in dogs. J Am Vet Med Assoc 1967; 150(4): 381-5.
[PMID: 6067829]

[17]　Parker A, Cusick P, Park R, Small E. Hemifacial spasms in a dog. Vet Rec 1973; 93(19): 514-6.
[http://dx.doi.org/10.1136/vr.93.19.514] [PMID: 4784121]

[18]　Lowrie M, Garosi L. Classification of involuntary movements in dogs: myoclonus and myotonia. J Vet Intern Med 2017; 31(4): 979-87.
[http://dx.doi.org/10.1111/jvim.14771] [PMID: 28557061]

[19]　Motta L, de Lahunta A. Canine hemifacial spasm: a misnomer? J Small Anim Pract 2015; 56(7): 480.
[http://dx.doi.org/10.1111/jsap.12376] [PMID: 26046370]

[20]　Cole L, Nuttall T. Clinical Techniques: When and how to do a myringotomy – a practical guide. Vet Dermatol 2021; 32(3): 302-e82.
[http://dx.doi.org/10.1111/vde.12966] [PMID: 33955092]

[21]　Strain GM. Aetiology, prevalence and diagnosis of deafness in dogs and cats. Br Vet J. 1996 Jan;152(1):17-36

[22]　Hermanson JW, De Lahunta A. Miller and Evans' Anatomy of the Dog-E-Book. Elsevier Health Sciences; 2018.

CHAPTER 19

Ototoxicity and its Clinical Management

J. Jyothi[1,*], **M. Bhavya Sree**[2] and **T. Jayanth Sai Kumar Reddy**[2]

[1] *Department of Veterinary Medicine, P.V. Narasimharao Telangana Veterinary University, Hyderabad, India*

[2] *P.V. Narasimharao Telangana Veterinary University, Hyderabad, India*

Abstract: The adverse effects of many medications used in veterinary treatment might cause hearing or balance problems in an animal. Although the predominance and ototoxicity pathways in both humans and lab animals have been well explored, significantly less research has been done on domestic dogs and cats. Since these adverse effects are universal among species, one can extrapolate from them and provide the veterinarian with details regarding possible chemotherapeutic side effects.

Keywords: Aminoglycosides, Cochlear toxicity, Hearing loss, Ototoxicity, Vestibular toxicity.

INTRODUCTION

Many medications used in veterinary care have adverse effects that can impair an animal's ability to hear or balance. It is noteworthy that all these side effects, including the important discoveries on the ototoxicity (harm to hearing and balance) of cisplatin, aminoglycoside antibiotics and other drugs occurred in the 20th century, were first identified in humans [1].

In veterinary medicine, the main medications that might be problematic include loop diuretics like furosemide, the anticancer medication cisplatin, and the antimicrobial aminoglycoside antibiotics gentamicin and amikacin, which cause ototoxicity. Certain medications, such the antibiotic erythromycin and the anthelmintic arsenical melarsomine, may also be somewhat ototoxic when taken occasionally or infrequently (Figs. **1**, **2** and **3**). Lastly, environmental factors—like elderly age and even being around loud near kennels. We should not be disregarded when examining possible reasons why animals might lose their hearing.

---

* **Corresponding author J. Jyothi:** Department of Veterinary Medicine, P.V. Narasimharao Telangana Veterinary University, Hyderabad, India; E-mail: jyothirvm1027@gmail.com

Tanmoy Rana (Ed.)

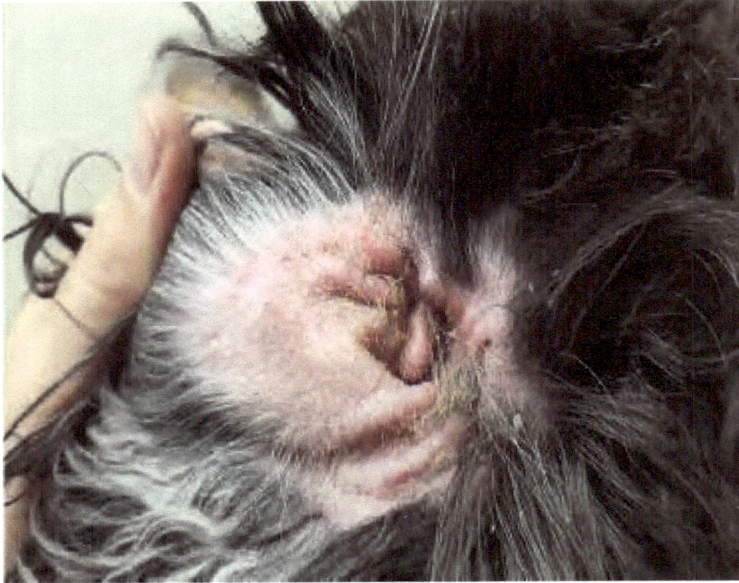

Fig. (1). Otitis externa (showing crusty lesions).

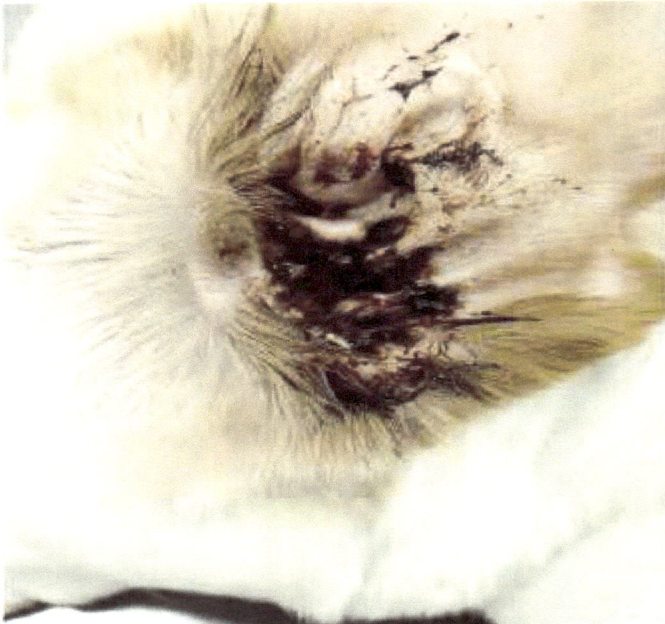

Fig. (2). Otitis interna (pus oozing from inner ear).

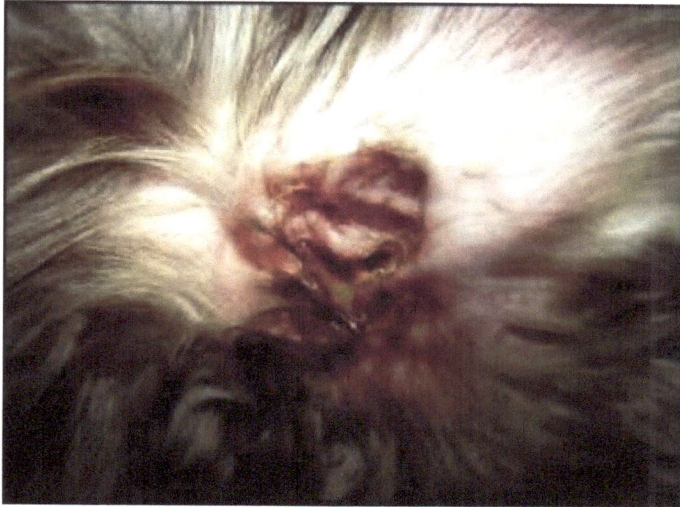

Fig. (3). Otitis interna (blood mixed with pus from inner ear).

INNER EAR PATHOLOGY

Long-term usage of aminoglycoside affects several types of internal ear cells, but the medications' main target is the sensory cells, namely the hair cells.

As the lesions deepen, the hair cells which are not regenerative start disappearing towards the middle and apical turns of the cochlear spiral, and disappears in the basal region.

Additionally, vestibular lesions and the resulting behavioural abnormalities can be caused by aminoglycoside drugs. The loss of sensory hair cells in the vestibule, also results in a compromised sense of balance [2].

The cells first disappear in the cristae ampullaris, the structure in charge of detecting angular acceleration and deceleration. Some areas of the maculae in the sacculus and utricle may also sustain the damage. The impact of cisplatin on the internal ear seems to be more complicated than that of aminoglycosides, affecting a range of cell types, even though loss of hair cells is a clinical characteristic feature (Table **1**).

Table 1. showing potential causes of hearing loss in dogs.

Aminoglycoside Antibiotics	Streptomycin, Neomycin, Gentamicin
Antineoplastics	Cisplatin, carboplatin
Diuretics	Ethacrynic acid, furosemide
Metallo Compounds	Arsenical, mercurial

(Table 1) cont.....

Aminoglycoside Antibiotics	Streptomycin, Neomycin, Gentamicin
Antimalarial	Quinine
Analgesics, Antipyretics	Salicylates
Polypeptide Antibiotics	Viomycin, vancomycin
Macrolide Antibiotics	Erythromycin

The stria vascularis driving power is necessary for the conversion of an auditory input and the nerve impulses to go to the brain, and is the audiological findings in addition to hearing loss at higher frequencies. Increased thresholds for the cochlea and compound action potentials suggest impaired function of hair cells and vestibulocochlear nerve fibres, respectively. Furosemide and other diuretics mainly affect the non-sensory tissues of the internal ear which can be identified by extensive physiological tests [3].

A reduced capacity of cochlear stimulation has been observed mainly in cats and dogs. Furosemide also reduces the amplitude of the vestibulocochlear nerve action in the dog and the cat. Moreover, cochlear microphonic is impacted.

Incidence

The majority of the drug's activity is specific to prokaryotes because aminoglycosides' therapeutic targets, are bacterial ribosomes, which are different from those of mammals. Aminoglycoside antibiotics may find a way to target comparable subunits in mammalian mitochondrial RNA. Amikacin, may target the cochlea more than gentamicin that affects both senses with a preference for balance.

Between 15 and 50 percent of animals are thought to be affected by ototoxicity.

The ability of aminoglycoside antibiotics is to get through the placental barrier and perhaps deafen the foetus. The majority of the pathophysiological harm caused by cisplatin that cannot be reversed. Most of the hearing system is impacted. The hearing loss is severe and occurs bilaterally. Its intensity is dose-dependent, and may become worse even after the medication has been started.

It is reasonable to anticipate a clinical incidence of diuretic ototoxicity, where the side effects are contingent upon the dosage and frequency of treatment. Only seldom has vertigo been reported as a side effect of furosemide medication. Drugs causing ototoxicity are Gentamicin, one of the antibiotics in the aminoglycoside class, which works against gram- negative bacteria. These medications are applied topically to treat ear infections in dogs and cats. They are also used in treating certain other conditions related to reproductive and respiratory tract [4].

Aminoglycoside antibiotics are administered through many parenteral routes and topically. But the drug given through any route may cause ototoxicity. They cannot be given orally due to poor absorption. Action of aminoglycosides is multifaceted, but one of the main mechanism is inhibition of synthesis of proteins that can be achieved by binding of the antibiotic to 30s subunit of ribosome of the bacteria.

Nephrotoxicity is a clinically serious side effect of cisplatin that can result in irreparable kidney damage. Sufficient pre- and post-treatment hydration as well as concurrent diuresis can effectively minimize nephrotoxicity. The avoidance of ototoxicity and neurotoxicity are the two other common side effects of cisplatin. When applied to cancer cells, cisplatin primarily inhibits the replication of DNA and finally causing apoptosis [3].

Although cisplatin is effective, there are certain mechanisms that cause resistance to apoptosis.

The most popular loop diuretic, furosemide, works on the kidney's loop of Henle epithelial cells. It is the medication of choice for treating certain conditions like oedema and hypertension, among other diseases. Furosemide alters the amount of electrolytes in the blood and the body's overall fluid content, which makes electrolytic disorders [5].

Unlike aminoglycosides and cisplatin, furosemide can cause ototoxicity that is typically transient and infrequently persistent. Even at individually safe dosages of the two medications, furosemide has the capacity to amplify the hearing loss caused by cisplatin and aminoglycoside to the point where combination therapy may result in total deafness.

PREVENTION OF OTOTOXICITY

Administration of antioxidants or similar ROS scavengers efficiently inhibits ROS generation and the ensuring cell death in the cochlea. For instance, ototoxicity caused due to aminoglycosides may be cured. Antioxidants are effective counteragents against aminoglycoside ototoxicity, as the production of ROS is causally linked to the pathways leading to cell death. Because antioxidant supplements are readily available, safe, and inexpensive. Aminoglycoside antibiotics may have adverse effects due to antioxidants. Some of the antioxidants are mostly helpful in reducing the side effects of kidney due to gentamicin in the pets [2].

Perhaps the most popular supplements are the antioxidants which are believed to boost immunity, lessen the toxicity of chemotherapy, and even directly treat the disease. In veterinary medicine, antioxidants have been utilized as a cancer treatment or as a supplement to drugs. Antioxidant therapy can prevent furosemide ototoxicity. However, it has been demonstrated that a number of other substances can lessen the ototoxicity that includes potassium sparing diuretics and some other drugs like organic acids that may help in some immunity [3].

CONCLUDING REMARKS

Aminoglycosides, diuretics, and cisplatin are the main culprits that affect domestic animals that cause ototoxicity in similar fashion. It can be challenging to diagnose the early symptoms caused due to these drugs. Similarly, early signs of hearing loss might not be noticeable during day-to-day activity because of the selective effect of the medication's on the auditory system.

Administration of excess aminoglycosides to dogs or cats during pregnancy may cause hearing impairments in their off springs. Mostly diuretic-induced ototoxicity is very temporary, careful monitoring of the correct dose may prevent long-term harm to the inner ear. Animals that are older or newborns are more susceptible to ototoxicity. When diuretics are used with cisplatin or aminoglycoside antibiotics, it can intensify the hearing loss to a greater extent in the animals.

So, the drugs that cause ototoxicity should be used with utmost care to prevent the damage caused by them. To reduce the pain, palliative treatment can be advised to dogs and cats.

REFERENCES

[1]   Schacht J, Hawkins JE. Sketches of otohistory. Part 11: Ototoxicity: drug-induced hearing loss. Audiol Neurotol 2006; 11(1): 1-6.
        [http://dx.doi.org/10.1159/000088850] [PMID: 16219991]

[2]   Scheifele P, Martin D, Clark JG, Kemper D, Wells J. Effect of kennel noise on hearing in dogs. Am J Vet Res 2012; 73(4): 482-9.
        [http://dx.doi.org/10.2460/ajvr.73.4.482] [PMID: 22452494]

[3]   Schatz A, Bugle E, Waksman SA. Streptomycin, a substance exhibiting antibiotic activity against gram-positive and gram-negative bacteria. Exp Biol Med (Maywood) 1944; 55(1): 66-9.
        [http://dx.doi.org/10.3181/00379727-55-14461]

[4]   Weinstein MJ, Luedemann GM, Oden EM, *et al.* Gentamicin, a new antibiotic complex from micromonospora. J Med Chem 1963; 6(4): 463-4.
        [http://dx.doi.org/10.1021/jm00340a034] [PMID: 14184912]

[5]   Magnet S, Blanchard JS. Molecular insights into aminoglycoside action and resistance. Chem Rev 2005; 105(2): 477-98.
        [http://dx.doi.org/10.1021/cr0301088] [PMID: 15700953]

CHAPTER 20

Para-aural Abscess and its Management

Urfeya Mirza[1,*], **Uiase Bin Farooq**[2], **Habbu Aishwarya Sunder**[3] and **Priyanka Pandey**[1]

[1] *Department of Veterinary Surgery and Radiology, Khalsa College of Veterinary and Animal Sciences, Amritsar Punjab, India*

[2] *MR College of Veterinary and Animal Sciences, Jhajjar, Haryana, India*

[3] *Central Institute for Research on Buffaloes (CIRB), Nabha, Punjab, India*

Abstract: Para-aural abscessation refers to the extension of purulent inflammation and infection outside the deeper parts of the external ear canal or the middle ear cavity, into the surrounding soft tissues. It can arise from trauma, neoplasia, foreign bodies, chronic otitis externa and previous ear surgery. Clinical signs of pain upon opening the mouth, para-aural swelling and the development of draining tracts in the region of the ear base and parotid gland can appear followed by signs of otitis interna such as ataxia and head tilt toward the affected side, and of facial nerve paralysis. Otoscopy will usually allow recognition of obstruction; however, large abscesses can be opened and drained if indicated before definitive treatment. Apart from contrast radiography (fistulograms), CT imaging is recommended as a diagnostic technique as it provides useful information with respect to the cause of the condition and the recommended surgical approach. Various diagnostic procedures and surgical approaches recommended for the treatment of para-aural abscessation have been elaborated in this chapter. The success and outcome of a surgical procedure does not only depend on the knowledge, experience and instrument and tissue handling of the surgeon, but also on the best peri- and postoperative care. In this chapter, peri- and postoperative analgesia, peri- and postoperative antibacterial therapy, postoperative nutritional management and postoperative dressings and wound management of patients undergoing ear surgery will be discussed under different headings.

Keywords: Abscess, Antibiotics, Auricle, Bandage, Cat, Dog, Ear, Otoscopy, Pain, Pus, Surgery.

INTRODUCTION

The term "para-aural abscessation" describes the spread of purulent inflammation and infection into the soft tissues around the external ear canal or middle ear

* **Corresponding author Urfeya Mirza:** Department of Veterinary Surgery and Radiology, Khalsa College of Veterinary and Animal Sciences, Amritsar Punjab, India; E-mail: urfeyamirza@gmail.com

Tanmoy Rana (Ed.)

cavity. Compared to cats, dogs, particularly Cocker Spaniels, are more likely to develop para-aural abscesses [1 - 3]. Trauma, neoplasia, foreign objects, chronic otitis externa, and previous ear surgery are all potential causes of infection spreading outside the ear canal and/or middle ear cavity [4, 5]. Blockage and stenosis of the external ear canal as well as subsequent abscessation are caused by the traumatized separation of the auricular and annular cartilages [6 - 8]. Even though it is a rare occurrence, congenital atresia of the external ear canal should be taken into consideration when making a diagnosis of para-aural abscessation in young animals [1]. When suppurative secretions collect in the deeper region of the ear canal and penetrate the otic cartilage due to neoplastic obstruction of the external ear canal, para-aural abscessation may develop [9]. However, inadequate debridement of the epithelial lining of the external bone meatus during prior total ear canal ablation (TECA) is the most frequent cause of para-aural abscessation [5, 10]. In a series of 17 dogs with para-aural abscessations, Lane and Watkins [1] observed that 50% of the cases had previously had otic surgeries. Recurrent deep infection rates are still as high as 2-10% even with wide lateral bulla osteotomy (LBO) [11 - 15].

Recurrent deep infection rates are close to 50% when surgery is done for an auditory cholesteatoma [16, 17]. Inadequate middle ear drainage through the auditory tube, osteomyelitis of the ossicles, retained infected ear canal cartilage, incomplete removal of the secretory epithelium lining the tympanic bulla, and damage to the parotid salivary gland are all factors that may contribute to the a etiopathogenesis [2, 3, 10, 14, 15, 18]. There is no decreased risk of deep infection when TECA is performed using Ventral bulla osteotomy (VBO) rather than Long bulla osteotomy (LBO) [11]. After TECA-LBO, clinical symptoms such as pain when opening the mouth, para-aural edema, and the emergence of draining tracts around the parotid gland and ear base may manifest 1 month to many years later [2, 3, 10, 18]. Additionally, there could be symptoms of facial nerve paralysis and otitis interna, including ataxia and a head tilt to the affected side [2, 3].

Usually, otoscopy will enable blockage recognition [1]. FNAB can produce purulent material in a closed abscess that can be used for sensitivity testing and culture. If necessary, large abscesses might be opened and drained before receiving final treatment. Usually, a probe will allow exploration of any draining pathways to determine if the discharge is coming from the middle or external ear [1]. Although fistulograms (contrast radiography), particularly those with lateral oblique views, may be useful for diagnosing [2, 3], CT imaging is suggested as it offers useful evidence regarding the reason of the state and the suggested surgical methodology. A lateral approach is preferred if diagnostic imaging shows indications of residual tissue from the horizontal ear canal or tissue that may indicate retained epithelium within the external bone meatus. It relies on the surgeon's preference in all other circumstances [2, 10]. The risks of facial nerve neuropraxia or retroglenoid vein hemorrhage are raised when doing VBO on dogs, as well as when taking a lateral approach in the absence of external ear canal landmarks [2, 13]. TECA with concurrent bulla osteotomy is also likely the preferred course of treatment in cases that arise spontaneously, unless avulsions of the ear canal can be corrected or blockages of the ear canal are repaired [1].

MANAGEMENT

A lateral approach to the middle ear or a ventral bulla osteotomy are two surgical options that may be used to treat a para-aural abscess that occurred after prior surgery [1, 2, 10, 18].

Total Ear Canal Ablation (TECA)

Surgery should be viewed as just one component of the total therapy strategy for dogs and cats with otitis externa, a complex, frequently systemic condition. The occurrence of generalized skin disorders, endocrine dysfunction, allergy diseases, and concomitant otitis media should be carefully taken into account. The success rate of the surgery will improve with appropriate treatment of underlying illnesses. TECA is reserved for:

• Cases where the recommended medical course of action has not been successful (often in the case of chronic ulcerative otitis externa or end-stage proliferative otitis externa with a *Pseudomonas* spp. superinfection).

• Para-aural abscessation.

• Chronic ear canal avulsions.

• Ear canal neoplasia [5, 15, 17, 19 - 30].

In earlier investigations, TECA had an overall complication rate of 82%, with chronic deep wound infection, abscessation, and severe fistula formation occurring in 10% of cases [13, 15, 31, 32]. Since then, it has been demonstrated that the primary cause of the majority of persistent infections was persistent epithelium within the bony ear canal and/or tympanic bulla [3, 8, 12, 18, 33 - 35]. As a result, for the past 20 years, TECA with extensive tympanic cavity exposure has been regarded as the gold standard treatment for end-stage ear canal illness [8, 34]. However, it has emerged in recent years that less invasive bulla osteotomies do not result in higher complication rates, provided that the whole epithelium lining of the ear canal up to and including the tympanic membrane is removed. The Venker-van Haagen procedure for reshaping the auricle provides great cosmetic results without compromising the quantity of tissue removed, making it the method of choice for preserving ear carriage [4, 36]. It is possible to combine an LBO with the TECA technique, which will be more detailly covered below.

Surgical Technique

After the patient has been draped and the entire auricle and surrounding area have been surgically prepared:

• From the intertragic incisure to the perceptible ventral limit of the vertical ear canal and from the tragohelicine incisure to the same ventral point, a V-shaped incision is made in the skin [4, 22].

• At this stage, the triangular skin flap is lifted with Adson forceps, dissected free towards the tragus at the level of the dermis, and retracted dorsally with Allis forceps [4, 22].

• By cutting through the subcutaneous tissue and muscles using blunt and sharp scissors, the cranial, lateral, and caudal aspects of the distal vertical ear canal are revealed. To prevent needless bleeding, this dissection should be done slowly and as close to the cartilage as possible. Continue cutting until powerful Mayo-Noble dissecting scissors can be advanced from the cranial and caudal side of the vertical ear canal under the cartilage of the auricle on the medial side.

• The remaining auricular cartilage is then separated from the skin and cartilage of the medial wall of the ear canal using these forceful scissors in an inverted U-V form [4, 22]:

• From the cranial side of the exposed vertical ear canal, one leg extends in the direction of a point just above all diseased tissue, which is typically near the anthelix.

• The second leg also leads to the same location, beginning on the caudal side of the vertical ear canal.

• In order to liberate the vertical ear canal of all fascial and muscular attachments, the vertical ear canal is now dissected in a circular motion to the level of the horizontal ear canal.

• To regulate haemorrhage electrocoagulation is compulsory.

• From this point on, the facial nerve in this region should be avoided with the utmost care. To accomplish this, utilize Kelly scissors and try to remain as near to the cartilage of the ear canal as possible [5, 10, 30].

• In order to reach the external acoustic meatus, which can be felt when manipulating the ear canal, the dissection is continued by releasing the horizontal portion of the ear canal from the surrounding tissues.

• Using scissors in a caudal to cranial direction, the cartilaginous part is divided from the osseous part while the facial nerve is preserved.

• A small curette, Adson-Brown tissue forceps, and Kelly scissors can be used to completely remove all of the skin containing ceruminous glands lining the osseous external ear canal, which is necessary for the treatment to be successful [5, 10, 22, 30].

• The external acoustic meatus should be flushed repeatedly for optimal visibility. Once the tympanic membrane has been removed, the surgery is finished with just bone visible and no secretory tissues left.

• In the event that this is done correctly and there is no chronic otitis media, no LBO is required [4, 22]. From this point forward, an LBO is done when there is chronic otitis media and an accumulation of inflammatory tissue or thick exudate in the middle ear cavity.

• The auricle must first be remodeled to complete closure:

• The most natural folding point at the pinna's base is used as the point of rotation as the caudal section of the pinna is folded forward toward the cranial part [4, 22].

• Starting at this point of folding, these pieces are then stitched together using monofilament absorbable suture material (2-0), leaving the ends of the sutures long to make removal easier later.

• The external auditory meatus is then separated from the skin by a Penrose drain, which is positioned 1 cm ventral to the incision.

• Next, two continuous layers of monofilament absorbable suture material (3-0) are used to seal the subcutaneous tissue.

• Using monofilament absorbable suture material (4-0) in a continuous pattern or non-absorbable suture material (4-0) in an interrupted pattern, the skin beneath the pinna is stitched and sealed up.

• After 3-5 days following surgery, when drainage has subsided to only minor amounts of serous discharge, the drain is typically removed.

• It is advised to wear an Elizabethan collar during the initial postoperative healing period.

Lateral Bulla Osteotomy

With or without a TECA, one can execute a lateral approach to the bulla. However, because the principal issue is in the ear canal, the treatment is most frequently done in conjunction with TECA, especially in dogs with chronic otitis externa and media [5, 14, 15, 33, 37, 38]. Therefore, the signs are comparable to those for TECA. A ventral approach to the bulla is advised for treating cats with primary middle ear illness. When remaining epithelial tissue in the region of the external bony meatus is suspected in dogs with recurrent fistulation or abscessation following TECA, likewise a lateral approach to the bulla is the advised strategy [2]. In order to augment residual hearing in animals with hearing loss, a lateral approach to the bulla without TECA can be used for surgery on the middle ear ossicles or for the placement of middle ear implants [39].

Surgical Technique

Following TECA, an LBO is carried out as follows when there is chronic otitis media and an accumulation of inflammatory tissue or thick exudate in the middle ear cavity.

• In order to protect the facial nerve and branches of the external carotid artery that run immediately ventral to the bulla, the tissues from the lateral aspect of the bulla are bluntly dissected as close to the bone as feasible using small periosteal elevators or raspatories [4, 5, 22, 37].

• With Bohler, Kerrison, and/or Zaufal-Jansen rongeurs, the lateral and ventral aspects of the bulla can now be removed, but only to the extent necessary to provide a clear view of the middle ear chamber.

• There is no requirement for subtotal bulla ostectomies or extensive bone resections.

• It is now possible to get samples for cytology, histopathology, susceptibility testing, and culture [4, 5, 22, 37]. The auditory ossicles and cochlea on the dorsomedial side of the bulla are protected by using a bone curette to gently remove any leftover epithelium or debris from inside the bulla.

• The tympanic chamber is liberally lavaged with warm saline after curettage.

• Closure and postoperative treatment follow TECA guidelines.

VENTRAL BULLA OSTEOTOMY

For the treatment of feline middle ear conditions such chronic otitis media, inflammatory polyps, or abscesses, the ventral bulla osteotomy (VBO) technique is frequently used. For polyps that protrude into the nasopharynx or that protrude through the tympanic membrane into the ear canal, traction-avulsion methods, nasopharyngotomy, or a lateral approach to the ear canal may be used to remove them. A more intrusive surgical procedure is advised when diagnostic imaging reveals extensive middle ear involvement or when polyp development returns after simple excision [40 - 45].

A more thorough excision of inflammatory polyps and aberrant mucosal lining is possible with the ventral approach to the bulla because it offers better exposure of the middle ear components. However, it prevents access to the external meatus to allow for the excision of diseased tissue. A LBO, either with or without a TECA, is suggested wherever LBO is suggested. Otitis media in dogs typically develops as a side effect of otitis externa, hence TECA-LBO is the surgical procedure used to treat this species' concomitant otitis media and middle ear ailment [10, 34, 43].

For the treatment of cholesteatoma and recurrent fistulation following TECA-LBO, several publications suggest a ventral approach to the middle ear in dogs [10, 18]. Dogs use a similar but more challenging strategy than cats do. In cats, ventral osteotomy complications can include Horner syndrome and the emergence of vestibular symptoms [10, 40, 43, 44, 46]. In between a few days and a few weeks, Horner syndrome symptoms typically go away. Vestibular symptoms that develop after surgery are typically iatrogenic, the result of excessive curettage, or they might be brought on by caloric damage. After any other acute inner ear injury and peripheral vestibular ataxia, these symptoms disappear in a similar way.

Surgical Technique

• Surgery preparation includes aseptically clipping the ventral neck and intermandibular region [43, 46, 47]. In order to maximize the exposure of the bullae, the patient is positioned in dorsal recumbency with a cervical support to extend the neck.

• Avoid over extending the neck at all costs, which can restrict blood flow to the brain and cause serious neurological damage. Therefore, the tip of the nose should never be perpendicular to the operating table and should always point slightly upward.

• The ipsilateral caudal margin of the mandible is 1 to 2 cm caudomedially from the ventral bullae.

• Halfway down the mandible, to the level of the atlas, a parallel incision is made, with the centre of the cut 2-3 cm to the affected side [44, 46, 47].

• If necessary, the linguofacial and maxillary veins are retracted, and the platysma and sphincter colli muscles are incised.

• When the bulla can be felt, the incision is deepened by blunt dissection between the digastricus muscle and the hypoglossal and styloglossal muscles [44, 46, 47]. The dissection site can be held in place with two small Senn retractors, two small Weitlaner retractors, or Gelpi retractors.

• A minor incision can be made over the bulla periosteum after the bulla has been discovered and the hypoglossal nerve has been recognized and preserved. The periosteal layer that covers the intended site for the osteotomy or ostectomy may be removed using small elevators.

• Alternately, a tiny osteotome can be used in place of a Steinmann pin to create a hole on the ventral surface. Using a little rongeur or Kerrison punch, the opening can be made larger [44, 46, 47].

• Initially, the broad ventral hypotympanic cavity is opened.

• Material is gathered for histopathology, cytology, sensitivity testing, culture, and other purposes.

• A tiny osteotome or Kerrison punches can be used to identify and open the bony septum dividing the ventral cavity from the dorsolateral compartment once this compartment has been cleaned [44, 46, 47].

• Once more, a small currette is used to empty this compartment, with special attention paid to removing polypous tissue from the auditory tube's opening and internal bone meatus.

• Typically, polypous tissue can be removed and then picked up with tiny mosquito forceps. The entire polyp may typically be entirely removed with the aid of the little curette and a tight yet careful hold on the polyp.

• Particularly close to the stapes and the circular window, aggressive curettage should be avoided.

• Depending on the preference of the surgeon, the cavity is cleansed and drained with a Penrose drain.

• The skin is closed intradermally with the same material, and the muscles do not need to be closed individually. Instead, the subcutaneous tissues are reapposed continuously using monofilament absorbable suture material.

PERIOPERATIVE MANAGEMENT

Following surgery, patients may experience pain, nausea, regurgitation, vomiting, and ileus, stress-induced catabolism, reduced pulmonary function, higher cardiac demands, and a risk of thrombosis. These issues, in addition to a potential surgical site infection, may result in serious complications and, at the very least, a requirement for a lengthy hospital stay. Anorexic or hyporexic patients are even more likely to suffer perioperative morbidity and mortality. The success and outcome of a surgery depend on the otorhinolaryngological surgeon's expertise, experience, and handling of the instruments and tissue, as well as on close coordination with nurses and anesthetists to give the finest pre- and postoperative care. The following requirements must be met for a positive result:

• Better pain management by early multimodal analgesia intervention

• Using techniques to provide regional anesthesia and minimize stress

• Appropriate antibiotic usage

• Providing dietary assistance

• Care for the wound.

Peri- And Postoperative Analgesia

The life of an organism depends on its capacity to recognize unpleasant stimuli. The nervous system responds to severe stimulation from thermal and mechanical stimuli or environmental and endogenous chemical irritants by detecting and interpreting noxious sensations (nociception) [48]. Two major kinds of nociceptors, Aδ afferents and C-fibre afferents, have been found in addition to specialized nerve terminals reacting to touch, vibration, movement, and proprioception [48 - 50]:

• Type I Aδ nociceptors have a relatively high heat threshold yet respond to both mechanical and chemical stimuli.

• Type II have a very high mechanical threshold but a much lower heat threshold.

The receptors for tissue damage do not revert to their pre-stimulus condition following activation, in contrast to other senses like vision. Additionally, following injury, the sensitivity of damage-detecting sensory nerve endings may change, and their synaptic connections within the central nervous system (CNS) may drastically change and reorganize (CNS plasticity) [51, 52]. The clinical ramifications include that, once pain has been established, analgesic medications are substantially less effective, and over time, even with continuous nociceptive stimulation, the animal experiences more pain. It is the ethical duty of the veterinary surgeon to attempt to avoid (pre-emptive analgesia) [53, 54] and/or alleviate pain in our companion animals who are undergoing surgery (using multimodal or balanced analgesia) [55, 56]. Additionally, the veterinary surgeon needs to be aware that tissue trauma, which is impacted by the surgeon's expertise and surgical method choices, affects the degree of postoperative discomfort [48, 57].

Principles of Effective Pain Management

Preoperative pain management is followed postoperatively by continuous pain assessment based on objective pain grading methods. The Glasgow Composite Pain measure (GCPS) is the most used and best-validated pain measure for canines (http://www.gla.ac.uk/media/media_233876_en.pdf.) [58]. For measuring postoperative pain in cats, the UNESP-Botucatu Multidimensional Composite Pain Scale [59] is rather easy to apply (http://www.animalpain.com.br/en-us/) [60]. Alternately, the Feline Acute Pain Scale from Colorado State University also can be applied.

• Employ a multimodal analgesia strategy. It is understood that compared to utilizing a unimodal method, analgesia regimens containing various types of analgesic medications that act on various receptor and neurotransmitter targets are more effective [55, 56]. Additionally, more thorough analgesia can be offered *via* multimodal approaches. For instance, systemic opioids typically have a short half-life (1-6 hours) but a rapid beginning of effect. Nonsteroidal anti-inflammatory medications (NSAIDs) on the other hand have a lengthy duration of action (24 hours), although they take between 30 and 60 minutes after administration to start working [61].

• If at all possible, use loco-regional approaches to support systemic (opioid-based) analgesia. These methods enable a balanced anesthesia technique, a lower concentration of volatile anesthetic agent during anesthesia, and a greater contribution to postoperative analgesia while reducing the severity of the surgical stress reaction [61]. They permit the use of lower opioid doses in the initial postoperative period or may permit the administration of a partial μ-agonist opioid rather than a full μ-agonist opioid, which is typically linked with less adverse effects such drowsiness and mild hypothermia.

• Opioids are the foundation of analgesic regimes [48, 61]; they are effective and have little to no haemodynamic impact. They are very adaptable medications, and the dose and dosing interval can be changed to offer each patient the best possible pain relief. Some opioids, such as morphine and fentanyl, can be given by continuous rate infusion (CRI), which can be more effective in relieving pain while using at overall lower amount of the medication than bolus administration.

• NSAIDs are an important part of perioperative analgesia regimes and offers a good relief from acute pain [54]. If an NSAID is not contraindicated in a specific patient, give it to surgical patients, particularly before any tissue damage is caused by the surgery.

• Adjunctive analgesics, such as ketamine, lidocaine, and dexmedetomidine, can be helpful for patients experiencing moderate to severe pain that is difficult to manage with opioids and NSAIDs [61] (some patients with extremely painful ear conditions, such as after bilateral total ear canal ablation with lateral bulla osteotomy (TECA-LBO)), or in patients experiencing extreme anxiety and stress where panting can exacerbate postoperative swelling of the air. Studies showing analgesic efficacy are weak, and there exists a poor evidence base that could aid in the justification of the dose [61].

• Typically, these medications must be infused intravenously by CRI; careful patient monitoring (pain, sedation) is crucial. If no solid history of opioid analgesia has been established, they should not be started.

Even though oral tramadol is not approved for use in animals, its use in dogs and cats for the treatment of acute pain has increased. Tramadol may be helpful in dogs and cats, according to a small number of studies [62, 63] and [64, 65] respectfully. However, analgesia in these species varies widely, and adverse effects (such as dysphoria, drowsiness, and nausea) are frequent. If at all possible, an NSAID should be used instead of tramadol; in addition, most studies have failed to demonstrate that oral tramadol combined with an NSAID provides greater analgesia than an NSAID alone; for these reasons, routine administration of tramadol and an NSAID is usually unnecessary in animals. Most cats cannot tolerate oral tramadol because it is so bitter, even whether it is given in food or in the form of gelatin capsule.

Endoscopic Procedures

To prevent patient reaction to the treatment, strong anesthesia or profound analgesia are needed for rhinoscopic and video-otoscopic procedures [66]. Butorphanol should not be used as a premedication instead of a μ-opioid [66]. To reduce reaction after inserting the scope in the nasal vestibule, lidocaine may be injected through the nares [66]. Spraying the soft palate and endoscope with lidocaine may help to lessen the jerking, twisting, or gagging that frequently occurs when the scope is retroflexed for nasopharyngoscopy. The patient response to this operation is greatly reduced by bilateral lidocaine maxillary nerve blocks, administered at a dose of roughly 1 mg/kg per side [67]. The great auricular nerve, which innervates the caudolateral region of the ear, can be blocked to prevent otoscopy and ear flushing in ears that are in excruciating pain. The auriculotemporal nerve, which innervates the cranial section of the vertical canal, can also be disrupted [68]. NSAIDs used postoperatively for two to three days will be enough analgesic for the majority of endoscopic procedures.

Surgical Procedures

The length of time and dosage of systemic opioid analgesia during the postoperative phase are mostly determined by the results of the pain evaluation, any side effects that are noticed, and the length of hospitalization prior to eventual discharge. The majority of animals who have invasive ear or nose surgery (ablation of ear canals, bulla osteotomy, rhinotomy) profit from local blocks given prior to surgery in the same manner as for endoscopic procedures, as well as from opioid and NSAID analgesia given postoperatively [22]. In general, if an animal has been receiving a full μ-opioid agonist postoperatively (such as methadone), it is prudent to switch to a partial μ-opioid agonist (such as buprenorphine) before terminating opioid therapy completely [61]. Therefore, the majority of animals will receive 1-2 days of methadone, then 1 day of buprenorphine, before being released.

There are significant variations across veterinary surgeons and practices, and there are currently very few data outlining the ideal time frame for NSAID administration following routine procedures. Additionally, it is critical to keep in mind that side effects are linked to both ineffective pain relief (without NSAIDs) and effective pain relief (with NSAIDs) [69], making it risky to administer NSAIDs without a need for them or to stop using them altogether. The invasiveness of the procedure, anticipated level of inflammation, and time frame needed for tissue recovery should all be taken into consideration when making decisions. Invasive ear and nose operations in dogs and cats call for NSAID therapy both during hospitalization and for up to seven to fourteen days after surgery in the home setting. NSAIDs must be used for three to five days after less invasive surgeries involving the throat that do not include bone resection.

Peri- And Postoperative Antibacterial Therapy

A major complication that could lead to the failure of the surgery is infection of a wound after surgery. Additionally, the healing process may take longer, the wound may dehisce, and infections in the wound may worsen the local inflammation (pain, redness, and swelling) brought on by the first operation and result in systemic sickness (fever, anorexia, and lethargy) [70]. There are times when a generalized infection can induce septic shock, which can impair the operation of important organs such the liver, kidneys, heart, and lungs and potentially result in death [71].

By classifying surgical incisions according to their contamination levels, it is possible to predict the incidence of postoperative infection [70, 71]:

• The reported infection rate for Category I clean wounds is 0-4.4%.

• The likelihood of a wound infection in Category II (clean-contaminated wounds) ranges between 5 and 10% on average.

• There is a 6-29% incidence of infection in Category III (contaminated wounds).

• The risk of infection is 30% higher in Category IV (unclean wounds).

Most small animal ear treatments would be categorized as contaminated or even dirty (inflammatory process present with purulent discharge), and surgical wounds where the aero-digestive tract is penetrated are considered to be clean-contaminated at best. In the human literature, there is level I evidence to support the use of prophylaxis in clean-contaminated head and neck procedures (where the aero-digestive tract is opened) and tonsillectomy, while level II evidence does not support the use of prophylaxis in clean head and neck procedures like salivary gland resection and thyroidectomy [72 - 74]. The highest infection rates in animals are identified after otological procedures [10], while in one report the lowest rate of surgical site infection was observed after otosurgical procedures (6%) and the highest rate (13%) after head and neck (HN) procedures [73]. In a study on HN cancer surgery, antibiotic prophylaxis was found to be successful in decreasing the frequency of surgical site infections; however, patients undergoing contaminated or clean procedures only benefited from perioperative antibiotic prophylaxis limited to the first 24 hours after surgery. Its prolongation past these 24 hours had no discernible advantage [75].

Infection rates of up to 40% [10, 12 - 15, 30, 32, 76, 77] have been reported for dogs undergoing otic surgery, but in cats surgical site infection appears to be less of a problem [78 - 80]. Although early reports have consistently advised wound drainage following TECA-LBO with active or passive drains to prevent incisional complications, no difference in wound complication rates was observed when TECA-LBO procedures were closed predominantly with or without drainage [77]. Therefore, the surgeon's preference will determine whether or not drains are used after TECA-LBO. Surgical site infections are uncommon in small animals and are hardly ever described, but several problems might develop during and after rhinotomy or pharyngolaryngeal surgery [81].

Antimicrobial Prophylaxis

Although antimicrobial agents are crucial for the prevention and treatment of surgical infections, effective surgical technique is still the most important goal, and pathogen contamination is minimized by strict adherence to aseptic procedures. To better the patient's condition, steps must also be taken to reduce other risk factors as much as feasible [70]. Antimicrobial prophylaxis is typically defined as the use of antibiotics during surgery to reduce the quantity of microorganisms to a level that the patients defense mechanisms can successfully destroy in order to prevent a surgical site infection that has already developed. The surgical site must have sufficiently high levels of antibiotics present at the time of contamination in order to receive an appropriate antimicrobial prophylaxis during an operation.

Due to this, it is recommended to start the intravenous antibiotic administration 30 to 60 minutes before to the start of the incision [71]. However, after being administered intramuscularly, several antibiotics soon acquire a suitably high content. Due to the potential for tissue irritation at the site of the wound and the more reliable and effective antibiotic plasma levels that are acquired after intravenous treatment, local prophylaxis is not indicated [71]. It is not required for tissue antibiotic levels to remain high in the body after surgery; often, a few hours are enough, unless there is a strong reason to persist (such as in the case of infection). When this occurs, it is considered antimicrobial therapy rather than prevention against bacteria.

In most cases, it is advised to use antibiotics as prophylactic in Category II (clean-contaminated wounds) [72 - 74]. The sort of bacteria that is most likely to be the main contaminant will determine which antibiotic should be used. The majority of patients undergoing ear surgery will have had cultures performed as part of the diagnostic process, and based on the results of the culture and sensitivity tests, a specific prophylactic antibiotic can be chosen. The pathogens *Staphylococcus pseudintermedius*, *Escherichia coli*, *Proteus mirabilis* and *Pseudomonas aeruginosa* are generally the most likely to be encountered. *Staphylococcus* spp., *Streptococcus* spp., and gram-negative bacteria can be detected in the respiratory tract [70]. In Category III and IV wounds, antimicrobial prophylaxis should be administered; however, additional precautions to reduce the level of contamination are advised, including thorough lavage of the area, debridement of necrotic or severely inflamed tissue, removal of foreign material, and drainage of the wound through the implantation of surgical drains. Parenteral prophylaxis with either potentiated amoxicillin (amoxicillin with clavulanic acid) or cephalosporins is recommended for patients undergoing ENT surgery, unless otherwise stated by a specific culture result. Beyond how many hours [71] hours after surgery, there is no evidence-based justification for continuing prophylactic antibiotics.

Postoperative Antibiotic Treatment

In Category III and IV wounds, the antimicrobial treatment is continued after surgery until the wound is healing properly (7–28 days after surgery) [70]. Prophylaxis alone might be sufficient for Category II wounds if the recovery went well and, for instance, no regurgitation had taken place that might have caused aspiration pneumonia. However, a postoperative course of antibiotics is also recommended in individuals with pre-existing diseases, such as low-grade bronchopneumonia, which is frequently observed in brachycephalic dogs.

Postoperative Nutritional Management After Surgery

A consistent correlation has been found between malnutrition and subpar clinical outcomes in humans, where nutritional status is a significant predictor of postoperative recovery [82]. It is considered that nutritional supplementation is similarly important for the recovery of severely ill dogs and cats since starvation causes similar metabolic effects in animals [83]. In order to maximize the likelihood of a quick and painless recovery, veterinary surgical patients receive pre- and postoperative care. This includes oxygen, fluids, anti-inflammatory drugs, and other medications to ensure a patient is haemodynamically and metabolically stable both during and after the surgical process. However, the therapeutic plan should take into account both nutritional assessment and management [84].

Every surgical patient should have their nutritional status evaluated at every consultation or evaluation since nutrition is essential for preserving patients' health and for enhancing their capacity to respond to illness and damage [84]. The WSAVA website (http://www.wsava.org/guidelines/global-nutrition-guidelines)

provides criteria for evaluating nutritional status of the patient [85]. The 'ebb/flow' paradigm states that animals undergoing surgery exhibit:

• A first hypometabolic reaction (the "ebb phase").

• Accompanied by an extended period of hypermetabolism (the "flow phase") [84, 86].

The ebb phase is typically characterized by a period of haemodynamic instability, which is accompanied by a decline in energy expenditure, hypothermia, modest protein catabolism, a reduction in cardiac output, and poor tissue perfusion. Without treatment, this could develop into a condition known as refractory or irreversible shock [86 - 88], which is characterized by severe lactic acidosis, decreased tissue perfusion, multiple organ failure, and death. These issues can be resolved by carefully monitoring the patient while under anesthesia and using intravenous fluids and medications as needed.

Patients enter the flow phase, during which significant metabolic changes take place, following a successful procedure with a stable anesthesia. The hallmarks of this response include profound protein catabolism, as well as increases in cardiac output, energy expenditure, glucose generation, and insulin and glucagon concentrations [89, 90]. Protein will be catabolized (used for energy and gluconeogenesis) and used for the production of acute-phase proteins and immunoglobulins that are required for wound healing due to the impact of inflammatory cytokines in this state of hypermetabolism. Given this hypermetabolic condition, early nutritional supplementation that provides energy and protein to encourage recovery is crucial [84].

To transition from a catabolic to anabolic state, one often needs nutritional support (l-glutamine, arginine, taurine, omega-6 fatty acids, and omega-3 fatty acids) for at least three days [84]. This not only demands postoperative food intake that is necessary but also that is of a good caliber. Patients can become hyporexic if sufficient analgesia is not given, especially after painful ear surgeries such as painful mastication (otitis media) or painful deglutition (throat surgery), thus this issue should be addressed and fixed immediately. Forced feeding won't increase spontaneous food intake in anorexic animals; instead, enteral or parenteral nutrition should be given [91]. The need for alternative assisted feeding approaches, which are more invasive and stressful, may be reduced in hyporectic animals by stimulating spontaneous food intake. However, alternative aided feeding approaches should be used to assure the administration of sufficient amounts of nutrients during the aforementioned hypermetabolic, postoperative phase if stimulation of spontaneous food intake does not result in an adequate amount of food intake [84].

Nutrients can be administered *via* nasoesophageal, oesophageal, or gastric tubes if necessary, although enteral nutrition delivery is always preferred to parenteral nutrition delivery. It is crucial to provide food and encourage spontaneous food consumption every day to monitor the restoration of appetite because it is a symptom of recovery. It is crucial to provide a peaceful and comfortable setting with adequate and attentive care, as hospitalization is frequently unpleasant for an animal [84]. Additionally, a light cycle that corresponds to the season should be used to promote food intake. Opiates, antimicrobials, diuretics, immunosuppressives, and chemotherapeutic drugs are only a few examples of pharmaceuticals that can have an inhibitory influence on food intake [89, 92]. A hyporexic animal at a hospital will usually consume the food it gets at home, but you can make it more appealing by adding moisture, heating it to body warmth, or giving it fresh food. Higher moisture content also aids in rehydrating patients and hastens the exit of nutrients from the stomach, decreasing the likelihood of vomiting or regurgitation [93]. This is crucial for those who have had throat surgery, including brachycephalic animals that have undergone staphylectomy.

Foods in cans have high levels of moisture, fat, and protein, all of which improve flavor. These are perfect for the first two weeks following throat surgery. Soft canned foods also have the potential advantage of reducing surgery site trauma in the intrapharyngeal and intralaryngeal regions. Giving patients with cancer cachexia and sarcopenia (loss of lean body mass that happens with aging in the absence of disease) foods that are higher in calorie density and higher in protein concentration can also help prevent further loss of lean body mass [94].

Postoperative Dressings And Wound Management

Following ENT surgery, there are several reasons [95 - 97] to cover your wound with a bandage:

- Environment-based wound protection.

- Defense against the patient's licking, biting, *etc.*, of the wounds.

- Assimilate exudate.

- Get rid of empty space.

- Apply pressure or release it.

- Dispense drugs topically.

- By immobilizing soft tissues, reduce discomfort.

In the majority of situations, bandages are used to treat a combination of these symptoms. Bandages are not typically applied to patients following nasal surgery due to the difficulty to eat, drink, or see due to the shape of the head, either due to long, tapering noses or due to the absence of a nose in brachycephalic animals. Putting the animal an Elizabethan collar will prevent auto mutilation in the surrounding areas. Following throat surgery, bandages are also not advised since they frequently slip or are put on excessively tightly, obstructing lymphatic and venous drainage. No bandages are ordinarily used in this area, with the exception of covering a drain in the neck region, which is typically secured with tie-over bandages. As long as they are not covering the surgical wound, large Elizabethan collars are acceptable.

After ear surgery, bandages are typically applied, especially after othaematoma correction or TECA-LBO, the technique for which will be covered here. Cats do not respond well with bandages, however after ventral bulla osteotomy, a little Elizabethan collar can be given if necessary, even though the majority of cats are unlikely to scratch the surgical site. To minimize unintentional removal of drains or sutures or damage to the incision, ears of the dog should be dressed following major ear surgery [98 - 102]. Instead of being taped to the local skin, the auricle is traditionally reflected back over the head [33, 103, 104]. To ensure proper ventilation of the ear canals and the ability to apply topical treatment as needed, this bandage should be replaced every day. Absorbent material can be applied over the surgical site and departing drain following TECA-LBO, folded over the ipsilateral auricle, and then firmly fastened.

CONCLUDING REMARKS

The term of para-aural abscess is applied to describe the condition when suppuration was extended from the external ear canal or the middle ear cavity into the surrounding soft tissues of the ear. Diagnosis is to be performed on otoscopic observation. Radiographic observation denotes a disruption of the normal air opacity of the affected ear canal. Drainage is to be performed also by creating a separate opening for the horizontal ear canal, or total ear canal ablation and lateral bulla osteotomy (TECA/LBO) for the better resolution of the clinical signs.

REFERENCES

[1]   Lane JG, Watkins PE. Para-aural abscess in the dog and cat. J Small Anim Pract 1986; 27(8): 521-31.
       [DOI: 10.1111/j.1748-5827.1986.tb02158.x].
       [http://dx.doi.org/10.1111/j.1748-5827.1986.tb02158.x]

[2]   Holt D, Brockman DJ, Sylvestre AM, Sadanaga KK. Lateral exploration of fistulas developing after
       total ear canal ablations: 10 cases (1989-1993). J Am Anim Hosp Assoc 1996; 32(6): 527-30.
       [http://dx.doi.org/10.5326/15473317-32-6-527] [PMID: 8906731]

[3]   Smeak DD, Crocker CB, Birchard SJ. Treatment of recurrent otitis media that developed after total ear

canal ablation and lateral bulla osteotomy in dogs: nine cases (1986–1994). J Am Vet Med Assoc 1996; 209(5): 937-42.
[http://dx.doi.org/10.2460/javma.1996.209.05.937] [PMID: 8790545]

[4]   Venker-van Haagen, A.J. (2005) The ear. In: Throat, and Tracheobronchial Diseases in Dogs and Cats. Venker-van Haagen AJ (ed) (edited by Ear & Nose). Schlutersche Verlagsgesellschaft: Hannover, Germany, pp. 1–50.

[5]   Bacon NJ. Pinna and external ear canal. In: Tobias KM, Johnston SA, Eds. Veterinary Surgery Small Animal. St Louis: Elsevier Saunders 2012; pp. 2059-77.

[6]   Boothe HW, Hobson HP, McDonald D. Treatment of traumatic separation of the auricular and annular cartilages without ablation: results in five dogs. Vet Surg 1996; 25(5): 376-9.
[http://dx.doi.org/10.1111/j.1532-950X.1996.tb01430.x] [PMID: 8879108]

[7]   Connery NA, McAllister H, Hay CW. Para-aural abscessation following traumatic ear canal separation in a dog. J Small Anim Pract 2001; 42(5): 253-6.
[http://dx.doi.org/10.1111/j.1748-5827.2001.tb02031.x] [PMID: 11380020]

[8]   McCarthy PE, Hosgood G, Pechman RD. Traumatic ear canal separations and para-aural abscessation in three dogs. J Am Anim Hosp Assoc 1995; 31(5): 419-24.
[http://dx.doi.org/10.5326/15473317-31-5-419] [PMID: 8542360]

[9]   Rogers KS. Tumors of the ear canal. Vet Clin North Am Small Anim Pract 1988; 18(4): 859-68.
[http://dx.doi.org/10.1016/S0195-5616(88)50086-4] [PMID: 3264960]

[10]   Smeak DD. Management of complications associated with total ear canal ablation and bulla osteotomy in dogs and cats. Vet Clin North Am Small Anim Pract 2011; 41(5): 981-94.
[http://dx.doi.org/10.1016/j.cvsm.2011.05.011] [PMID: 21889696]

[11]   Doyle RS, Skelly C, Bellenger CR. Surgical management of 43 cases of chronic otitis externa in the dog. Ir Vet J 2004; 57(1): 22-30.
[http://dx.doi.org/10.1186/2046-0481-57-1-22] [PMID: 21851652]

[12]   Smeak DD, Dehoff WD. Total ear canal ablation clinical results in the dog and cat. Vet Surg 1986; 15(2): 161-70. [DOI: 10.1111/j.1532-950X.1986.tb00197.x].
[http://dx.doi.org/10.1111/j.1532-950X.1986.tb00197.x]

[13]   Matthieson DT, Scavelli T. Total ear canal ablation and lateral bulla osteotomy in 38 dogs. JAAHA 1990; 26: 257-67.

[14]   Beckman SL, Henry WB Jr, Cechner P. Total ear canal ablation combining bulla osteotomy and curettage in dogs with chronic otitis externa and media. J Am Vet Med Assoc 1990; 196(1): 84-90.
[http://dx.doi.org/10.2460/javma.1990.196.01.84] [PMID: 2295558]

[15]   Mason LK, Harvey C, Orsher RJ. Total ear canal ablation combined with lateral bulla osteotomy for end-stage otitis in dogs. Results in thirty dogs. Vet Surg 1988; 17(5): 263-8.
[http://dx.doi.org/10.1111/j.1532-950X.1988.tb01012.x] [PMID: 3227638]

[16]   Marino DJ, MacDonald JM, Matthiesen DT, Patnaik AK. Results of surgery in cats with ceruminous gland adenocarcinoma. JAAHA 1994; 30: 54-8.

[17]   Williams JM, White RAS. Total ear canal ablation combined with lateral bulla osteotomy in the cat. J Soc Adm Pharm 1992; 33: 225-7. [DOI: 10.1111/j.1748-5827.1992.tb01121.x].

[18]   Hardie EM, Linder K, Pease AP. Aural cholesteatoma in twenty dogs. Vet Surg 2008; 37(8): 763-70.
[http://dx.doi.org/10.1111/j.1532-950X.2008.00455.x] [PMID: 19121172]

[19]   Lanz OI, Wood BC. Surgery of the ear and pinna. Vet Clin North Am Small Anim Pract 2004; 34(2): 567-99.
[http://dx.doi.org/10.1016/j.cvsm.2003.10.011] [PMID: 15062625]

[20]   Elkins AD. Surgery of the external ear canal. Probl Vet Med 1991; 3(2): 239-53. [PubMed: 1802251].
[PMID: 1802251]

[21] Smeak DD, Kerpsack SJ. Total ear canal ablation and lateral bulla osteotomy for management of end-stage otitis. Semin Vet Med Surg (Small Anim) 1993; 8(1): 30-41. [PubMed: 8456202].
[PMID: 8456202]

[22] ter Haar G. Basic Principles of Surgery of the External Ear (Pinna and Ear Canal). In: Kirpensteijn J, Klein WR, Eds. The Cutting Edge: Basic Operating Skills for the Veterinary Surgeon. London: Roman House Publishers 2006; pp. 272-83.

[23] Bojrab MJ, Constantinescu GM. Treatment of Otitis Externa. In: Bojrab MJ, Ed. Curr Tech Small Ani Surg. Baltimore, USA: Williams & Wilkins 1998; pp. 98-101.

[24] Bradley RL. Surgical management of otitis externa. Vet Clin North Am Small Anim Pract 1988; 18(4): 813-9.
[http://dx.doi.org/10.1016/S0195-5616(88)50083-9] [PMID: 3264957]

[25] Harvey CE. Ear canal disease in the dog: medical and surgical management. J Am Vet Med Assoc 1980; 177(2): 136-9. [PubMed: 7429946].
[PMID: 7429946]

[26] Phil Hobson H. Surgical management of advanced ear disease. Vet Clin North Am Small Anim Pract 1988; 18(4): 821-44.
[http://dx.doi.org/10.1016/S0195-5616(88)50084-0] [PMID: 3264958]

[27] McCarthy PE, McCarthy RJ. Surgery of the Ear. Vet Clin North Am Small Anim Pract 1994; 24(5): 953-69.
[http://dx.doi.org/10.1016/S0195-5616(94)50110-4] [PMID: 7817495]

[28] White RAS. The ear: surgery for chronic otitis. Vet Q 1998; 20(sup1) (Suppl. 1): S7-9.
[http://dx.doi.org/10.1080/01652176.1998.10807381] [PMID: 9651977]

[29] Doyle RS, Skelly C, Bellenger CR. Surgical management of 43 cases of chronic otitis externa in the dog. Ir Vet J 2004; 57(1): 22-30.
[http://dx.doi.org/10.1186/2046-0481-57-1-22] [PMID: 21851652]

[30] White RAS, Pomeroy CJ. Total ear canal ablation and lateral bulla osteotomy in the dog. J Small Anim Pract 1990; 31(11): 547-53. [DOI: 10.1111/j.1748-5827.1990.tb00683.x].
[http://dx.doi.org/10.1111/j.1748-5827.1990.tb00683.x]

[31] Anders BB, Hoelzler MG, Scavelli TD, Fulcher RP, Bastian RP. Analysis of auditory and neurologic effects associated with ventral bulla osteotomy for removal of inflammatory polyps or nasopharyngeal masses in cats. J Am Vet Med Assoc 2008; 233(4): 580-5.
[http://dx.doi.org/10.2460/javma.233.4.580] [PMID: 18710312]

[32] Sharp NJH. Chronic otitis externa and otitis media treated by total ear canal ablation and ventral bulla osteotomy in thirteen dogs. Vet Surg 1990; 19(2): 162-6.
[http://dx.doi.org/10.1111/j.1532-950X.1990.tb01159.x] [PMID: 2333689]

[33] Smeak DD, Kerpsack SJ. Total ear canal ablation and lateral bulla osteotomy for management of end-stage otitis. Semin Vet Med Surg (Small Anim) 1993; 8(1): 30-41. [PubMed: 8456202].
[PMID: 8456202]

[34] Smeak DD, Inpanbutr N. Lateral approach to subtotal bulla osteotomy in dogs. Compend Contin Educ Vet 2005; 27: 377-84.

[35] Doust R, King A, Hammond G, *et al.* Assessment of middle ear disease in the dog: a comparison of diagnostic imaging modalities. J Small Anim Pract 2007; 48(4): 188-92.
[http://dx.doi.org/10.1111/j.1748-5827.2007.00295.x] [PMID: 17381763]

[36] Venker-van Haagen AJ. Managing Diseases of the Ear. In: Kirk RW, Ed. Current Veterinary Therapy. Philadelphia, USA: W. B. Saunders 1983; pp. 47-52.

[37] Smeak DD. Total ear canal ablation and lateral bulla osteotomy. In: Bojrab MJ, Ed. Current Techniques in Small Animal Surgery. Baltimore, USA: Williams & Wilkins 1998; pp. 102-8.

[38] Mathews KG, Hardie EM, Murphy KM. Subtotal ear canal ablation in 18 dogs and one cat with minimal distal ear canal pathology. J Am Anim Hosp Assoc 2006; 42(5): 371-80.
[http://dx.doi.org/10.5326/0420371] [PMID: 16960041]

[39] Ter Haar G, Mulder JJ, Venker-van Haagen AJ, van Sluijs FJ, Smoorenburg GF. A surgical technique for implantation of the vibrant soundbridge middle ear implant in dogs. Vet Surg 2011; 40(3): 340-6.
[http://dx.doi.org/10.1111/j.1532-950X.2011.00806.x] [PMID: 21361989]

[40] Faulkner JE, Budsberg SC. Results of ventral bulla osteotomy for treatment of middle ear polyps in cats. JAAHA 1990; 26: 496-9.

[41] Trevor PB, Martin RA. Tympanic bulla osteotomy for treatment of middle-ear disease in cats: 19 cases (1984-1991). J Am Vet Med Assoc 1993; 202(1): 123-8.
[http://dx.doi.org/10.2460/javma.1993.202.01.123] [PMID: 8420899]

[42] Ader PL, Boothe HW. Ventral bulla osteotomy in the cat. JAAHA 1979; 15: 757-62.

[43] Booth HW. Ventral Bulla Osteotomy: Dog and Cat. In: Bojrab MJ, Ed. Current Techniques in Small Animal Surgery. Baltimore, USA: Williams & Wilkins 1998; pp. 109-12.

[44] Donnelly KE, Tillson DM. Feline inflammatory polyps and ventral bulla osteotomy. Compendium on the Continuing Education for the Veterinary Practitioner 2004; 26: 446-54.

[45] Gotthelf LN. Diagnosis and treatment of otitis media in dogs and cats. Vet Clin North Am Small Anim Pract 2004; 34(2): 469-87.
[http://dx.doi.org/10.1016/j.cvsm.2003.10.007] [PMID: 15062620]

[46] White RAS. Middle and inner ear. In: Tobias KM, Johnston SA, Eds. Veterinary Surgery Small Animal. St Louis: Elsevier Saunders 2012; pp. 2078-89.

[47] Fossum TW. Surgery of the Ear. In: Fossum TW, Hedlund CS, Hulse DA, Eds. Small Animal Surgery. 3rd ed. St Louis, USA: Mosby Elsevier 2007; pp. 289-316.

[48] Lascelles BD. Surgical pain: Pathophysiology, assessment, and treatment strategies. In: Tobias KM, Johnston SA, Eds. Veterinary Surgery Small Animal. St Louis: Elsevier Saunders 2012; pp. 237-47.

[49] Brainard BM, Hofmeister EH. Anesthesia Principles and Monitoring. In: Tobias KM, Johnston SA, Eds. Veterinary Surgery Small Animal. St Louis: Elsevier Saunders 2012; pp. 248-91.

[50] Gurney MA. Pharmacological options for intra-operative and early postoperative analgesia: an update. J Small Anim Pract 2012; 53(7): 377-86.
[http://dx.doi.org/10.1111/j.1748-5827.2012.01243.x] [PMID: 22747730]

[51] Lascelles XBD, Cripps JP, Jones A, Waterman EA. Post-operative central hypersensitivity and pain: the pre-emptive value of pethidine for ovariohysterectomy. Pain 1997; 73(3): 461-71.
[http://dx.doi.org/10.1016/S0304-3959(97)00141-3] [PMID: 9469538]

[52] Lascelles BDX, Waterman AE, Cripps PJ, Livingston A, Henderson G. Central sensitization as a result of surgical pain: investigation of the pre-emptive value of pethidine for ovariohysterectomy in the rat. Pain 1995; 62(2): 201-12.
[http://dx.doi.org/10.1016/0304-3959(94)00266-H] [PMID: 8545146]

[53] Welsh EM, Nolan AM, Reid J. Beneficial effects of administering carprofen before surgery in dogs. Vet Rec 1997; 141(10): 251-3.
[http://dx.doi.org/10.1136/vr.141.10.251] [PMID: 9308151]

[54] Lascelles BDX, Cripps PJ, Jones A, Waterman-Pearson A. Efficacy and kinetics of carprofen, administered preoperatively or postoperatively, for the prevention of pain in dogs undergoing ovariohysterectomy. Vet Surg 1998; 27(6): 568-82.
[http://dx.doi.org/10.1111/j.1532-950X.1998.tb00533.x] [PMID: 9845221]

[55] Williams VM, Lascelles BDX, Robson MC. Current attitudes to, and use of, peri-operative analgesia in dogs and cats by veterinarians in New Zealand. N Z Vet J 2005; 53(3): 193-202.

[http://dx.doi.org/10.1080/00480169.2005.36504] [PMID: 16012589]

[56]   Corletto F. Multimodal and balanced analgesia. Vet Res Commun 2007; 31(S1) (Suppl. 1): 59-63.
[http://dx.doi.org/10.1007/s11259-007-0085-5] [PMID: 17682848]

[57]   Kristiansson M, Saraste L, Soop M, Sundqvist KG, Thörne A. Diminished interleukin-6 and C-reactive protein responses to laparoscopic *versus* open cholecystectomy. Acta Anaesthesiol Scand 1999; 43(2): 146-52.
[http://dx.doi.org/10.1034/j.1399-6576.1999.430205.x] [PMID: 10027020]

[58]   Available from: http://www.gla.ac.uk/media/media_233876_en.pdf

[59]   Brondani JT, Mama KR, Luna SPL, *et al.* Validation of the English version of the UNESP-Botucatu multidimensional composite pain scale for assessing postoperative pain in cats. BMC Vet Res 2013; 9(1): 143.
[http://dx.doi.org/10.1186/1746-6148-9-143] [PMID: 23867090]

[60]   Available from: http://www.animalpain.com.br/en-us/

[61]   Murell J, Hellebrekers LJ. Post-operative Care and Pain Management. In: Kirpensteijn J, Klein WJ, Eds. The Cutting Edge: Basic Operating Skills for the Veterinary Surgeon. London: Roman House Publishers 2006; pp. 222-9.

[62]   Kongara K, Chambers JP, Johnson CB. Effects of tramadol, morphine or their combination in dogs undergoing ovariohysterectomy on peri-operative electroencephalographic responses and post-operative pain. N Z Vet J 2012; 60(2): 129-35.
[http://dx.doi.org/10.1080/00480169.2011.641156] [PMID: 22352930]

[63]   Mastrocinque S, Fantoni DT. A comparison of preoperative tramadol and morphine for the control of early postoperative pain in canine ovariohysterectomy. Vet Anaesth Analg 2003; 30(4): 220-8.
[http://dx.doi.org/10.1046/j.1467-2995.2003.00090.x] [PMID: 12925179]

[64]   Cagnardi P, Villa R, Zonca A, *et al.* Pharmacokinetics, intraoperative effect and postoperative analgesia of tramadol in cats. Res Vet Sci 2011; 90(3): 503-9.
[http://dx.doi.org/10.1016/j.rvsc.2010.07.015] [PMID: 20708759]

[65]   Steagall PVM, Taylor PM, Brondani JT, Luna SPL, Dixon MJ. Antinociceptive effects of tramadol and acepromazine in cats. J Feline Med Surg 2008; 10(1): 24-31.
[http://dx.doi.org/10.1016/j.jfms.2007.06.009] [PMID: 17765590]

[66]   Hernandez SM. Anaesthesia of the dog. In: Clark KW, Trim CM, Hall LW, Eds. Veterinary Anaesthesia. 11th ed. London: Elsevier 2013; pp. 405-98.

[67]   Cremer J, Sum SO, Braun C, Figueiredo J, Rodriguez-Guarin C. Assessment of maxillary and infraorbital nerve blockade for rhinoscopy in sevoflurane anesthetized dogs. Vet Anaesth Analg 2013; 40(4): 432-9.
[http://dx.doi.org/10.1111/vaa.12032] [PMID: 23534860]

[68]   Buback JL, Boothe HW, Carroll GL, Green RW. Comparison of three methods for relief of pain after ear canal ablation in dogs. Vet Surg 1996; 25(5): 380-5.
[http://dx.doi.org/10.1111/j.1532-950X.1996.tb01431.x] [PMID: 8879109]

[69]   Gowan RA, Lingard AE, Johnston L, Stansen W, Brown SA, Malik R. Retrospective case-control study of the effects of long-term dosing with meloxicam on renal function in aged cats with degenerative joint disease. J Feline Med Surg 2011; 13(10): 752-61.
[http://dx.doi.org/10.1016/j.jfms.2011.06.008] [PMID: 21906984]

[70]   Kummeling AK, Klein W. Surgical infections and antimicrobial prophylaxis. In: Kirpensteijn J, Klein WR, Eds. The Cutting Edge: Basic Operating Skills for the Veterinary Surgeon. London: Roman House Publishers 2006; pp. 89-95.

[71]   Cimino Brown D. Wound Infections and Antimicrobial Use. In: Tobias KM, Johnston SA, Eds. Veterinary Surgery Small Animal. St Louis: Elsevier Saunders 2012; pp. 135-9.

[72]   Fennessy BG, Harney M, O'Sullivan MJ, Timon C. Antimicrobial prophylaxis in otorhinolaryngology/head and neck surgery. Clin Otolaryngol 2007; 32(3): 204-7.
[http://dx.doi.org/10.1111/j.1365-2273.2007.01440.x] [PMID: 17550515]

[73]   Rasmussen S, Ovesen T. Insufficient reporting of infections after ear, nose and throat surgery. Dan Med J 2014; 61(1): A4735. [PubMed: 24393585].
[PMID: 24393585]

[74]   Girod DA, McCulloch TM, Tsue TT, Weymuller EA Jr. Risk factors for complications in clean-contaminated head and neck surgical procedures. Head Neck 1995; 17(1): 7-13.
[http://dx.doi.org/10.1002/hed.2880170103] [PMID: 7883554]

[75]   Garnier M, Blayau C, Fulgencio JP, *et al.* (Rational approach of antibioprophylaxis: systematic review in ENT cancer surgery). Ann Fr Anesth Reanim 2013; 32(5): 315-24.
[http://dx.doi.org/10.1016/j.annfar.2013.02.010] [PMID: 23566591]

[76]   Banks C, Beever L, Kaye B, Foo M, Ter Haar G, Rutherford L. Influence of extreme brachycephalic conformation on perioperative complications associated with total ear canal ablation and lateral bulla osteotomy in 242 dogs (2010-2020). Vet Surg. 2023 Jul; 52(5): 661-673.

[77]   Devitt CM, Seim HB III, Willer R, McPherron M, Neely M. Passive drainage *versus* primary closure after total ear canal ablation-lateral bulla osteotomy in dogs: 59 dogs (1985-1995). Vet Surg 1997; 26(3): 210-6.
[http://dx.doi.org/10.1111/j.1532-950X.1997.tb01486.x] [PMID: 9150559]

[78]   Ader PL, Boothe HW. Ventral bulla osteotomy in the cat. JAAHA 1979; 15: 757-62.

[79]   Beever L, Swinbourne F, Priestnall SL, Ter Haar G, Brockman DJ. Surgical management of chronic otitis secondary to craniomandibular osteopathy in three West Highland white terriers. J Small Anim Pract. 2019 Apr;60(4):254-260.

[80]   Pope ER. Feline inflammatory polyps. Semin Vet Med Surg (Small Anim) 1995; 10(2): 87-93. [PubMed: 7652218].
[PMID: 7652218]

[81]   Mercurio A. Complications of upper airway surgery in companion animals. Vet Clin North Am Small Anim Pract 2011; 41(5): 969-80.
[http://dx.doi.org/10.1016/j.cvsm.2011.05.016] [PMID: 21889695]

[82]   Stratton RJ, Elia M. Who benefits from nutritional support: what is the evidence? Eur J Gastroenterol Hepatol 2007; 19(5): 353-8.
[http://dx.doi.org/10.1097/MEG.0b013e32801055c0] [PMID: 17413283]

[83]   Chan DL. Metabolism and Nutritional Needs of Surgical Patients. In: Tobias KM, Johnston SA, Eds. Veterinary Surgery Small Animal. St Louis: Elsevier Saunders 2012; pp. 121-4.

[84]   Corbee RJ, Kerkhoven WJSV. Nutritional support of dogs and cats after surgery or illness. Open J Vet Med 2014; 4(4): 44-57.
[http://dx.doi.org/10.4236/ojvm.2014.44006]

[85]   Available from: http://www.wsava.org/guidelines/global-nutrition-guidelines

[86]   Chan DL. Nutritional requirements of the critically ill patient. Clin Tech Small Anim Pract 2004; 19(1): 1-5.
[http://dx.doi.org/10.1053/S1096-2867(03)00079-3] [PMID: 15025191]

[87]   Biffl WL, Moore EE, Haenel JB. Nutrition support of the trauma patient. Nutrition 2002; 18(11-12): 960-5.
[http://dx.doi.org/10.1016/S0899-9007(02)00987-5] [PMID: 12431718]

[88]   Wray CJ, Mammen JMV, Hasselgren PO. Catabolic response to stress and potential benefits of nutrition support. Nutrition 2002; 18(11-12): 971-7.
[http://dx.doi.org/10.1016/S0899-9007(02)00985-1] [PMID: 12431720]

[89]   Thatcher CD. Nutritional needs of critically ill patients. Compend Contin Educ Vet 1996; 18: 1303-9.

[90]   Biolo G, Toigo G, Ciocchi B, *et al.* Metabolic response to injury and sepsis: changes in protein metabolism. Nutrition 1997; 13(9) (Suppl.): 52S-7S.
        [http://dx.doi.org/10.1016/S0899-9007(97)00206-2] [PMID: 9290110]

[91]   de Aguilar-Nascimento JE, Bicudo-Salomao A, Portari-Filho PE. Optimal timing for the initiation of enteral and parenteral nutrition in critical medical and surgical conditions. Nutrition 2012; 28(9): 840-3.
        [http://dx.doi.org/10.1016/j.nut.2012.01.013] [PMID: 22554957]

[92]   Seike J, Tangoku A, Yuasa Y, Okitsu H, Kawakami Y, Sumitomo M. The effect of nutritional support on the immune function in the acute postoperative period after esophageal cancer surgery: total parenteral nutrition *versus* enteral nutrition. J Med Invest 2011; 58(1,2): 75-80.
        [http://dx.doi.org/10.2152/jmi.58.75] [PMID: 21372490]

[93]   Sachdeva P, Kantor S, Knight LC, Maurer AH, Fisher RS, Parkman HP. Use of a high caloric liquid meal as an alternative to a solid meal for gastric emptying scintigraphy. Dig Dis Sci 2013; 58(7): 2001-6.
        [http://dx.doi.org/10.1007/s10620-013-2665-2] [PMID: 23589143]

[94]   Freeman LM. Cachexia and sarcopenia: emerging syndromes of importance in dogs and cats. J Vet Intern Med 2012; 26(1): 3-17.
        [http://dx.doi.org/10.1111/j.1939-1676.2011.00838.x] [PMID: 22111652]

[95]   Swaim SF. Bandages and topical agents. Vet Clin North Am Small Anim Pract 1990; 20(1): 47-65.
        [http://dx.doi.org/10.1016/S0195-5616(90)50003-0] [PMID: 2405571]

[96]   Grambow Campbell B. Bandages and Drains. In: Tobias KM, Johnston SA, Eds. Veterinary Surgery Small Animal. St Louis: Elsevier Saunders 2012; pp. 221-30.

[97]   Campbell BG. Dressings, bandages, and splints for wound management in dogs and cats. Vet Clin North Am Small Anim Pract 2006; 36(4): 759-91.
        [http://dx.doi.org/10.1016/j.cvsm.2006.03.002] [PMID: 16787787]

[98]   Beckman SL, Henry WB Jr, Cechner P. Total ear canal ablation combining bulla osteotomy and curettage in dogs with chronic otitis externa and media. J Am Vet Med Assoc 1990; 196(1): 84-90.
        [http://dx.doi.org/10.2460/javma.1990.196.01.84] [PMID: 2295558]

[99]   McCarthy RJ. Surgery of the head & neck; total ear canal ablation with lateral bulla osteotomy. In: Lipowitz AJ, Caywood DD, Cann CC, Newton C, Schwartz A, Eds. Complications in Small Animals Surgery. Philadelphia, USA: Lippincott Williams & Wilkins 1996; pp. 118-28.

[100]   Haudequet PH, Gauthier O, Renard E. Total ear canal ablation associated with lateral bulla osteotomy with the help of otoscopy in dogs and cats: Retrospective study of 47 cases. Vet Surg 2006; 35: E1-E20.

[101]   Ahirwar V, Chandrapuria VP, Bhargava MK, Madhu S, Apra S, Shobha J. A comparative study on the surgical management of canine aural haematoma. Indian J Vet Surg 2007; 28: 98-100.

[102]   Kolata RJ. A simple method for treating canine aural haematomas. Canine Pract 1984; 11: 47-50.

[103]   Pope ER. Head and facial wounds in dogs and cats. Vet Clin North Am Small Anim Pract 2006; 36(4): 793-817.
        [http://dx.doi.org/10.1016/j.cvsm.2006.03.001] [PMID: 16787788]

[104]   Swaim SF, Henderson RA. Small Animal Wound Management. Philadelphia, USA: Williams & Wilkins 1997; pp. 133-50.

CHAPTER 21

Analgesia and Pain Management

Sanjiv Kumar[1,*], **Rajesh Kumar**[2] and **Ritesh Patel**[1]

[1] *Department of Veterinary Pathology, Bihar Veterinary College, Patna-14, Bihar, India*

[2] *Department of Veterinary Surgery and Radiology, Bihar Veterinary College, Patna-14, Bihar, India*

Abstract: Inflammation is the main cause of ear pain and it is termed as otitis. Pain is an entirely subjective experience and in animal species the assessment of pain is more challenging compared to humans. The pain should be recognized as early as possible in companion animals and should be treated accordingly, particularly the acute pain. Any types of tissue injury in the animals can be generator of pain. At times pain may occur in the absence of such causative factors also. Understanding the mechanisms of pain is very important for successful prevention and treatment. Assessment of pain is a vital and essential part of patient evaluation not only in individuals presented with a problem of pain but also in routine check-up individuals. Different classes of pharmacological agents are available and they are used for the management of pain. The chapter intends to present a practical and logical approach to the assessment and management of acute and chronic pain in animals.

Keywords: Canine, Otitis, Pain effects, Pain assessment, Pain management.

INTRODUCTION

Otitis is a term used for inflammation of the ear. Inflammation can affect external, middle or inner ear. Otitis externa is inflammation of the external part; Otitis media is inflammation of the middle parts and Otitis interna is inflammation of the inner ear. However, Otitis externa is the most common of these three infections. Pain is an entirely subjective experience and it is not even possible to accurately assess two individuals who are experiencing a common level or depth of pain. In animal species the assessment of pain is more challenging compared to humans [1].Verbal communication regarding the alleviation of pain in human helps in effective selection and use of analgesic agents. In animals, the lack of such verbal communication not only confounds the diagnosis and characterization of the experience of pain but also challenges the evaluation and selection of the

* **Corresponding author Sanjiv Kumar:** Department of Veterinary Pathology, Bihar Veterinary College, Patna-14, Bihar, India; E-mail: mrsanvet@rediffmail.com

analgesic therapy. Pain can diminish well-being of animals due to its aversive nature. Distress arising from the pain sensations, and the secondary effects due to pain may adversely affect the quality of life in the animals. Pain may affect appetite, intestinal function, sleep habits, grooming, and ability to experience normal pleasures, temperament and may

prolong the time needed for recovery from the underlying condition (McMillan, 2003; Gruen, 2022; Demirtas, 2023). Untreated pain may also result in systemic problems like hepatic lipidosis as a result of inappetence and inadequate caloric intake [2].

Pain is generally associated with trauma, either accidental or surgical, in addition, the onset of acute pain may be associated with some infectious diseases. Animals possess the same neuronal pathways and neurotransmitter receptors as humans, so it is expected that their perceptions of painful stimuli will be similar, and this is a basis for the use of laboratory animals for selection of analgesics for human use. Thus, the standard human pain control strategies may be applied to animals. Analgesics, local anesthetics, non-steroidal anti-inflammatory drugs that are commonly used in humans are also effective in animal condition. Differences in metabolism and distribution between various species, as well as financial considerations, may limit their use [3].

TYPES OF PAIN

Any types of tissue injury in the animals can be generator of pain. Sometimes pain may occur in the absence of such causative factors also. Understanding the mechanisms of pain is very important to successful prevention and treatment. Pain can be classified based on its duration of action: acute or chronic and physiologic or pathologic. Neuropathic pain occurs due to damage to the peripheral nervous system or central nervous system. Acute pain has been defined as pain that exists during the period of inflammatory response. It can include nociceptive pain (pain caused by direct activation of special sensory pain neurons) and neuropathic pain [4].

Pain generally arise from inflammation and massive tissue damage where a certain degree of peripheral and central sensitization is associated with extensive injury. This pain can be diffuse, disproportionate of injury potential, debilitative and often continues beyond the resolution of the inflammatory process [5, 6]. Pathologic pain is generally classified into inflammatory pain (somatic or visceral) of either an acute or chronic nature or neuropathic pain [7]. Chronic pain is defined as pain that exists beyond the expected duration. Chronic pain can develop from a variety of conditions and can be present in varying severities in individuals as mild to excruciating, periodic to constant, or uncomfortable to fully debilitating (Table 1).

Table 1. Showing pain scoring systems and their limitations.

Pain Scoring System	Limitation
Simple descriptive scale	• Significant variation between different observations • Absence of selection criteria for behavior record • Low sensitivity • Cannot identify small changes in pain response
Multidimensional scoring system	• Time consuming • No selection criteria for behavior change
Numerical rating scale	• Significant variation in between different observation • Evaluates one aspect of pain severity • Difference in pain severity between categories are undefined and inconsistent • It only evaluates pain experienced in the last 24 hours or average pain intensity"
Visual analogue scale	• Significant variation in between different observation • Sensitivity depends upon observer training and experience
Composite scoring system	• Time consuming • Few validated tool in small animals

THE NEGATIVE EFFECTS OF PAIN

• Pain stimulates inflammation, thus hampers wound healing.

• Pain stimulates sympathetic nerves which leads to decrease in peristaltic movement and therefore, prolongs repair of damages tissues.

• Pain causes patient suffering, which is also stressful for animal owners.

• Pain produces a catabolic state in the animals that may lead to wasting.

• The animal is more susceptible to infection as pain suppress the immune response.

• Pain cause release of stress hormones (Catecholamines), which can cause tachycardia and hypertension, which increase cardiac work and myocardial oxygen consumption [8].

PHYSIOLOGY OF PAIN

The pathway consists of four events: transduction of stimuli, its further transmission, modulation of information and finally the perception of pain.

• Transduction is the process of initially receiving the noxious stimulus like mechanical, chemical, or thermal and rapidly transforming it into electrochemical signal that can travel in the body. Peripheral nociceptors are free nerve endings located throughout the body and can receive this incoming information. This is the first step in the pain processing and it can be inhibited by local anesthetics [9].

• Transmission is the next step in the nociceptive pathway. This occurs *via* first-order neurons or primary afferent fibers. Transmission can be inhibited by local anesthetics like lignocaine used in a nerve block and can be influenced by medication such as alpha-2 adrenergic agonists.

• The modulation of pain involves the changing, inhibiting, or amplifying of the transmission impulses within the spinal cord. Numerous excitatory substances like substance P, glutamate, N-methyl-D-aspartate (NMDA), α-amino-3-hydroxy- 5-methyl4-isoxazolepropionic acid (AMPA), nerve growth factor (NGF), and transient receptor potential cation channel subfamily V member 1 (TrpV-1) promote and amplify incoming pain signals to reach the brain. At the same time, endogenous substances such as serotonin, norepinephrine, G-aminobutyric acid (GABA), cannabinoids, and endorphins attempt to depress the nociceptive response.

• Lastly, pain signals travel from the spinal cord to the brain *via* third-order neurons where perception occurs. This phase can be altered by opioids, alpha-2 adrenergic agonists, ketamine, sedatives, and NSAIDs. Although they do not provide analgesia, inhalant anesthetic agents, benzodiazepines, and phenothiazine's can block the perception of pain.

Pathway of Pain

Sensory neuron → send impluse along axon to spinal cord → thalmus → organise & send signals to sensory cortex → thalmus → organise upcoming information→ send impulse to spinal cord→ motor neuron at the affected site [10].

Etiology of Otitis

• Moisture in excess

• Allergies due to different allergens

• Infections due to bacteria, virus, fungus, parasites *etc.* (Fig. **1**).

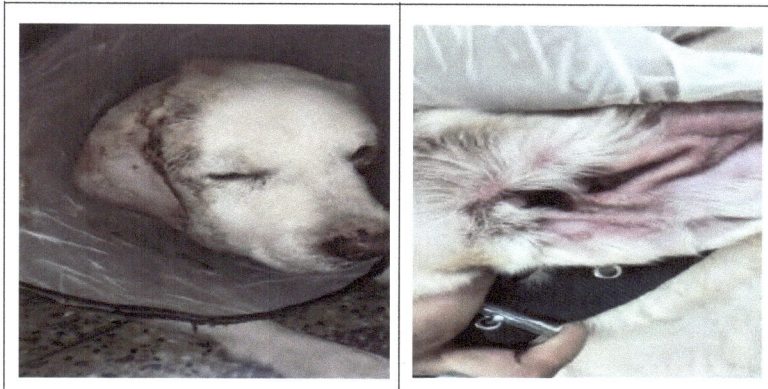

Fig. (1). Showing infection in ear of dogs.

• Tumours

• Wounds and Trauma by foreign bodies

• Haematoma *etc.* (Fig. **2**).

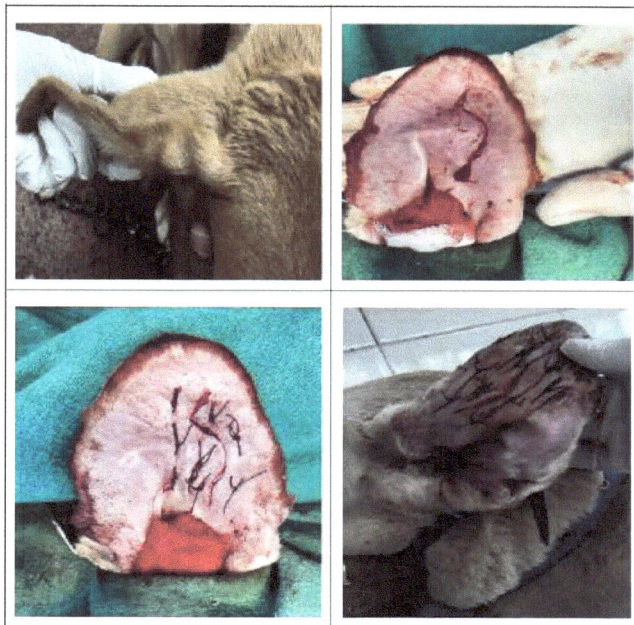

Fig. (2). Showing Haematoma and its surgical treatment in dog.

Symptoms

• Itching and scratching around and in the ears by foot.

• Head shaking, may be vigorous and consistent leading to head tilting (Fig. **3**).

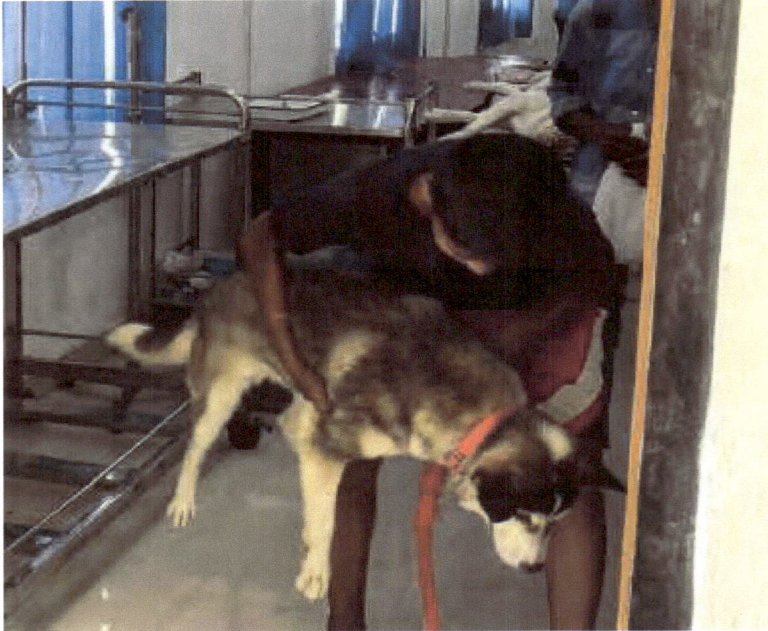

Fig. (3). Dog showing symptoms of tilting of head due to ear infection.

• Edematous and inflamed affected area.

• Foul discharge and smell

• Scabs over the skin due to deposition of inflammatory exudates.

PAIN MANAGEMENT

Effective treatment includes treatment of infection and inflammation by determining the underlying causes. For this cytological examination of the stained smear prepared from ear discharge swab will be useful. Cytological examination will also help to monitor response to therapy. Culture of the swabs from discharges will help in diagnosis of bacterial infections (Fig. **4**).

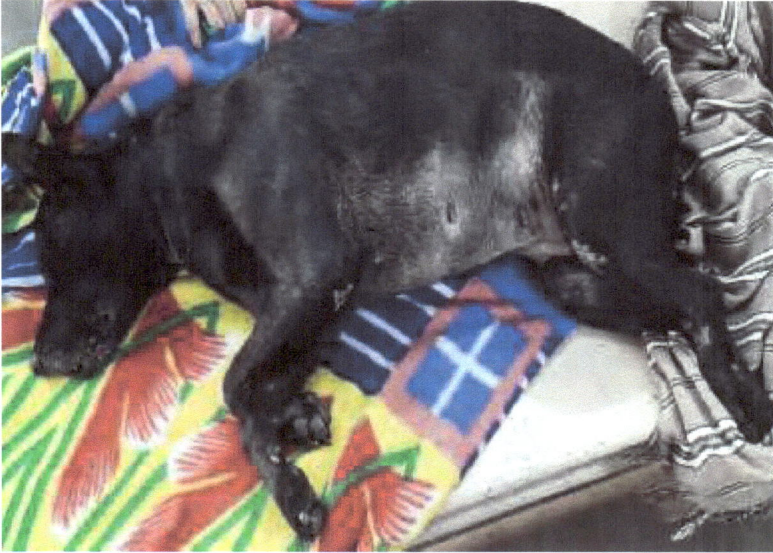

Fig. (4). Death of dog in complicated cases with secondary infections.

Simple ear infections can be cleared up simply at home by simple disinfection and washing of the ear, however, due care should be taken to prevent injury particularly of ear drum (Fig. **5**). Topical therapy is the important treatment for ear infection. A cleanser in combination with an ointment or eardrop can be used. Cleaning ears before topical therapy helps medicine to get deep into the ear canal. Depending on the severity of the infection, an oral medication may be used to help heal the infection. It is better not to use systemic antibiotic therapy for treatment of otitis externa as topical therapy can itself be of good use. Analgesia reflects the selective interruption of the transmission of injury signals. Different classes of pharmacological agents are available and they are used for the management of pain. The selection of these agents from different classes for the management of pain depends on the nature of pain and its threshold value. Surgical treatment in advanced cases may be needed to treat and cure the case (Fig. **6**). Homeopathic medications like Mullein Drops, Belladonna, Pulsatilla, Hepar Sulphuris can also be used alternatively. A follow-up examination must be ensured to confirm complete resolution [11].

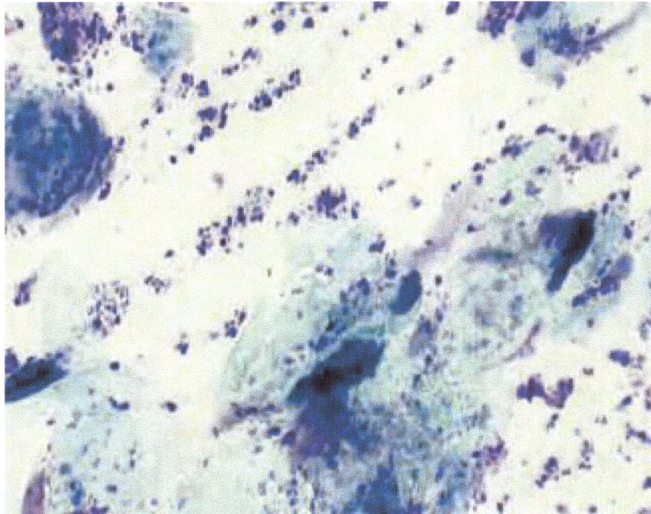

Fig. (5). Showing desquamated epithelial cells along with bacterial population in cytological examination of sample collected from infected ear.

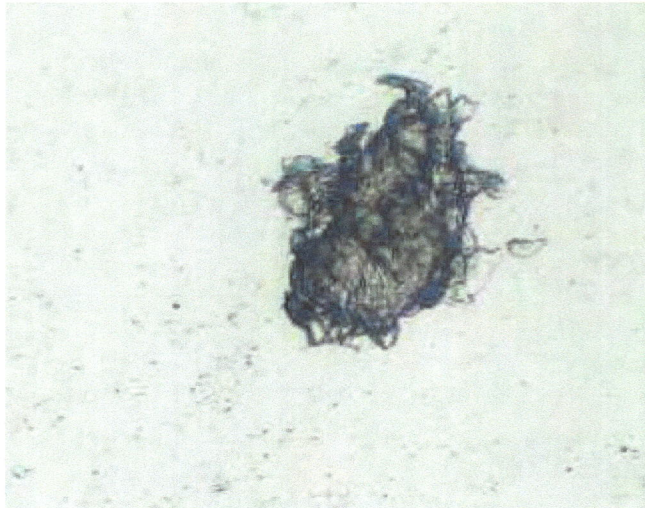

Fig. (6). Showing presence of ectoparasite in cytological examination of samples collected from infected ear.

PHARMACOLOGICAL AGENTS FOR CONTROL OF PAIN

Opioids produce analgesia by their actions on specific opioid receptors namely mu, kappa, and delta. Opioids may occasionally initiate panting in dogs. Respiratory depression is a common feature of opioids, however, if the drugs are used against the pain in incremental doses, it does not produce clinical problems. Pure agonist opioids produce more intensive analgesia than that of partial agonist drugs like pentazocine, nalorphine, butorphanol and buprenorphine [12].

At present buprenorphine, methadone, fentanyl *etc.* are widely used. Tramadol is a non-scheduled opioid with $1/100^{th}$ of the affinity for the receptor as morphine, it has also GABAergic and noradrenergic activity. It is very effective for management of short and medium duration of pain in dog at dose rate of 2-4 mg/kg twice day [13, 14]. Alpha-2 Adrenergic agents are also licensed for use in dogs (Fig. 7).

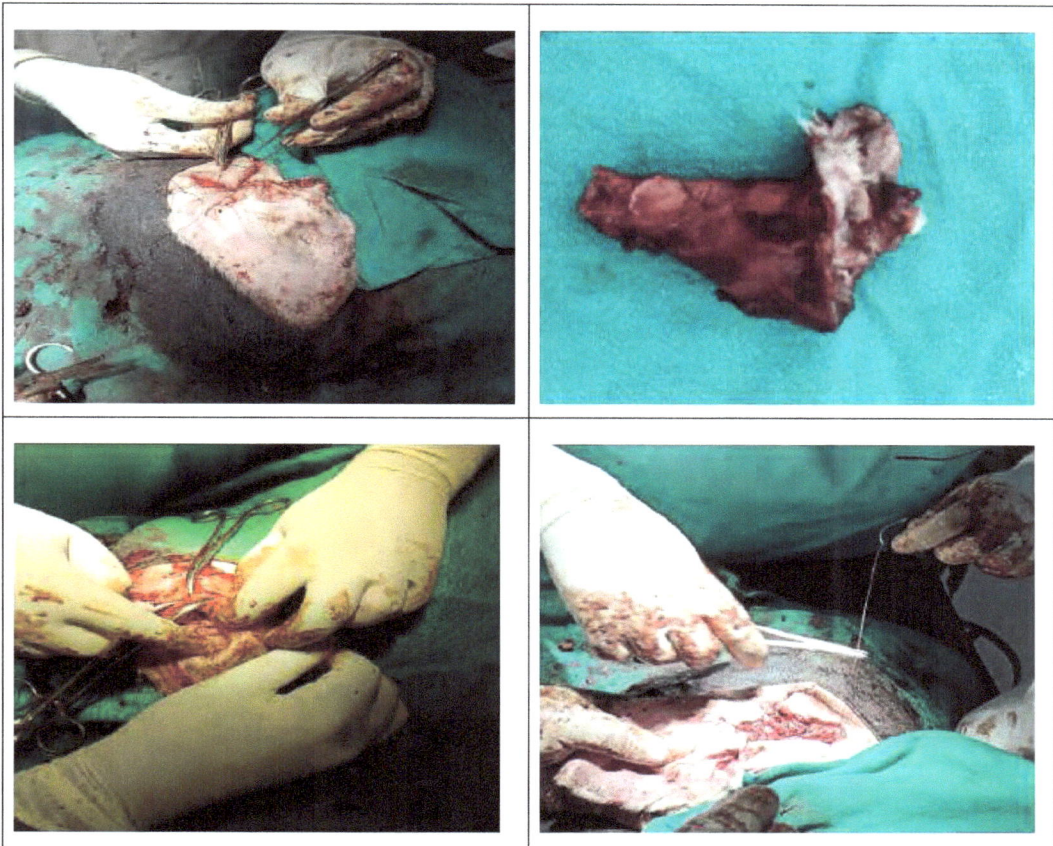

Fig. (7). Showing total ear canal resection by surgical-bulla osteotomy.

Local anesthetics reversibly bind sodium channels and block impulse conduction in nerve fibers. Local anesthetic agents spread more readily on axonal nerve membranes. These nerve membranes are highly lipid in composition and bind sodium channels with greater affinity. They produce desensitization and analgesia of skin surfaces (topical anesthesia), tissues (infiltration and field blocks), and regional structures (conduction anesthesia, IV regional anesthesia) [15].

Non-steroidal anti-inflammatory drugs (NSAIDs) are most commonly used for the relief of both acute and chronic inflammatory pain in veterinary medicine. NSAIDs have excellent therapeutic analgesic activity and an extended duration of action. NSAIDs exert analgesic effect by inhibition of the enzyme cyclooxygenase (COX), needed for algesia. The selective antagonists of COX-2 isoenzyme in canine have less potential to cause gastric ulcer and renal damage and are suitable for long term use. Loading dose of 0.1 mg/kg, followed on day 2-5 by 0.05 mg/kg and thereafter 0.05-0.1 mg/kg should be recommended. Paracetamol is used for chronic pain in dogs and have minimal gastrointestinal effects. Metamizole is a poor anti-inflammatory drug with analgesic and antipyretic properties acting *via* inhibiting cyclo-oxygenase enzymes. NSAIDs are administered in the perioperative period, as well as in other acute and chronic pain like osteoarthritis, cancer, and other inflammatory conditions. When used in chronic pain conditions, it must be used in lowest effective dose. These drugs have relatively long duration of action (12-24 hours) to agonists (xylazine, medetomidine, romifidine) when given systemically.It binds with adrenoceptors that are located in several areas within the spinal cord and brain stem concerned with analgesia and also cause muscle relaxation [14]. More selective COX-2, coxibs, such as firocoxib, mavacoxib, and robenacoxib drugs should be used in smaller pets [12]. Commonly used NSAIDs in dogs include carprofen, meloxicam, deracoxib, and firocoxib.

Corticosteroids

Administration of some corticosteroids has risk for abortion and immune suppression, which must be considered before use. The anti-inflammatory effect of the drug is mediated through prevention of arachidonic acid release and cyclo-oxygenase-2 inhibition [15]. This make corticosteroid potentially suitable in some cases of lameness associated with obvious inflammation.

Adjunctive Drugs

Adjunctive analgesic therapies are agents or techniques that control pain other than the traditional analgesics (opioids, nonsteroidal anti-inflammatory drugs, and local anesthetics). It may be pharmacologic or non-pharmacologic in nature. There are multiple drugs that are considered as adjunct analgesics, including antidepressants [16], NMDA receptor antagonists, and anticonvulsants. Palmitoylethanolamide is considered as dietary management of chronic pain in dogs. Adjunctive analgesics are mainly used to manage pain that is refractory to traditional analgesics and reduce the dose of traditional analgesics in order to lessen side effects. It is also used to treat symptoms other than pain.

CONCLUDING REMARKS

Common symptoms of ear infections of dogs include excessive continuous itching and scratching at the ear with shaking of head, swelling and redness around the ear canal, bad odor with discharge, and scabs or crusted over the skin in the ear. Ear infection leads to pain sensation and dog refuges to hold its ear. Proper ear cleaning and tropical application of antibiotics with steroid can cure the ear of dogs.

REFERENCES

[1]   Mota-Rojas D, Marcet-Rius M, Ogi A, *et al.* Current advances in assessment of dog's emotions, facial expressions, and their use for clinical recognition of pain. Animals (Basel) 2021; 11(11): 3334.
[http://dx.doi.org/10.3390/ani11113334] [PMID: 34828066]

[2]   McMillan FD. A world of hurts—is pain special? J Am Vet Med Assoc 2003; 223(2): 183-6.
[http://dx.doi.org/10.2460/javma.2003.223.183] [PMID: 12875442]

[3]   Gruen ME, Lascelles BDX, Colleran E, *et al.* AAHA Pain management guidelines for dogs and cats. J Am Anim Hosp Assoc 2022; 58(2): 55-76.
[http://dx.doi.org/10.5326/JAAHA-MS-7292] [PMID: 35195712]

[4]   Demirtas A, Atilgan D, Saral B, *et al.* Dog owners' recognition of pain-related behavioral changes in their dogs. J Vet Behav 2023; 62: 39-46.
[http://dx.doi.org/10.1016/j.jveb.2023.02.006]

[5]   Mathews KA. Pain assessment and general approach to management. Vet Clin North Am Small Anim Pract 2000; 30(4): 729-55.
[http://dx.doi.org/10.1016/S0195-5616(08)70004-4] [PMID: 10932822]

[6]   Hellyer P, Rodan I, Brunt J, Downing R, Hagedorn JE, Robertson SA. AAHA/AAFP pain management guidelines for dogs and cats. J Feline Med Surg 2007; 9(6): 466-80.
[http://dx.doi.org/10.1016/j.jfms.2007.09.001] [PMID: 17997339]

[7]   Lamont LA, Tranquilli WJ, Grimm KA. Physiology of Pain. Vet Clin North Am Small Anim Pract 2000; 30(4): 703-728, v.
[http://dx.doi.org/10.1016/S0195-5616(08)70003-2] [PMID: 10932821]

[8]   Julius D. TRP channels and pain. Annu Rev Cell Dev Biol 2013; 29(1): 355-84.
[http://dx.doi.org/10.1146/annurev-cellbio-101011-155833] [PMID: 24099085]

[9]   Melzack R, Coderre TJ, Katz J, Vaccarino AL. Central neuroplasticity and pathological pain. Ann N Y Acad Sci 2001; 933(1): 157-74.
[http://dx.doi.org/10.1111/j.1749-6632.2001.tb05822.x] [PMID: 12000018]

[10]   Patel, N. B. Physiology of pain. Guide to pain management in low-resource settings, 2010, 13.

[11]   Brooks, W. DVM, DABVP: 9/30/2020 (revised) 1/1/2001 (published). Veterinary partner, ear infections (Otitis) in dogs.

[12]   Shaffran N. Pain management: the veterinary technician's perspective. Vet Clin North Am Small Anim Pract 2008; 38(6): 1415-28.
[http://dx.doi.org/10.1016/j.cvsm.2008.07.002] [PMID: 18954690]

[13]   Oliva A, Alvarado A, s A, Avalos I. Clinical pharmacology of tramadol and tapentadol, and their therapeutic efficacy in different models of acute and chronic pain in dogs and cats. J Adv Vet Anim Res 2021; 8(3): 404-22.
[http://dx.doi.org/10.5455/javar.2021.h529] [PMID: 34722739]

[14]   Xiao L, Cheng J, Zhuang Y, *et al.* Botulinum toxin type A reduces hyperalgesia and TRPV1 expression in rats with neuropathic pain. Pain Med 2013; 14(2): 276-86.
[http://dx.doi.org/10.1111/pme.12017] [PMID: 23301515]

[15]   Flecknell PA, Liles JH, Williamson HA. The use of lignocaine-prilocaine local anaesthetic cream for pain-free venepuncture in laboratory animals. Lab Anim 1990; 24(2): 142-6.
[http://dx.doi.org/10.1258/002367790780890121] [PMID: 2366511]

[16]   Wright-Williams SL, Courade JP, Richardson CA, Roughan JV, Flecknell PA. Effects of vasectomy surgery and meloxicam treatment on faecal corticosterone levels and behaviour in two strains of laboratory mouse. Pain 2007; 130(1): 108-18.
[http://dx.doi.org/10.1016/j.pain.2006.11.003] [PMID: 17196337]

CHAPTER 22

Diagnostic Perspectives

Deepak Kumar[1,*] and **Savita Kumari**[2]

[1] *Department of Veterinary Pathology, Bihar Veterinary College, Patna, Bihar Animal Sciences University, Patna-800014, India*

[2] *Department of Veterinary Microbiology, Bihar Veterinary College, Patna, Bihar Animal Sciences University, Patna-800014, India*

Abstract: Dogs can get affected with several ear infections like parasitic ear diseases, bacterial disease, hormonal dysfunction, auto immune diseases as well as otitis externa and treatment may be initiated even in the absence of the diagnostic imaging. Nevertheless, animals suffering from infections like recurrent or severe otitis, and those having pronounced symptoms of para-aural inflammation, discomfort in mouth, vestibular syndrome or facial paralysis, require comprehensive check-up of the middle ear and contiguous structures. The anatomical complication and comparative inaccessibility of these structures is best dealt with diagnostic imaging of radiography, ultrasonography, computed tomography or magnetic resonance imaging technique. This article highlights the applications of certain imaging techniques for ear infections of dogs and cats and exemplifies some of the more representative findings.

Keywords: Canine, Dog, External ear, Inner ear, Middle ear, Otitis.

INTRODUCTION

The ear is an organ of hearing and balance and the external ear consists of the concha, the external auditory meatus along with ceruminous glands. The pinna is designed to capture and carry sound waves through the ear canal to the eardrum. The size and shape of the pinnae can vary with the breeds of dogs and can move their pinnae move independently of each other. When compared to human beings, the ear canal of the dog is much deeper and presents as a better funnel to carry sound to the eardrum. In comparison to the average person, the dog can hear about 4 times better and also detect the sounds at higher frequencies. The middle ear comprises of eardrum and a air-filled chamber containing three small bones named hammer, anvil and stirrup. It also contains two muscles, the oval window, and the Eustachian tube (a thin tube that connects the middle of the ear with the

---

* **Corresponding author Deepak Kumar:** Department of Veterinary Pathology, Bihar Veterinary College, Patna, Bihar Animal Sciences University, Patna-800014, India; E-mail: drdeepakpath@gmail.com

Tanmoy Rana (Ed.)

back of the nose and allows air to flow through middle ear), whereas, the inner ear is a complicated structure responsible for hearing and balance and have cochlea (for hearing) and the vestibular system (for balancing). Ear infections forms one of the most frequently diagnosed complications in dogs and are generally not problematic to detect. Around 20-30% of the dog approach to the pet clinics for some sort of ear infections. The ear disease may comprise of external ear, middle ear or internal ear. There may be many diverse reasons and numerous treatment regimens to effect a cure [1]. Hygiene is one of the major factors both in curing the problem and prevention of recurrence of infection. Ear infections can easily develop as chronic problem. So appropriate therapy during the early course of the disease is of paramount importance along with long term assurance to keep the ears clean. A primary source is an actual provoking agent that causes ear disease by itself without predisposing or perpetuating causes (Fig. **1**).

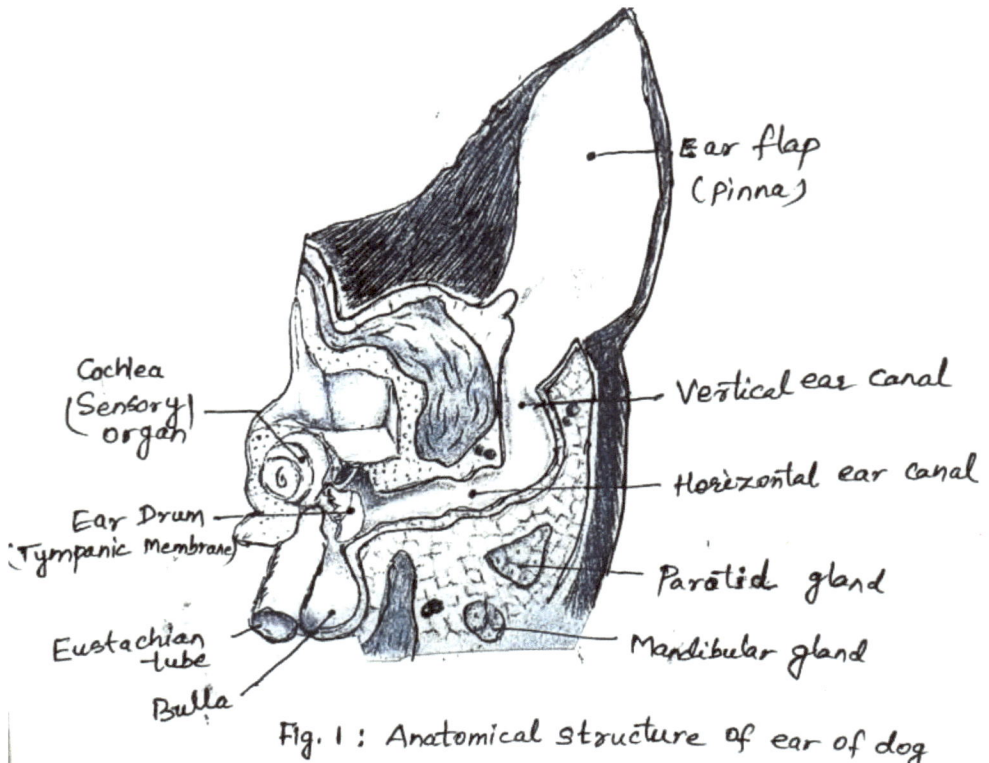

Fig. 1 : Anatomical structure of ear of dog

Fig. (1). Cytology examination of ear swab.

Parasites

Ticks, Ear mites (*Otodectescynotis*), several species of mites, namely *Demodex canis*, *Demodex cati*, *Sarcoptes scabiei*, *Notoedres cati* are some of the common parasites found in ears. Ear mites are frequently observed parasites in the ears and are responsible for more than 50% of all the ear diseases in cats and about 5-10% in dogs. Ear mites can cause itching because of an allergic reaction to them, not because of a small number of mites. Mite infections are very contagious. If your dog is asymptomatic, it is possible that your dog is re-infected with a parasite that causes persistent ear disease. Cats with chronic waxy ears are more likely to have a *Demodex cati* infection [2].

Micro-organisms

In the majority of cases, the bacteria and yeast are the cause and not the main cause of Otitis externa. The bacteria will only become harmful when it reaches the ear with the help of liquid media, such as swimming in unclean water.

Ringworm (Dermatophyte) is one of the most common causes of Earflap disease (pinna). Yeast infection is harmful and can be inoculated in a poor hygiene grooming saloon. Ear canals with warm, moist and dark conditions provides a favorable breeding surface for microbes like bacteria and yeast. Hence, it may be more important to change the conditions of the ear canal than to kill the bacteria or yeast.

Hypersensitivity (Allergies)

Allergy to airborne pollen (atopy), food and contact allergy, for example ear canal atopy, allergic contact dermatitis can be caused by drugs used in the ear [3].

Seborrhea

Seborrheic ailments are common in dogs and indicate a shortcoming of the standard skin maturation cycle along with an overproduction of oils. Cocker spaniels, Irish Setters, Beagles and Basset Hounds are breeds that are prone to seborrhea.

Hormonal Disorders

Hormonal disorders like hypothyroidism is one of the most common cause of hormonal dysfunction in ear infections. Other causes may include Male feminizing syndrome, Sertoli cell tumors and some ovarian imbalances in females.

Nasopharyngeal Polyp

Nasopharyngeal polyps are fleshy, benign masses of connective tissue that arise from the respiratory epithelium of the cat's nasopharynx, Eustachian tube, or tympanic cavity. Young cats get sick more often than older cats.

Auto Immune Diseases

Auto immune diseases comprises of rare diseases and are characterized by malfunction of self- immune system. In this, the immune system harms the normal body tissues and exposes for inflammation and ulcers. This type of reaction can also happen with ears.

Neoplasms: Ceruminous gland adenocarcinoma may be encountered.

Uncommon Causes

Rare causes of otitis externa in dogs or cats include immune-mediated skin infections such as pemphigus, lupus or juvenile cellulitis, drug side effects, erythema multiforme, distemper virus, and traumatic cartilage.

Otitis Externa

Otitis externa is classified as reactive or infectious in nature. Reactive is characterized by an acute erythematous reaction, as well as chronic proliferative and verrucous forms of the disease. In contrast, infectious diseases include acute and chronic infections, chronic ulcerative diseases, and parasitic or fungal infections. Inflammation of the external ear canal, otitis externa, can be seen as a symptom in many diseases. In cats, it is comparatively less common and usually involves ear mites [4]. In most chronic cases, the eardrum ruptures and the infection are expected to spread to the middle ear. This otitis media becomes a source of recurrence of otitis externa (Fig. **2**).

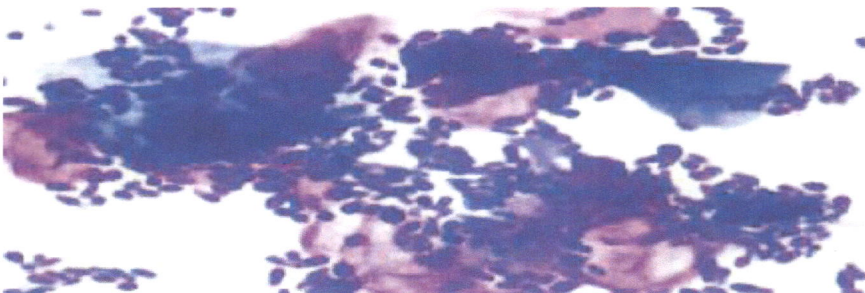

Fig. (2). Cytology examination of ear swab.

Otitis Media (Middle Ear Infection)

The middle ear comprises the area beyond the tympanic membrane, or eardrum. Inflammation and pus accumulation within the tympanic cavity can be challenging to address with local treatments and often serve as a persistent source of infection, potentially leading to the continuation of otitis externa. Middle ear disease usually causes calcification of the ear canal with build-up of debris in the middle ear and bulla. Surgical interventions are needed for the removal of these plugs. Other parts of mouth like temporomandibular joint also can show this inflammatory reaction, involving pain in the mouth while chewing, opening or touching the area. All chronic cases have one or more predisposing factors that prevent the healing of ear disease [5]. Persistent factors may lead to reduced response to treatment, irrespective of underlying predisposing factors or causes. Bacterial infections with *Pseudomonas* spp., *Proteus* spp., *Klebsiella* spp., *Escherichia coli, Staphylococcus intermediusetc.* can cause spontaneous inflammation and damage. Among fungal infections, *Malassezia pachydermatis* is considered as one of the common and persistent fungal infection. This yeast shapes like a sprouted peanut, a bottle, or a footprint and found in about one third of the ears of normal dogs. On the alterations of the microenvironment of the ear, it becomes pathogenic. Chronic inflammation in ear progresses the ear canal mucosa for a series of pathological alterations leading to persistent disease [6]. These changes include enlarged production of ear exudations (oils, waxes, sebum) along with overproduction of skin that folds, thickens and converts to hyperplastic. These changes lead to several difficulties for the animals like narrowing of the ear canal by thickened skin, prevention of effective cleaning and treatment of the ear canal due to excessive skin folds, accumulation of inflammatory debris including dead squamous cells and waxy discharge and also provide conducive environment for the growth of yeast and bacteria. accumulates in the ear canal. Many of these micro-organisms liberate toxins as metabolic derivatives that enhance the inflammatory changes encountered in chronic otitis media.

DIAGNOSIS

Otoscope cones used for the diagnosis should be kept clean and soaked in disinfectant between patients to prevent the spread of disease. Examination of the ear canal should start with the good ear, then the bad ear. Anesthesia may be required for observing the swollen and painful ear. Medicines are used to comfort from the inflammation. Discharge can help to assess the type of infection, *viz.* Black, crumbly discharge indicates mites' infestation. Dark brown, creamy, sweet-smelling discharge with itching represents yeast infection, whereas, red earlobe with little discharge indicates allergy. Golden to brown, creamy discharge (ceramic) are indicative of chronic, allergic, seborrheic or hormonal complications. In bacterial infections generally yellow purulent discharge is seen. Moist, painful, red, ulcerated ear canals with a thin layer of whitish discharge are acute moisture-related bacterial infection resulting from bathing or "swimmer's ear" [7]. To determine the abnormalities of a tympanic membrane, anesthesia is required and it is done with the help of a soft red rubber feeding tube inserted through the otoscope under direct visualization [1]. It is assessed that if the tip of the tube stops moving down the ear canal and the tip is still observable, then the eardrum is still present and if the end of the tube disappeared, the eardrum is missing and the tube has gone into the middle ear. It is difficult to evaluate the normality of the discharge membrane (tympanic membrane) [8]. As a result of the disease, the membrane loses the typical fish-like appearance and appears opaque, thickened and with a coloration of gray or brown. Sometimes a culture and sensitivity of the ear discharge is used to help determine which bacteria or fungi are causing the problem. Because many organisms are commonly grown in culture and some are common residents, this test is not always useful.

CONCLUSION

Otoscopic examination is one of the most prominent tool for determination of ear examination of dogs. Ear cytology before treatment and/or culture and repeat cytology at end of treatment will be beneficial for the better treatment of the diseases. CT/MRI Scan also provides useful diagnosis for the better treatment of the ear infection of dogs. Deep ear flushing with proper tropical application of proper drug are useful for the better efficacy of the treatment regimen.

REFERENCES

[1]   Peterson. S. Manual of Skin diseases of Dog and Cat. 2nd Ed. Blackwell Publication. 2008.

[2]   Scott. D.W., W.H. Miller and C.E. Griffin. Small Animal Dermatology. 6th Ed. Saunders.

[3]   Radostits. O.M., C.C. Gay, K.W. Hinchiliff and P.P. Constable. Veterinary Medicine. A Text Book of the Diseases of cattle, horses, sheep, pigs and goats. 10th Ed. Elsevier Publication, 2007.

[4]   Bischoff MG, Kneller SK. Diagnostic imaging of the canine and feline ear. Vet Clin North Am Small Anim Pract 2004; 34(2): 437-58.
[http://dx.doi.org/10.1016/j.cvsm.2003.10.013] [PMID: 15062618]

[5]   Garosi LS, Dennis R, Schwarz T. Review of diagnostic imaging of ear diseases in the dog and cat. Vet Radiol Ultrasound 2003; 44(2): 137-46.
[http://dx.doi.org/10.1111/j.1740-8261.2003.tb01262.x] [PMID: 12718347]

[6]   Garosi LS, Lamb CR, Targett MP. MRI findings in a dog with otitis media and suspected otitis interna. Vet Rec 2000; 146(17): 501-2.
[http://dx.doi.org/10.1136/vr.146.17.501] [PMID: 10887999]

[7]   Owen MC, Lamb CR, Lu D, Targett MP. Material in the middle ear of dogs having magnetic resonance imaging for investigation of neurologic signs. Vet Radiol Ultrasound 2004; 45(2): 149-55.
[http://dx.doi.org/10.1111/j.1740-8261.2004.04025.x] [PMID: 15072148]

[8]   Trower ND, Gregory SP, Renfrew H, Lamb CR. Evaluation of the canine tympanic membrane by positive contrast ear canalography. Vet Rec 1998; 142(4): 78-81.
[http://dx.doi.org/10.1136/vr.142.4.78] [PMID: 9491526]

Laser Surgery: A Practical Guide

Falguni Mridha[1,*]

[1] *Department of Veterinary Clinical Complex, Faculty of Veterinary & Animal Science, West Bengal University of Veterinary & Animal Sciences, Kolkata-700094, India*

Abstract: Surgeries where light beams are used for different operative procedures by absorbing laser energy and controlling reflection, scatter, and transmission are simply termed laser surgeries. Photobiomodulation (PBM) is extensively known for its therapeutic benefit in the safeguarding and regeneration of tissues by employing visible light to excite biological functions in a non-thermal and non-cytotoxic mode. By using a twenty-watt CO_2 laser with a straightened handpiece and a 1.4 mm metal grip, aural hematoma of canines and felines can be easily done. Lateral ear canal ablation by the Lacroix-Zepp technique is done using CO_2 laser surgery. Special laser-induced thermotherapy (LITT) can be used in interstitial spaced organs where tumor cells need to be treated. In throat cancer, Neodymium Yttrium Al garnet, popularly known as Nd-yag lasers, is used successfully. Some lasers, like argon, only pass the external layer of skin in laser therapy.

Keywords: Ear, Hematoma, Granuloma, Laser, Otitis, Surgery.

INTRODUCTION

A laser beam is an exclusive, potent type of energy for beneficial work on special sense organs like the ear [1]. Laser operation is a kind of operation that exploits a particular light beam as a substitute for appliances used for operative procedures by absorbing laser energy and controlling reflection, scatter, and transmission. Actually, laser means "Light (by) Amplification (by) Stimulated Emission (discharge) Radiation". The laser was initially used in surgery and therapeutics in the early 1960s.

New laser variation persists to have a huge impact on veterinary medicine and operative procedures. A huge portion of its use has been found in the management of different dermatological lesions and remedies in veterinary field conditions [2].

[*] **Corresponding author Falguni Mridha:** Department of Veterinary Clinical Complex, Faculty of Veterinary & Animal Science, West Bengal University of Veterinary & Animal Sciences, Kolkata-700094, India; E-mail: falgunimridha82@gmail.com

Some appropriate uses of lasers are indicated in various kinds of surgeries. The subsequent points are several general suggestions:

• For tumor surgery
• Haemostatic effect by sealing minute blood vessels
• Reduction of swelling by sealing lymph supply
• Decreasing the multiplication of tumor cells
• For treatment of some skin lesions by removing moles, warts, small masses, *etc.* [3] (Fig. **1**).

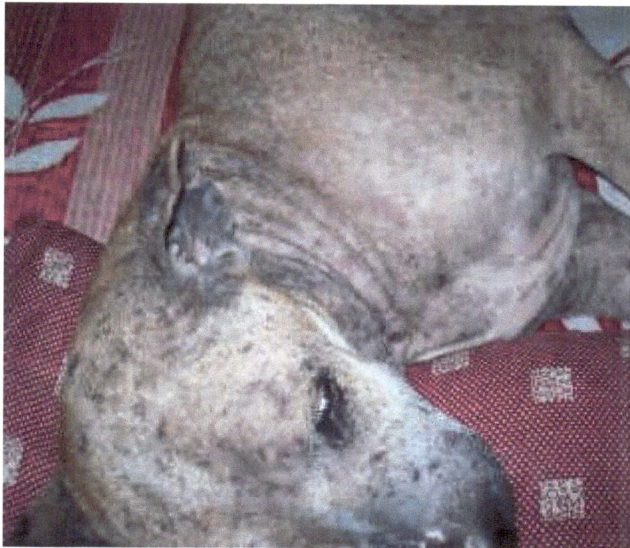

Fig. (1). Dog with otitis interna.

In spite of all the achievements made by scientists and veterinary practitioners, it has been noted that no single surgical procedure can act as an ideal procedure. Though the surgical procedure with which the operator is most familiar is probably the safest, adaptation to other techniques has a good prospect for successful outcomes of surgical maneuvers. Moreover, with variable sizes and shapes of the ear and with variable outcomes in different species or individuals in ear surgery, it is necessary to use the best possible procedure, like laser surgery, as the latest standard procedure in routine application [4] (Fig. **2**).

Photobiomodulation (PBM) is extensively known for its therapeutic potential to safeguard and regenerate tissues. PBM can reduce pain and inflammation and improve cancer management. It stimulates healing and tissue repair. The understanding of how PBM achieves its biological impact has identified endogenous photo acceptors that are widely expressed in special cell types, including skin cells, as well as in the extracellular matrix [5]. PBM is defined by the employment of visible light to excite biological functions in a non-thermal and non-cytotoxic mode. Relationship between light and these photo acceptors have been established to modulate biological processes, including inflammation, the control of bacteria, angiogenesis, and signal transduction pathways that employ transcription factors activating several genes involved in multiple aspects of cell biology [6].

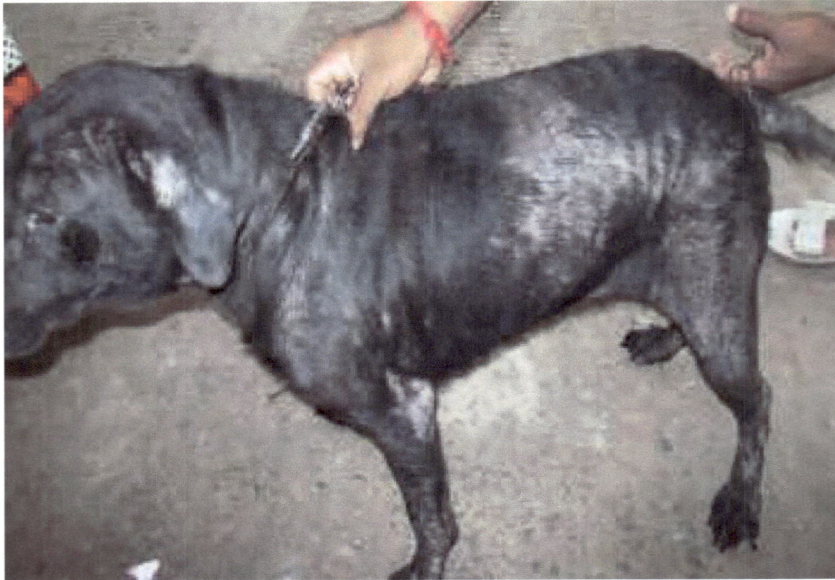

Fig. (2). Dog with granuloma on ear before laser surgery.

Fluorescence biomodulation (FB), a form of PBM that distinctively employs fluorescence light energy (FLE), has been verified to advance the healing of both acute and chronic wounds. A study has established that acute incisional wounds have reduced inflammation, along with more physiologic re-epithelization and collagen remodeling, resulting in better quality and less visible scars [7].

The LED-illuminated gel (*LIG*) consists of two parts: a light source comprised of blue light emitting diodes (LEDs; peak wavelength between 440 and 460 nm) and a topical substrate including chromophores. These FB substrates are generally constructed of silicone- or nylon-based membranes or amorphous hydrogels, optimized for different therapeutic uses and delivery of photonic energy [8] (Fig. 3).

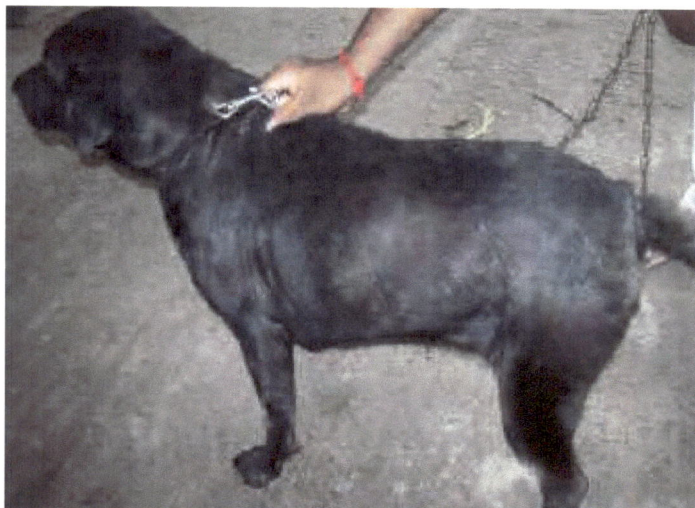

Fig. (3). Dog with granuloma on ear after laser surgery.

In vitro studies assessed the potential mechanisms of action behind FB technology and how they modulate cellular activity in inflammatory dermatological conditions [9]. FB using *LIG* showed a high capacity to increase collagen production in human dermal fibroblasts, attenuate the inflammatory reaction by significantly decreasing the release of tumor necrosis factor-alpha (TNF-α) and interleukin-6 (IL-6) from both human dermal fibroblast and human embryonic kidney cells, and enhance angiogenesis in human aortic endothelial cells, increasing both microvascular tube and branching points formation, similar to vascular endothelial growth factor (VEGF), a potent angiogenic factor [10]. Furthermore, in biopsies from canine chronic deep pyoderma treated with *LIG*, an increase in the number and size of mitochondria occurred, demonstrating an augment in mitochondrial activity.

Recent studies have shown that *LIG* has a beneficial effect on wound healing in canine; an excellent safety profile and efficacy have also been shown in canine pyoderma and otitis [11].

The topical *LIG* is beneficial in the management of canine otitis externa. The use of *LIG* has a positive effect on otitis externa in dogs.

Laser Surgery to Treat Canine Aural Haematoma

An aural hematoma is a blood-filled subcutaneous fluctuant swelling on either side of the ear pinna formed when a traumatic break of the capillaries and severance of the auricular cartilage and skin occurs. It may be unilateral or bilateral. Hematoma can affect both canines and felines, though felines are much less commonly affected. Affected animals usually present with a record of head shaking or strong scratching of the ear. In the early stages, the hematoma is warm to the touch with the skin and may be erythematous, and the pet may experience discomfort [12].

Procedure: Incision and drainage holes are made on the inner surface of the affected ear.

Some sutures are made to obliterate the empty area and assist in adherene of ear cartilage with skin.

Type of anesthesia: Ggeneral anesthesia

Apparatus: Twenty-wattage CO_2 laser with a 0.4 mm stick handpiece with a metallic or golden grip

Laser setting:

Point distance:0.4mm

Electric outlet:8 - 10 W

Light outlet: SP

Technique: The animal is controlled in lateral recumbency, keeping the affected ear upwards. The area is washed from debris with dried powdered material for aseptic surgery. Then, CO_2 laser is applied to obliterate the superficial granulated tissues over the desired area of aural hematoma [13].

A straight hand bit is directed upright over the area for suitable focal space. Drainage openings are made in the middle to permit sufficient draining of hematoma. Blood clots, along with fibrins, are removed by Allis Tissue Forceps and sterile forceps. Simple interrupted sutures are positioned properly. Interrupted suture must penetrate the full thickness of the ear and be tied over the outer side of the affected ear. Branches of the greater auricular artery must be avoided. Interrupted sutures must be tight enough to eliminate the dead area or space of hematoma with a pocket of hematoma cavity [14] (Fig. **4**).

Closure: Light pressure wrap is preferred.

Post-operative evaluation:

1. The ear canal is flushed properly.

2. Proper medication is done at the site of operation.

3. The bandage should be removed after 8 to 10 days according to healing.

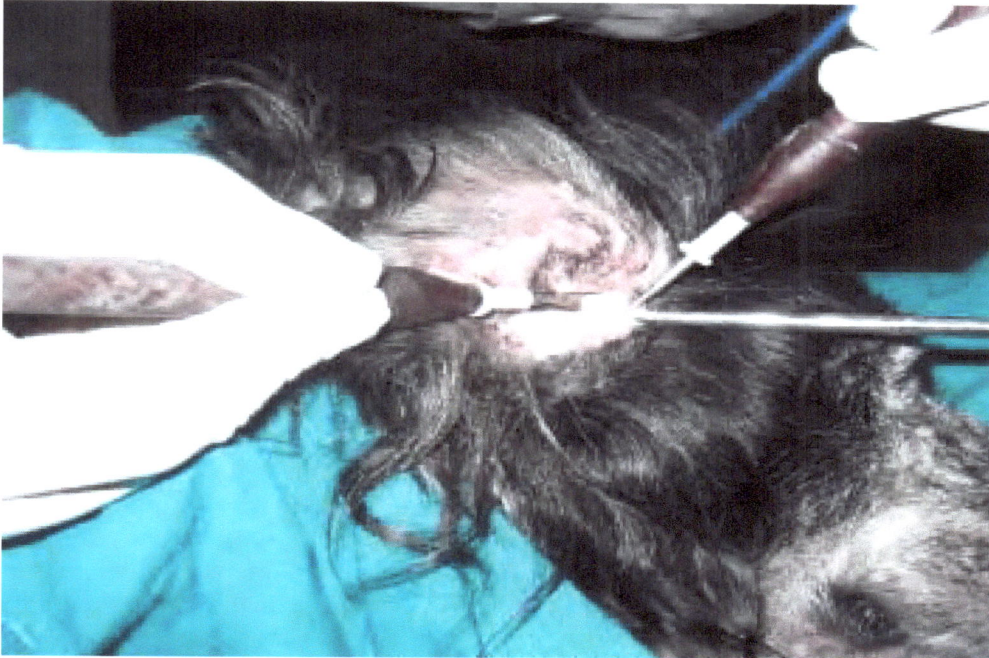

Fig. (4). Dog with ear tumor.

Laser Surgery to Treat Feline Aural Haematoma

An aural hematoma is a blood-filled subcutaneous fluctuant swelling on either side of the ear pinna. Due to trauma, numerous auricular vessels rupture, and blood accumulates between the skin and layer of cartilage [15]. It may be unilateral or bilateral in feline. Hematoma can affect felines, though felines are much less commonly affected. Affected felines usually present with a record of head shaking or strong scratching of the ear. In the early stages, the hematoma is warm to the touch with the skin, may be erythematous, and the pet may experience discomfort. A variety of techniques are used to treat small feline hematomas. Aspiration with an 18G needle is the most common, but due to repeated aspiration, this procedure is not commonly used among felines [16].

Procedure: An incisional drainage hole is made on the medial surface of the ear pinna. Stay sutures are placed to obliterate the dead space and facilitate the readherence of auricular cartilage to the skin.

Anesthesia: General anesthesia

Equipment: 20-watt CO_2 laser with a straight handpiece and a 0.4 mm metal or gold grip

Laser setting:

Point distance:0.4mm

Electric outlet:6-8 W

Light outlet: CW

Technique: The animal is controlled in lateral recumbency, keeping the affected ear upwards. The area is properly cleaned from any debris and dried crusted material for the aseptic surgery. The CO2 laser is applied to remove the overlying granulation tissue at the affected area of the haematoma [17]. The laser handpiece is used for the direction perpendicular to the skin for appropriate focal distance. The drainage holes are kept equidistant from each other to allow adequate and proper drainage for hematoma. The clotted blood and fibrin are also removed by using tissue forceps and hand forceps. Stay sutures in mattress patterns are generally applied for the proper placement. The suture must be applied for the proper penetration of the full thickness of the ear and tied on the convex surface of the ear. Branches of the greater auricular artery should be avoided. Sutures must be sufficient to obliterate dead space and pockets of the hematoma cavity [18].

Closure: Light pressure wrap is preferred.

Post-operative evaluation:

1. The ear canal is flushed properly.

2. Proper medication is done at the site of operation

3. The bandage should be removed after 8 to 10 days according to healing

4. Self-mutilation must be avoided by neck shields and bandaging

Laser surgery for lateral ear canal resection

Due to chronic otitis or otorrhoea, drainage is necessary. The lesions can be surgically removed. Patients usually present with a record of head shaking or strong scratching of the ear.

Procedure: Ablation by Lacroix-Zepp technique.

Anesthesia: General anesthesia

Apparatus: Twenty-wattage CO_2 laser with a stick handpiece, a mechanical scanner with a 3mm pattern scan, and a 1.4 mm metallic grip [19].

Laser setting:

Point distance:0.4mm

Electric outlet:8 - 10 W

Light outlet: SP

Procedure: Ear canal is lavaged. The outer and inner surfaces of the ear flap are arranged for operation. Pinna and skin are prepared for surgery. The proper positioning handpiece should be upright from the affected area to the rostral, along with the caudal border of the skin, with a proper incision given above the upright ear duct exploiting metal tip. The incision is joined vertically to the affected area [20]. The affected covering flaps are carefully picked up and utilized like a lever to pertain pressure over subcutis and perpendicular aural cartilage. The used handpiece is then positioned at right angles to the lateral surface. Then, nearly two-thirds of portions of the auricle flaps are cut out from the surface. Then, the residual portion is positioned in a descending manner, and sutures are carefully placed under the border of lower incision sites, like a "drainboard". The ablation or vaporization of hyperplastic inflammatory tissue is generally done on the inner side of an upright auditory tube [21].

Closure: No bandaging is needed.

Post-operative evaluation:

1. Removal of the suture 7 to 14 days after healing.

2. Antibiotic coverage for 14 days, locally and systematically.

3. Retreatment of the area to avoid recurrence.

Laser Surgery to Treat Aural Granuloma

Single or multiple lesions of canine leproid granuloma syndrome can be found on dorsal ear folds caused by mycobacteria, transmitted by biting insects. It is commonly found in breeds such as Boxer, Doberman Pinschers, *etc.* [15]. The lesions can be surgically removed. It may be unilateral or bilateral. Patients usually present with a record of head shaking or strong scratching of the ear. Surgery: Ablating and vaporizing of granulation tissue over the skin.

Anesthetic protocol: General anesthesia

Apparatus: Twenty-wattage CO_2 laser with a stick handpiece and a 1.4 mm metallic grip.

Laser setting:

Point distance:1.4mm

Electric outlet:15- 20 W

Light outlet: 20Hz at 50msec SP

Procedure: The animal is controlled in lateral recumbency, keeping the affected ear upwards. The area is cleared from dried tissues and foreign bodies for aseptic surgery. Twenty-wattage CO_2 laser is applied to clear the superficial newly formed granulating tissue at the desired area. The granulating tissue removal procedure from the epidermal, dermal layer of skin, as well as the nearer area, must be small for the desired outcome. The resultant char with the laser is flushed to remove dried tissues and foreign bodies. After completion, the remaining char is cleaned from the surface [17].

Closure: Wound management dressing is preferred for 48 hours.

Post-operative evaluation:

4. Ensure complete healing up to 6 weeks.

5. Retreatment of the area to avoid recurrence.

Laser Surgery for Ablation of Skin Mass Over Ear

The following types are some of the special lasers used for ear tumor treatment:

CO_2 Lasers

These types of lasers are capable of taking out a lean coat of tissue, particularly from the face of the skin devoid of the lower layer. This type of laser can be utilized to eliminate coat malignancy and a few premalignant cells [4],

Laser Setting

Point distance: 0.8mm

Electric output:12 to15 W

Beam production: CW

Interstitial Thermotherapy by Laser or LITT

Laser-induced interstitial thermotherapy (LITT) applies lasers to warm definite regions of the patient. Generally, tumors between organs are targeted. The laser particularly enhances the temperature of a tumor. It causes shrinkage, damage, or destruction of malignant cells [9].

Nd-YAG Lasers

Neodymium yttrium aluminum garnet laser is generally known as the Nd-YAG laser. These lasers are able to penetrate the lowest into body parts and cause quick coagulation of blood. Optical fibers are used to carry the laser light to internal organs. In the case of throat cancer, its application can be easily seen.

Ar Laser or Argon Lasers

It passes through the outer layer of tissue or skin. In the treatment of cancer cells, photodynamic therapy or PDT is used by activating chemicals in malignant cells

Recent Advances in Laser Aural Surgery

Lasers have been exploited in ear surgery for decades. CO_2 fiber delivery in laser surgery makes it more effective now. For progress in hearing and elimination of infection, fiber delivery system laser surgery is unique as the procedure is precise.

The next points summarize the application of the laser in current aural surgery [18].

Laser-Assisted Myringotomy

The surgeon utilizes a laser in place of a surgical blade to make an incision in the eardrum to permit proper drainage of infection. Decreased scarring of the surgical site or eardrum may occur compared to a normal procedure. This procedure also requires less time to heal. There is no necessity for a ventilation tube after surgery. Actually, this procedure is best in acute otitis.

Laser Stapedectomy, Laser Ear Surgery in Otosclerosis:

In stapedectomy, the lasers are applied to support the surgery. In this procedure, pathologic fixed bone is generally removed by the rational use of a laser by the surgeon to improve hearing. Less trauma also occurs in this type of surgery. Different kinds of lasers are used, but CO_2 lasers are the best for this type of surgery. The CO_2 fiber delivery system uses a CO2 laser with a flexible handpiece instrument, which is very sound, accurate, and safe for the patient [1, 4].

Chronic Middle Ear Disease and Cholesteatoma

For the elimination of persistently thickened mucosal and scarred tissue in patients with chronic infections in the ear, lasers can be used successfully. Cholesteatoma or infected ear cysts can also be eliminated through laser surgery. Minimal cauterization during cholesteatoma surgery is the most appreciable advantage over routine surgery. Minimal mucosal swelling and minimal bleeding during surgery are other advantages that make the procedure safe to perform with the exact removal of mass [12].

Laser Surgery to Treat Canine Otitis

Laser therapy is useful as it helps **to reduce the inflammation and pain**caused by otitis. In addition, laser therapy presents an antimicrobial effect on some of the microorganisms involved in the pathology, such as *Pseudomonas aeruginosa*. It has also been observed that it helps to speed up the healing procedure and reduces scar tissue in cases of tympanic perforation [8].

Ear Tumor Surgery by Laser

Obliteration of tumors from the middle ear or inner ear can easily be achieved by the CO_2 fiber delivery system. Vascular tumor surgery from the inner ear is very challenging in routine surgery. In the case of laser, bleeding and the duration of surgery both can be reduced dramatically. Acoustic neuromas can be easily operated with CO_2 fiber delivery system laser surgery [7].

CONCLUDING REMARKS

Laser ear surgery has become the new horizon for pet owners for various conditions. The current development with this innovative expertise is now exploited for the enhancement of surgical intervention through a secure technique to perform ear operations and make them more accurate. In addition, it has allowed us to increase the application of the laser in other fields and develop fruitful outcomes with ear operations in these fields.

REFERENCES

[1]   Avci P, Gupta A, Sadasivam M, *et al.* Low-level laser (light) therapy (LLLT) in skin: stimulating, healing, restoring. Semin Cutan Med Surg 2013; 32(1): 41-52. (PMC free article). (PubMed). (Google Scholar).
        [PMID: 24049929]

[2]   Bacon NJ. Pinna and external ear canal. In: Tobias KM, Johnston SA, Eds. Veterinary surgery: small

animal. St. Louis: Elsevier Saunders 2012; pp. 2059-77. (Google Scholar)

[3]   Baxter GD, Liu L, Petrich S, *et al.* Low level laser therapy (Photobiomodulation therapy) for breast cancer-related lymphedema: a systematic review. BMC Cancer 2017; 17(1): 833.
[http://dx.doi.org/10.1186/s12885-017-3852-x] [PMID: 29216916]

[4]   Buback JL, Boothe HW, Carroll GL, Green RW. Comparison of three methods for relief of pain after ear canal ablation in dogs. Vet Surg 1996; 25(5): 380-5.
[http://dx.doi.org/10.1111/j.1532-950X.1996.tb01431.x] [PMID: 8879109]

[5]   Berger N, Eeg PH. Veterinary laser surgery-apractical guide. 2006 blackwell publishing professional, 2121 State Avenue, Ames, Iowa.

[6]   Cole LK. Anatomy and physiology of the canine ear. Vet Dermatol 2010; 21(2): 221-31.
[http://dx.doi.org/10.1111/j.1365-3164.2009.00849.x] [PMID: 20230592]

[7]   Coleman KA, Smeak DD. Complication rates after bilateral *versus* unilateral total ear canal ablation with lateral bulla osteotomy for end-stage inflammatory ear disease in dogs: 79 ears. Vet Surg 2016; 45(5): 659-63.
[http://dx.doi.org/10.1111/vsu.12505] [PMID: 27357276]

[8]   da-Palma-Cruz M, da Silva RF, Monteiro D, *et al.* Photobiomodulation modulates the resolution of inflammation during acute lung injury induced by sepsis. Lasers Med Sci 2019; 34(1): 191-9.
[http://dx.doi.org/10.1007/s10103-018-2688-1] [PMID: 30443882]

[9]   Hamblin MR. Photobiomodulation or low-level laser therapy. J Biophotonics 2016; 9(11-12): 1122-4.
[http://dx.doi.org/10.1002/jbio.201670113] [PMID: 27973730]

[10]   Hamblin MR. Photobiomodulation, photomedicine, and laser surgery: a new leap forward into the light for the 21st century. Photomed Laser Surg 2018; 36(8): 395-6.
[http://dx.doi.org/10.1089/pho.2018.29011.mrh] [PMID: 30089079]

[11]   Hill PB, Lo A, Eden CAN, *et al.* Survey of the prevalence, diagnosis and treatment of dermatological conditions in small animals in general practice. Vet Rec 2006; 158(16): 533-9.
[http://dx.doi.org/10.1136/vr.158.16.533] [PMID: 16632525]

[12]   Jacobson LS. Diagnosis and medical treatment of otitis externa in the dog and cat : review article. J S Afr Vet Assoc 2002; 73(4): 162-70.
[http://dx.doi.org/10.4102/jsava.v73i4.581] [PMID: 12665128]

[13]   Kulkarni S, Meer M, George R. Efficacy of photobiomodulation on accelerating bone healing after tooth extraction: a systematic review. Lasers Med Sci 2019; 34(4): 685-92.
[http://dx.doi.org/10.1007/s10103-018-2641-3] [PMID: 30311084]

[14]   Langella LG, Casalechi HL, Tomazoni SS, *et al.* Photobiomodulation therapy (PBMT) on acute pain and inflammation in patients who underwent total hip arthroplasty—a randomized, triple-blind, placebo-controlled clinical trial. Lasers Med Sci 2018; 33(9): 1933-40.
[http://dx.doi.org/10.1007/s10103-018-2558-x] [PMID: 29909435]

[15]   Ngo J, Taminiau B, Fall PA, Daube G, Fontaine J. Ear canal microbiota – a comparison between healthy dogs and atopic dogs without clinical signs of otitis externa. Vet Dermatol 2018; 29(5): 425-e140.
[http://dx.doi.org/10.1111/vde.12674] [PMID: 30084115]

[16]   Noli C, Sartori R, Cena T. Impact of a terbinafine–florfenicol–betamethasone acetate otic gel on the quality of life of dogs with acute otitis externa and their owners. Vet Dermatol 2017; 28(4): 386-e90.
[http://dx.doi.org/10.1111/vde.12433] [PMID: 28295766]

[17]   Oliveira LC, Leite CA, Brilhante RS, Carvalho CBM. Comparative study of the microbial profile from bilateral canine otitis externa. Can Vet J 2008; 49(8): 785-8. (PMC free article). (PubMed). (Google Scholar).
[PMID: 18978972]

[18]   Rosser EJ Jr. Causes of otitis externa. Vet Clin North Am Small Anim Pract 2004; 34(2): 459-68.
[http://dx.doi.org/10.1016/j.cvsm.2003.10.006] [PMID: 15062619]

[19]   Saridomichelakis MN, Farmaki R, Leontides LS, Koutinas AF. Aetiology of canine otitis externa: a retrospective study of 100 cases. Vet Dermatol 2007; 18(5): 341-7.
[http://dx.doi.org/10.1111/j.1365-3164.2007.00619.x] [PMID: 17845622]

[20]   Scapagnini G, Marchegiani A, Rossi G, *et al.* Management of all three phases of wound healing through the induction of fluorescence biomodulation using fluorescence light energy. Proceedings volume 10863 of SPIE (Society of Photo-optical Instrumentation Engineers), Photonic diagnosis and treatment of infections and inflammatory diseases II, 108630W, 7 March 2019, San Francisco, California, US.
[http://dx.doi.org/10.1117/12.2508066]

[21]   Wolfe TM, Bateman SW, Cole LK, Smeak DD. Evaluation of a local anesthetic delivery system for the postoperative analgesic management of canine total ear canal ablation – a randomized, controlled, double-blinded study. Vet Anaesth Analg 2006; 33(5): 328-39.
[http://dx.doi.org/10.1111/j.1467-2995.2005.00272.x] [PMID: 16916355]

CHAPTER 24

Prevention and Control Strategy

Bhavanam Sudhakara Reddy[1,*], **Sirigireddy Sivajothi**[1] and **Kambala Swetha**[1]

[1] *College of Veterinary Science-Proddatur, Sri Venkateswara Veterinary University, Andhra Pradesh, India*

Abstract: Ear diseases are considered as one of the common disorders in small animal practice and the number one cause for veterinary visits among dog owners. Commonly reported clinical signs in dogs with ear disease were scratching or pawing at the ear, otitis, head tilting, head shaking, strong and unpleasant odour from the ears, abnormal ear discharges and pain evincing while palpation of ears. These ear infections can cause significant discomfort to the dogs as well as occurrence of recurrence. The first step in the control and prevention of ear infections is to identify the primary and/ or perpetuating factors. Followed by regular cleaning of the ears to facilitate the removal of debris, exudates, microbes and foreign bodies. In already existing ear diseases, to prevent further extension of the infection systemic and topical antimicrobial therapy is advised. Selection of the antibiotic must be based on the antibiotic sensitivity test in recurrent ear diseases, with the required dosage and duration of therapy. Most of the ear diseases, the combination of systemic and topical antimicrobial therapy along with steroids is advised to control the inflammation of the ear canal. In the case of ectoparasitic infestations, regular control measures are to be taken care of further by utilizing localized or generalized ectoparasiticidal drugs. Dogs who were allergic to grasses, trees and weeds should not allow for swimming in ponds and as a preventive measure always ear plugs should be applied while swimming and cleaning the ears with ear cleansers which will contain acetic acid. Dogs with *Malassezia pachydermatis* are more prone to the development of ear infections specifically dog breeds with high skin fold packets and it can be prevented by regular bathing with medicated shampoo containing the ketoconazole and chlorhexidine. Early diagnosis of adenocarcinoma, sebaceous gland tumour and basal cell tumour should be carried out by cytology and diagnostic imaging techniques. To maintain the immunity of the skin, nutrition supplements like omega-3 fatty acids, polyunsaturated fatty acids, linoleic acid, eicosapentaenoic acid and docosahexaenoic acid are advised.. To help prevent the recurrence of dermatological or ear diseases, it is recommended to provide food containing probiotics, essential amino acids, fatty acids, magnesium, pantothenic acid, pyridoxine, biotin and zinc. These nutrients play important roles in maintaining healthy skin and ear function, supporting the immune system, and reducing the likelihood of recurrent issues. Dogs with a history of atopic dermatitis can be offered a hypo-allergic diet and immunotherapy to prevent further development of ear infections. Breeds with

---

* **Corresponding author Bhavanam Sudhakara Reddy:** College of Veterinary Science-Proddatur, Sri Venkateswara Veterinary University, Andhra Pradesh, India; E-mail: bhavanmvet@gmail.com

Tanmoy Rana (Ed.)

floppy ears are more prone to ear diseases because of the presence of predisposing factors like floppy ears, hairy ear canal openings, perpetuating factors like easily inflammable ear canal glands and other common primary factors like high moisture and humidity. It can be controlled by frequent ear examinations, drying of the ears and early diagnosis of other dermatological issues. Dogs with endocrine disorders like hyperadrenocorticism and hypothyroidism can develop ear diseases more frequently than other dogs because these diseases can alter the dog's immunity, causing the thinning of the skin which is more susceptible to skin and ear infections.

Keywords: Control, Diagnosis, Ear diseases, Etiology, Prevention, Signs, Treatment.

INTRODUCTION

Ear diseases are considered one of the common disorders in small animal practice and they are the number one cause of veterinary visits among dog owners. Common clinical signs in dogs with ear diseases were: A. Scratching or pawing at the ear. During the beginning of the infection, dogs will exhibit this activity frequently and act as a resource for the development of secondary lesions. It is because of chronic itching around the ear or head region. During chronicity it may worse with time becomes as ear complications erythematic, oedema and pinnal disorders and otitis. In most of cases itchy ear is self-limiting and if it continues as such becomes otitis [1, 2]. B. Head tilting and shaking. Head shaking or tilting considered as one of the common clinical presentation to the clinic by the pets with ear infections and it is due to pressure building up in the ears from the infection as a result head tilting is noticed to relieve the pressure. Noticing only head tilt and head shaking is indicative of neurological problems in dogs which require further investigation to rule out the other causes [3]. C. Loss of balance. During chronic ear infections, dogs loss the balance may cause gait abnormalities and difficulty in going up and down stairs. D. Strong odour from the ears. The presence of an unpleasant and strong odour from the ears is indicative of otitis which originated from the ear exudates mixed with the bacteria [4, 5]. Swelling and redness of the ears. During the severity of infection from mild to moderate stage it can cause swelling of the ears and becoming red in colour which can be appreciated by physical examination and pain while handling [9, 10]. 6. Oozing of discharges from the ear. Oozing of the pus discharges from ears is indicative of infection and colour may from green, white, or brown (Fig. **1**) [5, 6].

Other documented signs of otitis were narrowing of the ear canal, development of the ear polyps, or loss of tympanic membrane integrity. If these conditions were not treated properly it leads to development of chronic pain and deafness.

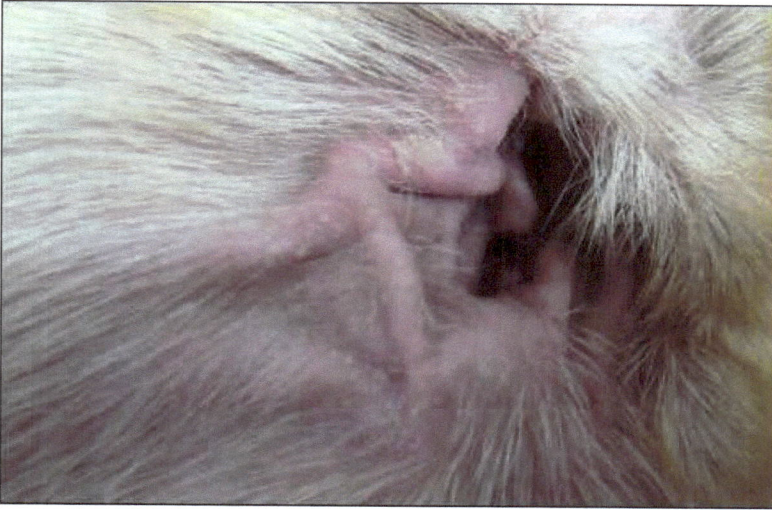

Fig. (1). Dog with otitis and exfoliations due to atopy.

Prevention and control of ear diseases can be carried out by:

- Identification of primary/predisposing factors and addressing the issue.
- Systemic therapy and topical therapy.
- Management of ectoparasites.
- To prevent swimmer's ear.
- Management of *Malassezia* infection.
- Management of neoplasia.
- Ear health supplementations.
- Management of allergic conditions.
- Removal of foreign bodies.
- Early intervention of hormonal disorders.
- Care of floppy ears breeds.

Identification of Primary/Predisposing Factors

Recurrent ear infections are very common in small animal practice. The first step in the prevention of ear infections is to identify the primary/perpetuating factors. In dogs, ear canals are combination of two types of secretory glands: sebaceous and ceruminous glands. During the process of epithelial cell migration, accumulated cerumen and debris transported from the tympanic membrane to the external ear canal which facilitates the self-cleaning process, helping eliminate the underlying causes of ear infections [7]. Ear diseases are caused by primary factors, perpetuating factors, predisposing factors and secondary complications. All the factors responsible for the development of the inflammation of the ear canal cause otitis and/or other ear diseases and provide the environment favourable for the growth of commensal organisms, principally *Malassezia* and *Staphylococcus* spp [8]. Further, it causes erythema, oedema, soft tissue swelling, and hyperplasia of epithelia and glandular structures [9, 10]. Ear examinations are carried out by the Otoscopy to visualize the ear canal, tympanic membranes and the presence of any predisposing factors for the development of ear diseases (Fig. **2**). Cytological examination of the ear discharges will provide the involvement of bacteria, yeast and type of neutrophils in the exudates (Fig. **3**). Before ear examination, cleaning of ears is helpful to visualize the ear canal, to eliminate the microbes, foreign bodies. Ear cleansers provide the beneficial affects like cerumenolytic, antimicrobial, astringent, and acidifying properties to prevent further accumulation of microbes [11, 12]. It is suggested that predisposition may be inherently affected by the ear type and amount of hair in the ear canal, amount of humidity or temperature within the ear canal [13, 14]. The list of different primary and secondary causes for ear infections are mentioned in Table **1**.

Systemic Therapy

Appropriate antimicrobial therapy can be carried out by both systemic and topical antimicrobials. Systemic antimicrobial therapy includes antibiotic therapy, antifungal therapy along with anti-inflammatory therapy.

Antibiotic Therapy

The selection of systemic antimicrobial agents must be based on the results of microbial culture and antibiotic sensitivity test of samples received from the ear canal and it may vary with the cytological findings of ear discharges [15].

Antifungal Therapy

Malassezia is considering the most common isolates from apparently healthy and dogs with ear disease. When dogs with ear disorders, assessment of intensity of the yeasts are important in different locations of the body as well as ears. Ketoconazole, fluconazole, terbinafine, iotraconazole are more commonly utilized antifungal agents in treating with yeast infection [16, 17].

Anti-inflammatory Therapy

These drugs are available in dogs with ear canal stenosis or severe inflammation to reduce the inflammation of the ear canal associated with primary ear diseases or secondary infections [18, 19].

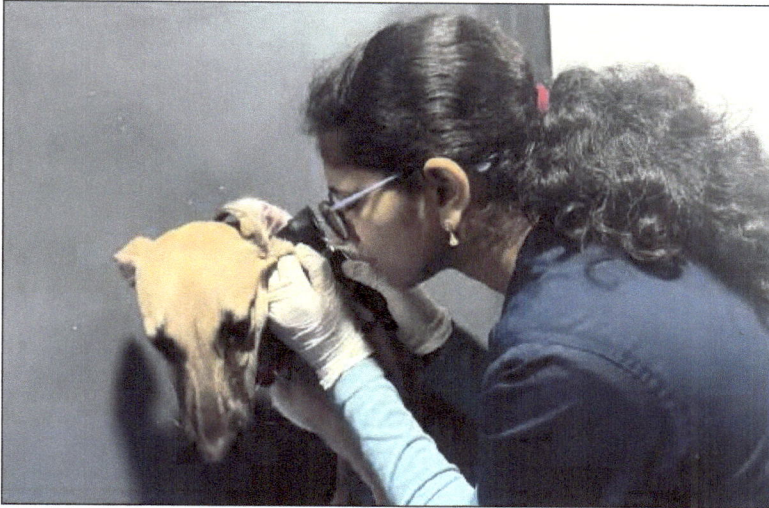

Fig. (2). Regular otoscopic examination of ears.

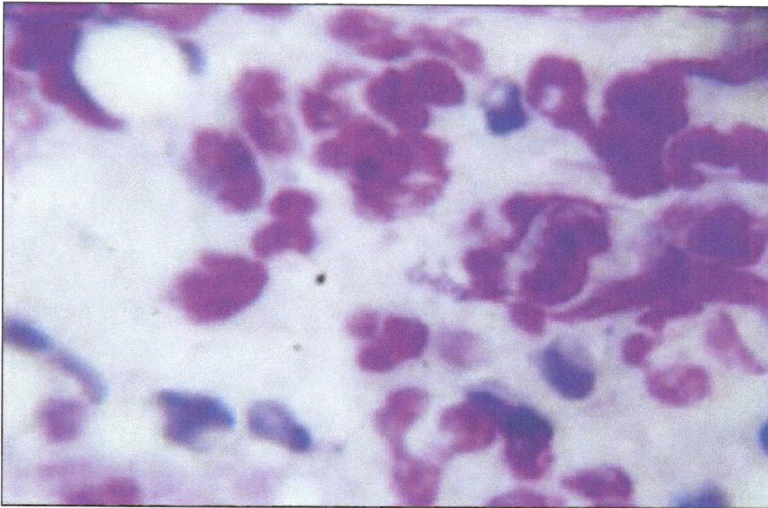

Fig. (3). Stained slide impression smears with neutrophils and *cocci* (1000x).

Table 1. Different etiological factors associated with ear diseases in dogs.

Cause	Examples
Primary causes of ear diseases in dogs	
Ecto parasites	Mites, Ticks, Lice
Fungal infections	*Microsporum canis, Trichophyton mentagrophytes*
Hypersensitivity	Environmental allergy, food allergy, flea allergy
Endocrine disorders	Hypothyroidism, hypercortisolism, sex hormone imbalances

(Table 1) cont.....

Cause	Examples
Primary causes of ear diseases in dogs	
Foreign bodies	Plant material, hair, sand, hardened medication
Glandular disorders	Ceruminous, sebaceous, apocrine gland hyperplasias; ceruminous cystomatosis
Tumours	Ceruminous gland adenoma, basal cell tumour, papilloma
Non – neoplastic growths	Inflammatory polyps
Secondary causes of ear diseases in dogs	
Bacteria	*Staphylococcus* and *Pseudomonas species*
Yeast	*Malassezia pachydermatis, Candida albicans*
Predisposing factors which increase the risk for development of ear diseases in dogs	
Conformation	Pendulous pinna, congenital stenosis, excessive hairs in ear canal
Breed disposition	Cocker spaniel, German shepherd, poodle, basset hound
Excessive moisture	Swimmer's ear
Immunosuppression	Medications, immunosuppressive diseases
Overtreatment	Excessive cleaning and moisture, physical trauma
Perpetuating factors responsible for ear diseases	
Progressive pathologic changes	Altered epithelial migration, proliferation, hyperplasia, stenosis, and calcification

Topical Therapy

Active ingredients in topical therapy of dogs with ear disease can be divided into the following categories:

• **Corticosteroids:** Corticosteroids are advised to reduce the pain, inflammation, and oedema of ear canal and associated structures. It is highly advisable as a solo therapy in managing allergic otitis. In cases of bacterial or fungal infection, it will be combined with antibiotics or antifungal agents to provide rapid relief of pain and uncomfortable symptoms. Hydrocortisone can potentially be used for chronic recurrent allergic otitis but is not usually beneficial in acute, exudative, or proliferative otitis [20, 21].

• **Antibiotics:** Choosing antibiotic therapy depends on the cytological examination of ear discharges and by carryout antibiotic sensitivity test. Amino glycosides are effective against a wide variety of gram-positive and gram-negative bacteria and consider first-line antibiotic selections and fluoroquinolones are broad spectrum of activity and consider second-line antibiotics.

• **Tris-EDTA:** Tris-EDTA is useful to increase the cell membrane permeability of the gram negative bacteria causing the weakening of it and usually combines with antibiotics when treating gram-negative bacterial infections.

• **Antifungal Medications:** Topical antifungal medications advised to treat the yeast infection and commonly used topical antifungal agents were miconazole, ketoconazole and clotrimazole.

• **Others:** Regular utilization of preparations containing acetic acid can be effectively used to prevent the recurrence of ear infections (Fig. **4**) [21]. The list of topical medications were mentioned in Table **2**.

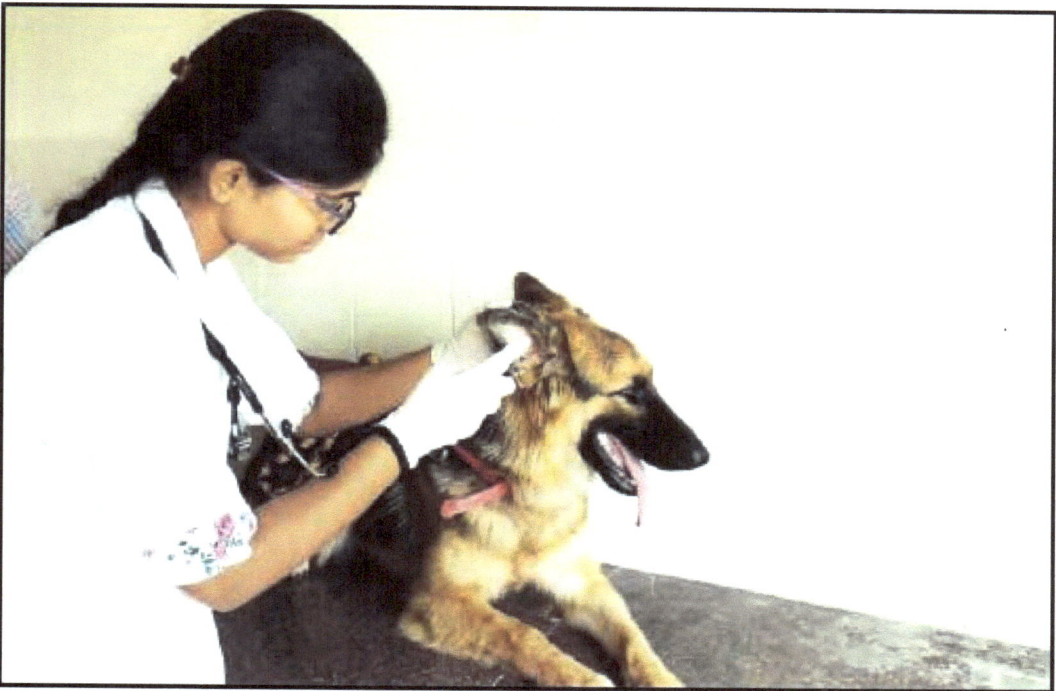

Fig. (4). Frequent topical application of ear medications.

Table 2. Topical medications employed for treating and preventing ear diseases.

Generic Name	Dose	Frequency	Description
Fluocinolone 0.01% DMSO 60%	4-6 drops	q12h initially, q48-72h maintenance	Potent corticosteroid anti-inflammatory
Hydrocortisone 1.0%	2-12 drops	q12h initially, q24-48h maintenance	Mild corticosteroid anti-inflammatory

(Table 2) cont.....

Generic Name	Dose	Frequency	Description
Hydrocortisone 1.0%, lactic acid	5-10 drops	q12h for 5 days	Mild corticosteroid anti-inflammatory, drying agent
Hydrocortisone 0.5%, sulfur 2%. acetic acid 2.5%	2-12 drops	q12-24h initially, q24-48h maintenance	Mild corticosteroid anti-inflammatory, astringent, germicidal
Chlorhexidine 2%	Dilute 1:4 in water	As necessary	Antibacterial & antifungal activity
Chlorhexidine 1.5%	Dilute 2% in propylene glycol	q12 h	Antibacterial & antifungal activity
Povidone –iodine 10%	Dilute 1:10-1:50 in water	As necessary	Antibacterial activity
Polyhydroxidine iodine 0.5%	Dilute 1:1-1:5 in water	As necessary q12 h once weekly	Antibacterial activity
Acetic acid 5%	Dilute 1:1-1:3 in water	As necessary q12h-24h for *Pseudomonas*	Antibacterial activity, lowers ear canal pH
Neomycin 0.25%, triamcinolone 0.1%, thiabendazole 4%	2-12 drops depending on ear size	q12h up to 7 days	Antibacterial & antifungal activity, parasiticide (mites), moderate corticosteroid anti-inflammatory
Neomycin 0.25%, triamcinolone 0.1%, nystatin 100,000 U/ml	2-12 drops depending on ear size	q12h to once weekly	Antibacterial & antifungal activity, moderate corticosteroid anti-inflammatory
Chloramphenicol 0.42% prednisone 0.17%, tetracaine2%, squalene	2-12 drops depending on ear size	q12h up to 7 days	Antibacterial activity, mild corticosteroid anti-inflammatory
Gentamicin 0.3%, betamethasone valerate 0.1%	2-12 drops depending on ear size	q12h for 7 to 14 days	Antibacterial activity, potent corticosteroid anti-inflammatory
Gentamicin 0.3%, betamethasone 0.1%, Clotrimazole 0.1%	2-12 drops depending on ear size	q12h for 7 days	Antibacterial & antifungal activity, potent corticosteroid anti-inflammatory
Gentamicin 0.3%, betamethasone valerate 0.1%, acetic acid 2.5%	2-12 drops depending on ear size	q12h for 7 to 14 days	Antibacterial activity, potent corticosteroid anti-inflammatory
Polymixin B 10,000 lU/ml, hydrocortisone 0.5%	2-12 drops depending on ear size	q12h	Antibacterial activity, mild corticosteroid anti-inflammatory,
Enrofloxacin 0.5%, silver sulfadiazine 1%	2-12 drops depending on ear size	q12h for 7 to 14 days	Antibacterial activity

(Table 2) cont.....

Generic Name	Dose	Frequency	Description
Isopropyl alcohol 90%, Boricacid 2%	Fill ear canal	As necessary	Drying agent
Acetic acid 2%, aluminum acetate	Fill ear canal	q12-48h	Drying agent, Antibacterial activity, Lowers ear canal pH Antibacterial & antifungal activity
Silver sulfadiazine	Dilute 1:1 with water, 1g powder in 100ml water	q12h for 14 days	Antibacterial & antifungal activity
Tris EDTA ± gentamicin 0.03%	2-12 drops depending on ear size	q12h for 14 days	1L distilled water, 1.2g Tris EDTA, 1ml glacial acetic acid; Antibacterial activity
Miconazol 1%; ± dexamethasone phosphate (4 mg /ml)	2-12 drops depending on ear size	q12-24h	Antifungal activity
Ivermectin 0.01%	0.5 ml per ear	Once	Parasiticide (mites)
Pyrethrins 0.15%, piperonyl butoxide 1.5%	2-12 drops depending on ear size	Twice at 7-day interval	Parasiticide (mites)

Management of Ectoparasites

Dogs with ectoparasitic infestations like ticks, mites and lice can cause ear diseases with severe aural irritation and discomfort. Parasitic infestations are small, motile appeared as white spots in the external ear canal; infestation is typically accompanied by a brown, waxy discharge (Figs. **5** and **6**) [21, 22]. During the early stage of infection, clinical signs are non-specific but few exhibit pruritus with ear scratching, rubbing and self-inflicted trauma and erythematous pinna. Diagnosis of the ectoparasites is done by direct visualization of ticks or lice and by visualization of the mites in ear discharges under microscopy. Management of ectoparasites is carried out by local administration of ear drops with acaricidal activity and/or with a systemic spot-on/oral product with frequent monitoring for re-infections [23, 24]. The available topical parasiticidal drugs were amitraz, rotenone and selamectin [25, 26]. Thorough cleaning of the environment and pet equipment, treatment of all household pets and whole-body therapy is necessary for a complete treatment [27, 28].

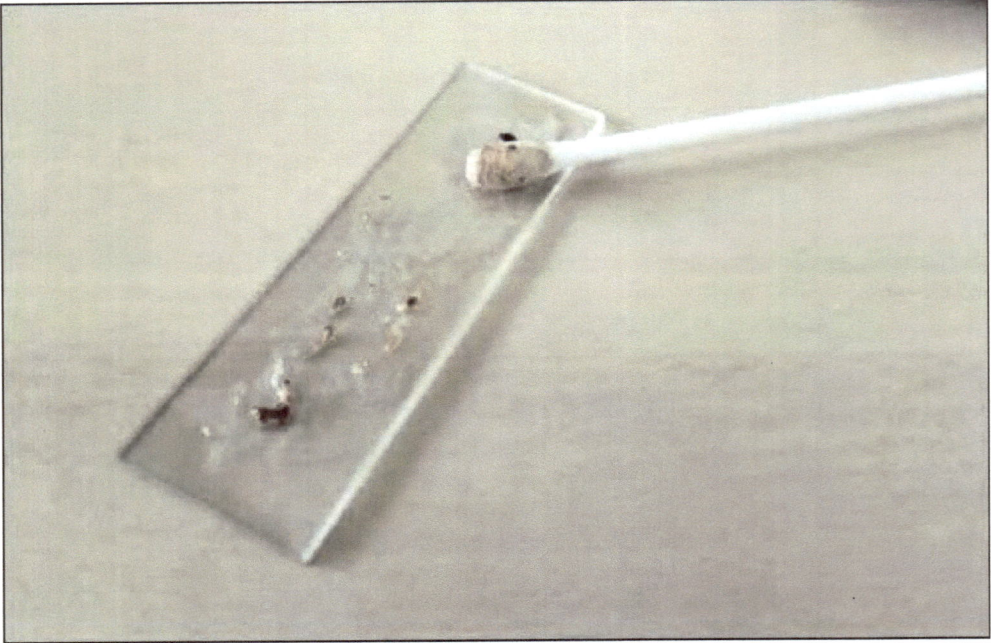

Fig. (5). Regular examination of type of ear discharges.

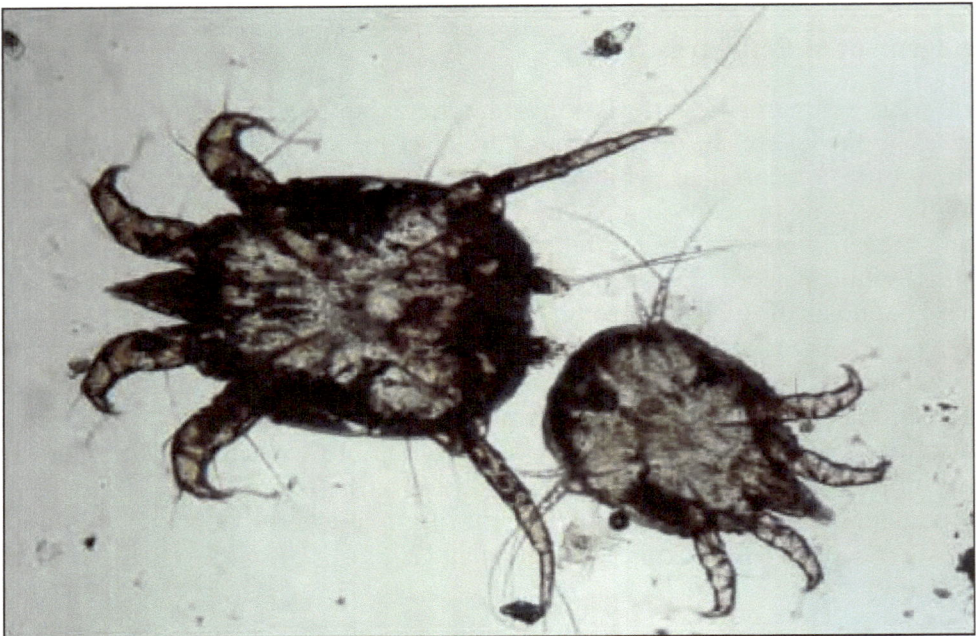

Fig. (6). Presence of mites in ear discharges (100x).

Swimmers Ear

The term, swimmer's ear is another term to describe inflammation in the outer ear canal caused by the trapping of ear canal for a long period. When the host fails to fight the microbial agents, organisms invade the ear canal and cause inflammation. Dogs which had the underlying allergy, dogs allergic to grasses, trees and weeds exhibiting itching and redness of the skin, paws and ears too. Dogs display clinical signs consistent with swimmer's ear such as head shaking, pawing at the head/ears, rubbing ears on objects, twitching of the ears and restlessness. Ear diseases can be prevented by avoiding swimming for dogs which are prone to ear infections, regularly keeping the ear plugs while swimming, frequent hair clipping in the ears to improve air circulation, regular cleaning of ears with a drying agent, such as a 1:1 blend of organic apple cider vinegar or white vinegar with sterile water. Vinegar also serves as an anti-bacterial and anti-fungal agent and balances the ear's pH to prevent yeast.

Management of *Malassezia* Infection

Malassezia pachydermatis is commensal yeast characterized by round to oval budding organisms and it is normally present in low numbers in the external ear canals and superficial muco-cutaneous sites in dogs (Fig. **7**) [28]. *Malassezia* dermatitis in dogs is usually a secondary problem due to an underlying skin disease such as an allergic disease like canine atopic dermatitis, flea allergy dermatitis, recurrent bacterial pyoderma and hypothyroidism [29]. Predisposing factors like high humidity, presence of skin folds, altered cutaneous pH levels; prolonged antibiotic and corticosteroid therapy are considered as common in dogs [30, 31]. *Malassezia pachydermatis* is thought to have a symbiotic relationship with commensal *Staphylococci*, which produces mutually beneficial growth factors and micro-environmental alterations [31, 32]. Recommending both systemic and topical therapy is adviced in dogs with *Malassezia* infection. Other component of medications was dietary elimination trials, antibiotic therapy, and antipruritic therapy which require administration up to 3 to 4 weeks period along with the evaluation of clinical efficacy and re-evaluation of intensity. Available topical medications were 2% ketoconazole, 2% miconazole, 2% climbazole, 2% chlorhexidine, 2% lime sulfur, 0.2% enilconazole, or 1% selenium sulfide is usually effective [33]. It is advisable topical shampoos which will contain the two different active ingredients may provide better efficacy than the single ingredient [30]. Medicated antifungal wipes or pads such as those containing 0.3% chlorhexidine, 0.5% climbazole, and Tris-EDTA solution are effective against *M. pachydermatis* [34]. For patients with generalized or multifocal lesions, oral antifungal therapy in combination with topical therapy is most effective. The available oral antifungal drugs were ketoconazole, fluconazole, terbinafine, and itraconazole [34, 35].

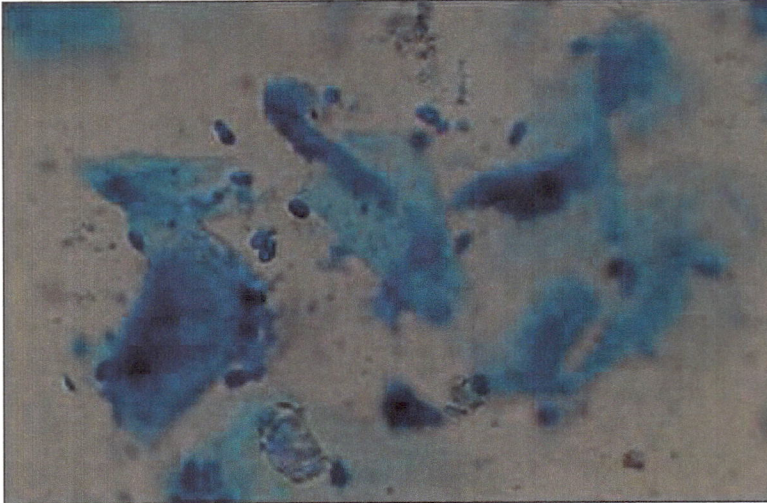

Fig. (7). Stained tape impressions smears revealed presence of *Malassezia* (1000x).

MANAGEMENT OF NEOPLASIA

Ear tumours including ceruminous gland adenoma or adenocarcinoma, sebaceous gland tumour and basal cell tumour are considering as chronic ear diseases conditions. Depending on the tumour type there may or may not be an underlying cause and chronic inflammation is considered as predisposing factor. Reportable signs were skin changes on the ear, crusts, ulcers or proliferative tissue, bleeding, odour, discharge, nodular masses, large growths filling the ear canal and vestibular signs. These tumours are diagnosed by assessing the complete blood count, radiography, CT scan and biopsy for a definitive diagnosis (Fig. **8**). Based on the tumour type, size, and location, surgical resection or removal is the treatment of choice. Prevention of ear tumours can be a difficulty but the early intervention of tumours can prevent ear infections further.

EAR HEALTH SUPPLEMENTATIONS

Skin is considered as the vital immunological structure of the body which is influenced by both the nutritional status of the individual and different host immunological factors [36, 37]. Canine dermatological issues predisposed by low levels of nutrition and/or changes in the epithelial barriers and hormonal imbalances. Nutritional supplementations in the prevention of ear diseases were:

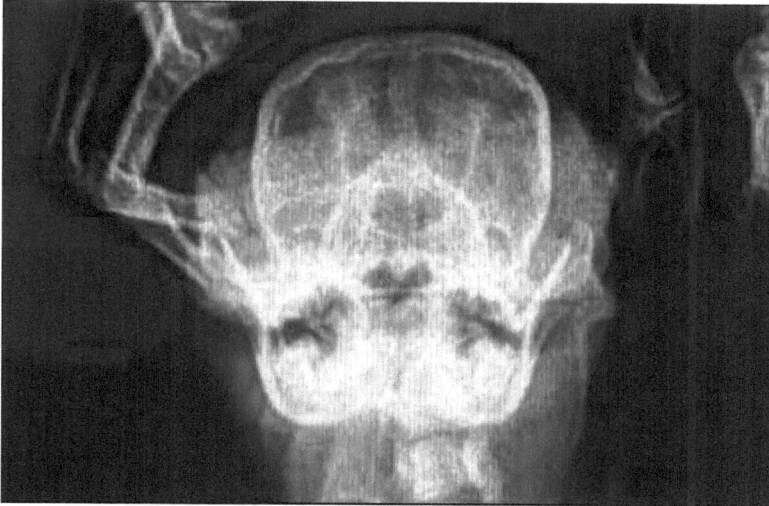

Fig. (8). Radiographic examination ears in dogs with recurrent otitis/neoplasia.

Polyunsaturated Fatty Acids

Omega 3 fatty acids are supposed to produce their beneficial effects by shifting the arachidonic acid cascade towards the production of less inflammatory mediators such as prostaglandins and leukotrienes [38 - 40]. Although supplementation of n-3 polyunsaturated fatty acids (PUFAs) is commonly recommended for a variety of pruritic and skin inflammatory diseases to reduce their clinical manifestations [41]. Linoleic acid (LA), an n-6 fatty acid, is crucial for maintaining the epidermal barrier function. Diets supplemented with LA have shown significant reductions in trans-epidermal water loss. Essential fatty acids (EFAs) from the n-6 gammalinolenic acid (GLA) and n-3 eicosapentaenoic acid (EPA) and docosahexaenoic acid (DHA) families possess anti-inflammatory effects and immunomodulating properties on the skin. While natural anti-inflammatory agents are often considered devoid of side effect [42, 43], Polyunsaturated fatty acids (PUFAs) have been demonstrated to potentially lead to side effects, such as: Impairment of platelet and immune function, possible interactions with medications and nutrients, gastrointestinal adverse effects, adverse effects on wound healing and weight gain [44].

Probiotics

An essential role of the gut microbiota is to serve as a vital component of the intestinal barrier, safeguarding the host against pathogens and regulating the immune system. Moreover, it contributes significantly to maintaining the structural and functional integrity of the gut [45].

Vitamins and Minerals

Alterations in skin and hair coat condition can result from various nutritional deficiencies. Optimal keratinization relies on an ample provision of multiple nutrients and micronutrients, encompassing vitamins and minerals [46]. Deficiencies in numerous essential amino acids, fatty acids, vitamins, and minerals can cause many types of modifications in skin structure or function which are prone to diseases.

Epidermal atrophy, hyperkeratosis, parakeratosis, acanthosis and zinc-responsive dermatosis are considered because of a deficiency of vitamins and minerals [47 - 50]. Supplementation of vitamin D and vitamin E is essential in the prevention of recurrent dermatological issues in dogs with atopic dermatitis [51 - 54].

MANAGEMENT OF ALLERGIC CONDITIONS

Atopic dermatitis is multifaceted in dogs, treatment option varies from the dog to dog and considered to be tailored to the individual patient and combined interventions should be used to improve outcomes. The cause of the allergy, stage of the disease condition, lesions distribution of lesions are essential in the formulation of treatment regimen [55, 56]. Dogs with recurrent dermatological disorders and ear diseases are frequently checked for the elimination of allergic triggers which includes:

Changes in the Diet

By elimination of known allergen from dogs diet on a routine basis.

Flea Allergies

It is mostly recorded in dogs with flea infestation and develops allergic reactions to the protein in the flea's saliva. Flea allergies can be controlled by frequent inspection of dogs coat for fleas and by application of flea repellents.

Inhalant Allergies

Allergy to mold, pollen, trees, weeds, and dust mites can cause inflammation of the skin.

Allergic Dermatitis

The specific treatment used for your dog's allergy will be determined by the specific allergen causing their symptoms. It is treated by immunotherapy by preparing the hyper-sensitizing injections that are specially manufactured for an individual dog and administered regularly which can take 6 to 12 months duration.

Bathing

Bathing with a nonirritating shampoo can relieve mild signs and symptoms [57].

Medications

Administration of topical and oral glucocorticoids, antihistamines and injectable recombinant interferons effectively reduce pruritus and skin lesions, while topical glucocorticoids and immunotherapy that target specific allergens can prevent recurrent dermatitis (Fig. **9**).

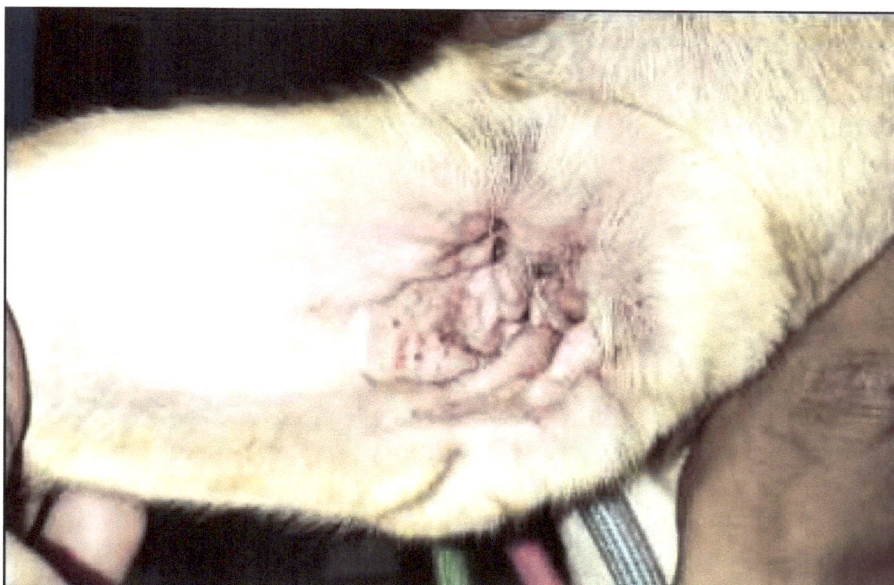

Fig. (9). Dog with hyperplasia and otitis.

REMOVAL OF FOREIGN BODIES

A foreign object in the ear can cause pain, infection and hearing loss. If there is any delay in the removal it can cause secondary complications. It can be prevented by a few instructions as follows. Never poke the objectives with sticks or ear buds it can push them deeper into the ears which can cause more damage. Removal by using tweezers. Washing the ear canal with water only if there is no damage to the eardrum. But never use the water if food or plant material is strucked.

EARLY INTERVENTION OF HORMONAL DISORDERS

Endocrine diseases are caused by an imbalance of the hormone levels in the body. Some of the endocrine disorders can cause the development of dermatological lesions and ear disorders.

Cushing's Disease (Hyperadrenocorticism)

This condition is indeed caused by an increase in circulating levels of the hormone cortisol, often resulting in recurrent skin lesions and thinning of the skin. Treatment typically involves medication to regulate the overproduction of cortisol by the adrenal glands, and in some cases, surgery to address issues with the adrenal glands.

Hypothyroidism

This condition is characterized by a decrease in thyroid hormone production by the thyroid glands and is commonly seen in middle-aged and older dogs. Skin and coat changes are typical symptoms, with the skin often becoming thickened and more pigmented, while the hair coat can become dull, dry, and sparse. Dogs with hypothyroidism are also prone to skin infections and may experience poor wound healing. Diagnosis is made through a thyroid hormone level blood test, and treatment typically involves administering oral thyroid supplements [58, 59].

CARE OF FLOPPY EARS BREEDS

Breeds with floppy ears are more prone to the ear diseases because of the presence of predisposing factors like floppy ears, hairy ear canal openings, perpetuating factors like easily inflammable ear canal glands and other common primary factors like high moisture and humidity. It can be controlled by frequent ear examinations, drying of the ears and early diagnosis of other dermatological issues. Dogs with long, floppy ears like hounds and spaniels can be at higher risk for ear infections. Indeed, the floppy ears of certain breeds can trap moisture, and many dogs may have narrower ear canals. Pendulous pinnal carriage, or drooping ears, has long been identified as a predisposing factor for otitis externa. This conformation can lead to heat and moisture retention within the ear canal and may also be more prone to retaining foreign material compared to other ear carriage types [60 - 63]. In addition, beagles, golden retrievers, poodles have dropped pinnae as identified as the risk of these breeds for getting frequent ear diseases (Fig. **10**). Obesity is indeed considered a predisposing factor for the development of otitis in dogs. Additionally, the sex of the dog can also play a role in the development of ear diseases. Androgen hormones in males may increase sebum production, which can predispose to flare-ups of latent otic infections and favor overgrowth of *Malassezia* spp. Conversely, estrogen hormones can have an opposite effect, drying the skin, which may promote secondary infections, especially in cases of allergic dermatitis [64].

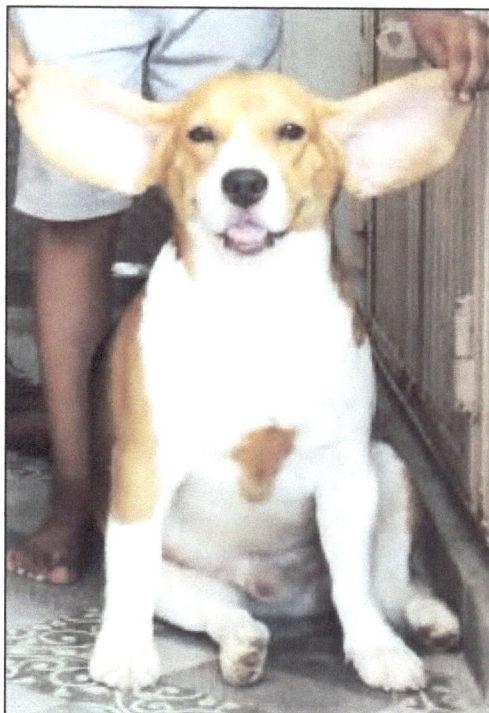

Fig. (10). Floppy ear dogs – More prone for Otitis.

CONCLUSION

The ear of dogs should be dry and clean with dog-safe commercial ear cleaning solution. Proper cleaning of ear is highly recommended for the prevention of ear infection. Trimming of hair around the ear is also beneficial for the prevention of ear infection. Allergies are a risk factor for the reoccurrence of ear infection. Proper allergy testing with dietary changes, lifestyle changes, and/or medication will help to manage the ear infection. Proper treatment and cleaning management will be beneficial to treat ear infection in dogs.

REFERENCES

[1]   Murphy KM. A review of techniques for the investigation of otitis externa and otitis media. Clin Tech Small Anim Pract 2001; 16(4): 236-41.
        [http://dx.doi.org/10.1053/svms.2001.27601] [PMID: 11793879]

[2]   Jacobson LS. Diagnosis and medical treatment of otitis externa in the dog and cat : review article. J S Afr Vet Assoc 2002; 73(4): 162-70.

[http://dx.doi.org/10.4102/jsava.v73i4.581] [PMID: 12665128]

[3]   Bugden DL. Identification and antibiotic susceptibility of bacterial isolates from dogs with otitis externa in A ustralia. Aust Vet J 2013; 91(1-2): 43-6.
        [http://dx.doi.org/10.1111/avj.12007] [PMID: 23356371]

[4]   Zur G, Lifshitz B, Bdolah-Abram T. The association between the signalment, common causes of canine otitis externa and pathogens. J Small Anim Pract 2011; 52(5): 254-8.
        [http://dx.doi.org/10.1111/j.1748-5827.2011.01058.x] [PMID: 21539570]

[5]   Hariharan H, Coles M, Poole D, Lund L, Page R. Update on antimicrobial susceptibilities of bacterial isolates from canine and feline otitis externa. Can Vet J 2006; 47(3): 253-5.
        [PMID: 16604982]

[6]   Lyskova P, Vydrzalova M, Mazurova J. Identification and antimicrobial susceptibility of bacteria and yeasts isolated from healthy dogs and dogs with otitis externa. J Vet Med A Physiol Pathol Clin Med 2007; 54(10): 559-63.
        [http://dx.doi.org/10.1111/j.1439-0442.2007.00996.x] [PMID: 18045339]

[7]   Colombo S, Cornegliani L, Vercelli A, Fondati A. Ear tip ulcerative dermatitis treated with oclacitinib in 25 dogs: a retrospective case series. Vet Dermatol 2021; 32(4): 363-e100.
        [http://dx.doi.org/10.1111/vde.12992] [PMID: 34250688]

[8]   Reinbacher E, Kneissl S, Hirt R, Spergser J, Panakova L. Myringotomy in dogs: Contamination rate from the external ear canal - a pilot study. Vet Anim Sci 2020; 10: 100125.
        [http://dx.doi.org/10.1016/j.vas.2020.100125] [PMID: 32734025]

[9]   Mohammaddavoodi A, Kneissl S, Hirt R, Spergser J, Aghapour M, Panakova L. A novel video-endoscope-guided myringotomy technique in dogs: Investigation in the value of vertical access to the tympanic membrane from beneath the patient - a pilot study. Vet Anim Sci 2021; 12: 100173.
        [http://dx.doi.org/10.1016/j.vas.2021.100173] [PMID: 33842734]

[10]   Cole LK, Kwochka KW, Kowalski JJ, Hillier A. Microbial flora and antimicrobial susceptibility patterns of isolated pathogens from the horizontal ear canal and middle ear in dogs with otitis media. J Am Vet Med Assoc 1998; 212(4): 534-8.
        [http://dx.doi.org/10.2460/javma.1998.212.04.534] [PMID: 9491161]

[11]   Rosychuck R. Challenges in otitis. Proceedings of the 7th World Congress of Veterinary Dermatology. Vancouver, BC, Canada. 2012; pp. 298-304.

[12]   Aslan J, Shipstone MA, Mackie JT. Carbon dioxide laser surgery for chronic proliferative and obstructive otitis externa in 26 dogs. Vet Dermatol 2021; 32(3): 262-e72.
        [http://dx.doi.org/10.1111/vde.12960] [PMID: 33830550]

[13]   Parnell-Turner H, Griffin CE, Rosenkrantz WS, Kelly Keating M, Bidot WA. Evaluation of the use of paired modified Wright's and periodic acid Schiff stains to identify microbial aggregates on cytological smears of dogs with microbial otitis externa and suspected biofilm. Vet Dermatol 2021; 32(5): 448-e122.
        [http://dx.doi.org/10.1111/vde.13009] [PMID: 34351013]

[14]   Reddy BS, Kumari KN, Rao VV, Rayulu VC. Cultural isolates and the pattern of antimicrobial sensitivity of whole cultures from recurrent pyoderma in dogs 2011, 7 (1): 40-42.

[15]   Reddy BS, Kumari KN, Rao VV, Rayulu VC. Efficacy of cefpodoxime with clavulanic acid in the treatment of recurrent pyoderma in dogs. 2014.

[16]   Reddy BS, Sivajothi S. Notoedric mange associated with *Malassezia* in cats. International Journal of Veterinary Health Science and Research 2014; 2: 101.

[17]   Mendelsohn CM. Topical antimicrobial for otitis. In: Bonagura JD, Twedt DC, Eds. Kirk's Current Veterinary Dermatology XV. St. Louis: Elsevier 2012; pp. 462-5.

[18]   Morris DO. Medical therapy of otitis externa and otitis media. Vet Clin North Am Small Anim Pract

2004; 34(2): 541-55.
[http://dx.doi.org/10.1016/j.cvsm.2003.10.009] [PMID: 15062623]

[19]   Rosenkrantz WS, Mendelsohn CL. Dermatologic therapy. In: Miller W, Griffin CE, Campbell K, Eds. Muller and Kirk's Small Animal Dermatology. 7th ed. St. Louis: Elsevier 2013; pp. 109-83.

[20]   Mendelsohn CL, Griffin CE, Rosenkrantz WS, Brown LD, Boord MJ. Efficacy of boric-complexed zinc and acetic-complexed zinc otic preparations for canine yeast otitis externa. J Am Anim Hosp Assoc 2005; 41(1): 12-21.
[http://dx.doi.org/10.5326/0410012] [PMID: 15634862]

[21]   Reeder CJ, Griffin CE, Polissar NL, Neradilek B, Armstrong RD. Comparative adrenocortical suppression in dogs with otitis externa following topical otic administration of four different glucocorticoid-containing medications. Vet Ther 2008; 9(2): 111-21.
[PMID: 18597249]

[22]   Harvey RG, Harari J, Delauche AJ. Ear diseases of the dog and cat. London: Manson Publishing Ltd 2001.

[23]   Wall R, Shearer D. Veterinary ectoparasites; biology, pathology and control. 2nd ed., London: Blackwell science 2001.
[http://dx.doi.org/10.1002/9780470690505]

[24]   Scott DW, Miller WH, Griffin CE. Muller and Kirk's small animal dermatology. 6th ed., Philadelphia: W.B. Saunders 2001.

[25]   Campbell KL. Other external parasites. In: Ettinger SJ, Feldman EC, Eds. Textbook of veterinary internal medicine. 6th ed. St. Louis, Missouri: Saunders Elsevier 2005; Vol. 1: pp. 66-7.

[26]   Reddy BS, Kumari KN. Canine scabies - Its therapeutic management and zoonotic importance. Intas Polivet 2013; 14: 292-4.

[27]   Reddy BS, Kumari KN. Demodicosis and its successful management in dogs. Ind J of Field Veterinarian 2010; 6(2): 48-50.

[28]   Radlinsky MG, Mason DE. Diseases of the ear. In: Ettinger SJ, Feldman EC, Eds. Textbook of veterinary internal medicine. 6th ed. St. Louis, Missouri: Saunders Elsevier 2005; Vol. 2: pp. 1171-4.

[29]   Hill P. Small Animal Dermatology: A practical guide to the diagnosis and managment of skin diseases in dogs and cats. Oxford, UK: Butterworth-Heinemann 2002; pp. 143-7.

[30]   Hnilca KA. Small Animal Dermatology: A color atlas and therapeutic guide. 3rd ed. Elsevier Saunders 2011; pp. 83-4.

[31]   Patterson AP, Frank LA. How to diagnose and treat *Malassezia* dermatitis in dogs. Vet Med 2002; 97: 612-23.

[32]   Cavana P, Petit JY, Perrot S, *et al.* Efficacy of a 2% climbazole shampoo for reducing *Malassezia* population sizes on the skin of naturally infected dogs. J Mycol Med 2015; 25(4): 268-73.
[http://dx.doi.org/10.1016/j.mycmed.2015.10.004] [PMID: 26603053]

[33]   Maynard L, Rème CA, Viaud S. Comparison of two shampoos for the treatment of canine *Malassezia* dermatitis: a randomised controlled trial. J Small Anim Pract 2011; 52(11): 566-72.
[http://dx.doi.org/10.1111/j.1748-5827.2011.01124.x] [PMID: 21985533]

[34]   Berger DJ, Lewis TP, Schick AE, Stone RT. Comparison of once-daily *versus* twice-weekly terbinafine administration for the treatment of canine *Malassezia* dermatitis – a pilot study. Vet Dermatol 2012; 23(5): 418-e79.
[http://dx.doi.org/10.1111/j.1365-3164.2012.01074.x] [PMID: 22823935]

[35]   Guillot J, Bensignor E, Jankowski F, Seewald W, Chermette R, Steffan J. Comparative efficacies of oral ketoconazole and terbinafine for reducing *Malassezia* population sizes on the skin of Basset Hounds. Vet Dermatol 2003; 14(3): 153-7.
[http://dx.doi.org/10.1046/j.1365-3164.2003.00334.x] [PMID: 12791049]

[36]   Marsella R, Olivry T, Carlotti DN. Current evidence of skin barrier dysfunction in human and canine atopic dermatitis. Vet Dermatol 2011; 22(3): 239-48.
[http://dx.doi.org/10.1111/j.1365-3164.2011.00967.x] [PMID: 21414049]

[37]   Woldemeskel M. Nutraceuticals in Veterinary Medicine. Springer; Cham, Switzerland: 2019. Nutraceuticals in dermatological disorders; pp. 563–568.

[38]   Olivry T, Mueller RS. Evidence-based veterinary dermatology: a systematic review of the pharmacotherapy of canine atopic dermatitis. Vet Dermatol 2003; 14(3): 121-46.
[http://dx.doi.org/10.1046/j.1365-3164.2003.00335.x] [PMID: 12791047]

[39]   Olivry T, Bizikova P. A systematic review of randomized controlled trials for prevention or treatment of atopic dermatitis in dogs: 2008–2011 update. Vet Dermatol 2013; 24(1): 97-117.e25, 6.
[http://dx.doi.org/10.1111/j.1365-3164.2012.01088.x] [PMID: 23331686]

[40]   Rees CA, Bauer JE, Burkholder WJ, *et al.* Effects of dietary flax seed and sunflower seed supplementation on normal canine serum polyunsaturated fatty acids and skin and hair coat condition scores. Vet Dermatol 2001; 12(2): 111-7.
[http://dx.doi.org/10.1046/j.1365-3164.2001.00234.x] [PMID: 11360337]

[41]   Nesbitt GH, Freeman LM, Hannah SS. Effect of *n* -3 fatty acid ratio and dose on clinical manifestations, plasma fatty acids and inflammatory mediators in dogs with pruritus. Vet Dermatol 2003; 14(2): 67-74.
[http://dx.doi.org/10.1046/j.1365-3164.2003.00328.x] [PMID: 12662263]

[42]   Abba C, Mussa PP, Vercelli A, Raviri G. Essential fatty acids supplementation in different-stage atopic dogs fed on a controlled diet. J Anim Physiol Anim Nutr (Berl) 2005; 89(3-6): 203-7.
[http://dx.doi.org/10.1111/j.1439-0396.2005.00541.x] [PMID: 15787996]

[43]   Noli C, Carta G, Cordeddu L, Melis MP, Murru E, Banni S. Conjugated linoleic acid and black currant seed oil in the treatment of canine atopic dermatitis: A preliminary report. Vet J 2007; 173(2): 413-21.
[http://dx.doi.org/10.1016/j.tvjl.2005.12.006] [PMID: 16495095]

[44]   Lenox CE, Bauer JE. Potential adverse effects of omega-3 Fatty acids in dogs and cats. J Vet Intern Med 2013; 27(2): 217-26.
[http://dx.doi.org/10.1111/jvim.12033] [PMID: 23323770]

[45]   Salem I, Ramser A, Isham N, Ghannoum MA. The gut microbiome as a major regulator of the gut-skin axis. Front Microbiol 2018; 9: 1459.
[http://dx.doi.org/10.3389/fmicb.2018.01459] [PMID: 30042740]

[46]   Hooda S, Minamoto Y, Suchodolski JS, Swanson KS. Current state of knowledge: the canine gastrointestinal microbiome. Anim Health Res Rev 2012; 13(1): 78-88.
[http://dx.doi.org/10.1017/S1466252312000059] [PMID: 22647637]

[47]   Feng W, Ao H, Peng C, Yan D. Gut microbiota, a new frontier to understand traditional Chinese medicines. Pharmacol Res 2019; 142: 176-91.
[http://dx.doi.org/10.1016/j.phrs.2019.02.024] [PMID: 30818043]

[48]   Klinger CJ, Hobi S, Johansen C, Koch HJ, Weber K, Mueller RS. Vitamin D shows *in vivo* efficacy in a placebo-controlled, double-blinded, randomised clinical trial on canine atopic dermatitis. Vet Rec 2018; 182(14): 406.
[http://dx.doi.org/10.1136/vr.104492] [PMID: 29419484]

[49]   Plevnik Kapun A, Salobir J, Levart A, *et al.* Vitamin E supplementation in canine atopic dermatitis: improvement of clinical signs and effects on oxidative stress markers. Vet Rec 2014; 175(22): 560.
[http://dx.doi.org/10.1136/vr.102547] [PMID: 25205675]

[50]   Plevnik Kapun A, Salobir J, Levart A, Tavčar Kalcher G, Nemec Svete A, Kotnik T. Plasma and skin vitamin E concentrations in canine atopic dermatitis. Vet Q 2013; 33(1): 2-6.
[http://dx.doi.org/10.1080/01652176.2012.758395] [PMID: 23323961]

[51] Tsoureli-Nikita E, Hercogova J, Lotti T, Menchini G. Evaluation of dietary intake of vitamin E in the treatment of atopic dermatitis: a study of the clinical course and evaluation of the immunoglobulin E serum levels. Int J Dermatol 2002; 41(3): 146-50.
[http://dx.doi.org/10.1046/j.1365-4362.2002.01423.x] [PMID: 12010339]

[52] Udenberg TJ, Griffin CE, Rosenkrantz WS, *et al.* Reproducibility of a quantitative cutaneous cytological technique. Vet Dermatol 2014; 25(5): 435-e67.
[http://dx.doi.org/10.1111/vde.12138] [PMID: 24898683]

[53] Plant JD, Gortel K, Kovalik M, Polissar NL, Neradilek MB. Development and validation of the canine atopic dermatitis lesion index, a scale for the rapid scoring of lesion severity in canine atopic dermatitis. Vet Dermatol 2012; 23(6): 515-e103.
[http://dx.doi.org/10.1111/j.1365-3164.2012.01113.x] [PMID: 23140318]

[54] Hill PB, Lau P, Rybnicek J. Development of an owner-assessed scale to measure the severity of pruritus in dogs. Vet Dermatol 2007; 18(5): 301-8.
[http://dx.doi.org/10.1111/j.1365-3164.2007.00616.x] [PMID: 17845617]

[55] Olivry T, DeBoer DJ, Favrot C, *et al.* Treatment of canine atopic dermatitis: 2015 updated guidelines from the International Committee on Allergic Diseases of Animals (ICADA). BMC Vet Res 2015; 11(1): 210.
[http://dx.doi.org/10.1186/s12917-015-0514-6]

[56] Cafarchia C, Gallo S, Capelli G, Otranto D. Occurrence and population size of *Malassezia* spp. in the external ear canal of dogs and cats both healthy and with otitis. Mycopathologia 2005; 160(2): 143-9.
[http://dx.doi.org/10.1007/s11046-005-0151-x] [PMID: 16170610]

[57] Griffin JS, Scott DW, Erb HN. *Malassezia* otitis externa in the dog: the effect of heat-fixing otic exudate for cytological analysis. J Vet Med A Physiol Pathol Clin Med 2007; 54(8): 424-7.
[http://dx.doi.org/10.1111/j.1439-0442.2007.00938.x] [PMID: 17877584]

[58] Miller W, Griffin C, Campbell K. Diseases of eyelids, claws, anal sacs, and ears. In: Miller WH, Griffin CE, Campbell KL, editors. Muller & Kirk's Small Animal Dermatology. 7. Elsevier Mosby; 2013. pp. 724–773.

[59] Angus JC. Otic cytology in health and disease. Vet Clin North Am Small Anim Pract 2004; 34(2): 411-24.
[http://dx.doi.org/10.1016/j.cvsm.2003.10.005] [PMID: 15062616]

[60] Terziev G, Borissov I. Prevalence of ear diseases in dogs – a retrospective 5-year clinical study. Bulg J Vet Med 2018; 21(1): 76-85.
[http://dx.doi.org/10.15547/bjvm.1075]

[61] Favrot C, Steffan J, Seewald W, Picco F. A prospective study on the clinical features of chronic canine atopic dermatitis and its diagnosis. Vet Dermatol 2010; 21(1): 23-31.
[http://dx.doi.org/10.1111/j.1365-3164.2009.00758.x] [PMID: 20187911]

[62] McGreevy PD, Wilson BJ, Mansfield CS, *et al.* Labrador retrievers under primary veterinary care in the UK: demography, mortality and disorders. Canine Genet Epidemiol 2018; 5(1): 8.
[http://dx.doi.org/10.1186/s40575-018-0064-x] [PMID: 30377534]

[63] Pegram C, Raffan E, White E, *et al.* Frequency, breed predisposition and demographic risk factors for overweight status in dogs in the UK. J Small Anim Pract 2021; 62(7): 521-30.
[http://dx.doi.org/10.1111/jsap.13325] [PMID: 33754373]

[64] O'Neill DG, Packer RMA, Lobb M, Church DB, Brodbelt DC, Pegram C. Demography and commonly recorded clinical conditions of Chihuahuas under primary veterinary care in the UK in 2016. BMC Vet Res 2020; 16(1): 42.
[http://dx.doi.org/10.1186/s12917-020-2258-1] [PMID: 32046714]

SUBJECT INDEX

www.ingramcontent.com/pod-product-compliance
Lightning Source LLC
Chambersburg PA
CBHW050519240326
41598CB00086B/95